2011
YEAR BOOK OF
OPHTHALMOLOGY®

The 2011 Year Book Series

Year Book of Anesthesiology and Pain Management™: Drs Chestnut, Abram, Black, Gravlee, Lien, Mathru, and Roizen

Year Book of Cardiology®: Drs Gersh, Cheitlin, Elliott, Gold, Graham, and Thourani

Year Book of Critical Care Medicine®: Drs Dellinger, Parrillo, Balk, Dorman, Dries, and Zanotti-Cavazzoni

Year Book of Dermatology and Dermatologic Surgery™: Dr Del Rosso

Year Book of Diagnostic Radiology®: Drs Osborn, Abbara, Elster, Manaster, Oestreich, Offiah, Rosado de Christenson, Stephens, and Walker

Year Book of Emergency Medicine®: Drs Hamilton, Bruno, Handly, Mullin, Quintana, and Ramoska

Year Book of Endocrinology®: Drs Schott, Apovian, Clarke, Eugster, Ludlam, Meikle, Schinner, Schteingart, and Toth

Year Book of Gastroenterology™: Drs Talley, DeVault, Harnois, Murray, Pearson, Philcox, Picco, and Smith

Year Book of Hand and Upper Limb Surgery®: Drs Yao and Steinmann

Year Book of Medicine®: Drs Barker, Garrick, Gersh, Khardori, LeRoith, Seo, Talley, and Thigpen

Year Book of Neonatal and Perinatal Medicine®: Drs Fanaroff, Benitz, Donn, Neu, Papile, Polin, and van Marter

Year Book of Neurology and Neurosurgery®: Drs Klimo and Rabinstein

Year Book of Obstetrics, Gynecology, and Women's Health®: Drs Dungan and Shulman

Year Book of Oncology®: Drs Arceci, Bauer, Chiorean, Gordon, Lawton, Murphy, Thigpen, and Tsao

Year Book of Ophthalmology®: Drs Rapuano, Cohen, Flanders, Fudemberg, Hammersmith, Milman, Myers, Nagra, Nelson, Penne, Pyfer, Sergott, Shields, Talekar, and Vander

Year Book of Orthopedics®: Drs Morrey, Beauchamp, Huddleston, Swiontkowski, and Trigg

Year Book of Otolaryngology-Head and Neck Surgery®: Drs Sindwani, Balough, Franco, Gapany, and Mitchell

Year Book of Pathology and Laboratory Medicine®: Drs Raab, Parwani, Bejarano, and Bissell

Year Book of Pediatrics®: Dr Stockman

Year Book of Plastic and Aesthetic Surgery™: Drs Miller, Gosain, Gurtner, Gutowski, Ruberg, Salisbury, and Smith

Year Book of Psychiatry and Applied Mental Health®: Drs Talbott, Ballenger, Buckley, Frances, Krupnick, and Mack

Year Book of Pulmonary Disease®: Drs Barker, Jones, Maurer, Raza, Tanoue, and Willsie

Year Book of Sports Medicine®: Drs Shephard, Cantu, Feldman, Jankowski, Khan, Lebrun, Nieman, Pierrynowski, and Rowland

Year Book of Surgery®: Drs Copeland, Behrns, Daly, Eberlein, Fahey, Huber, Klodell, Mozingo, and Pruett

Year Book of Urology®: Drs Andriole and Coplen

Year Book of Vascular Surgery®: Drs Moneta, Gillespie, Starnes, and Watkins

2011

The Year Book of
OPHTHALMOLOGY®

Editor-in-Chief
Christopher J. Rapuano, MD
Professor of Ophthalmology, Jefferson Medical College of Thomas Jefferson University; Director, Cornea Service; Co-Director, Refractive Surgery Department, Attending Surgeon, Wills Eye Institute, Philadelphia, Pennsylvania

Wills Eye®

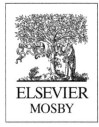

ELSEVIER
MOSBY

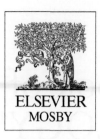

ELSEVIER
MOSBY

Vice President, Continuity: Kimberly Murphy
Editor: Yonah Korngold
Production Supervisor, Electronic Year Books: Donna M. Skelton
Electronic Article Manager: Mike Sheets
Illustrations and Permissions Coordinator: Dawn Vohsen

Composition by TNQ Books and Journals Pvt Ltd, India

Editorial Office:
Elsevier
1600 John F. Kennedy Blvd.
Suite 1800
Philadelphia, PA 19103-2899

International Standard Serial Number: 0084-392X
International Standard Book Number: 978-0-323-08421-5

Printed and bound by CPI Group (UK) Ltd, Croydon, CR0 4YY

Transferred to Digital Print 2011

Editorial Board

Table of Contents

Journals Represented

Journals represented in this YEAR BOOK are listed below.

Acta Ophthalmologica
American Journal of Ophthalmology
Annals of Plastic Surgery
Archives of Ophthalmology
British Journal of Ophthalmology
British Journal of Radiology
Clinical Endocrinology
Clinical Neurology and Neurosurgery
Cornea
Dermatologic Surgery
Epilepsy Research
Eye
Eye & Contact Lens
Human Pathology
Journal of American Association for Pediatric Ophthalmology and Strabismus
Journal of Cataract & Refractive Surgery
Journal of Computer Assisted Tomography
Journal of Pediatric Ophthalmology & Strabismus
Journal of Plastic, Reconstructive & Aesthetic Surgery
Journal of Refractive Surgery
Journal of the American Academy of Dermatology
Journal of the National Cancer Institute
Journal of the Neurological Sciences
Modern Pathology
Neurology
Neurosurgery
New England Journal of Medicine
Ophthalmic Plastic & Reconstructive Surgery
Ophthalmic Surgery, Lasers & Imaging
Ophthalmology
Radiology
Retina
Science
World Neurosurgery

STANDARD ABBREVIATIONS

The following terms are abbreviated in this edition: acquired immunodeficiency syndrome (AIDS), cardiopulmonary resuscitation (CPR), central nervous system (CNS), cerebrospinal fluid (CSF), computed tomography (CT), deoxyribonucleic acid (DNA), diopter (D), electrocardiography (ECG), health maintenance organization (HMO), human immunodeficiency virus (HIV), intensive care unit (ICU), intramuscular (IM), intravenous (IV), magnetic resonance (MR) imaging (MRI), ribonucleic acid (RNA), ultrasound (US), and ultraviolet (UV).

NOTE

The YEAR BOOK OF OPHTHALMOLOGY® is a literature survey service providing abstracts of articles published in the professional literature. Every effort is made to assure the accuracy of the information presented in these pages. Neither the editors nor the publisher of the YEAR BOOK OF OPHTHALMOLOGY® can be responsible for errors in the original materials. The editors' comments are their own opinions. Mention of specific products within this publication does not constitute endorsement.

To facilitate the use of the YEAR BOOK OF OPHTHALMOLOGY® as a reference tool, all illustrations and tables included in this publication are now identified as they appear in the original article. This change is meant to help the reader recognize that any illustration or table appearing in the YEAR BOOK OF OPHTHALMOLOGY® may be only one of many in the original article. For this reason, figure and table numbers will often appear to be out of sequence within the YEAR BOOK OF OPHTHALMOLOGY®.

1 Cataract Surgery

The Effect of α_1-Adrenergic Receptor Antagonist Tamsulosin (Flomax) on Iris Dilator Smooth Muscle Anatomy

Santaella RM, Destafeno JJ, Stinnett SS, et al (Duke Univ Med Ctr, Durham, NC; et al)

Ophthalmology 117:1743-1749, 2010

Purpose.—To characterize and determine the effect of tamsulosin (Flomax) on the human iris dilator muscle anatomy.

Design.—Retrospective, case-control study.

Participants.—This study comprised 51 cadaveric eyes from 27 patients (14 with a history of tamsulosin use and 13 control patients) who underwent autopsy at the Duke University Medical Center, Durham, North Carolina.

Methods.—Patients' records were reviewed, and age, medical, surgical, and ocular history; gender; medications; and duration and dosage of tamsulosin were recorded. Specimens were sectioned through the pupillary axis in the horizontal meridian and reviewed by light microscopy. A morphometric analysis was performed to measure the maximum and minimum iris dilator muscle thickness and the iris stromal thickness (micrometers) at 6 points in each eye. All microscopic evaluations and measurements were performed by the same masked observer.

Main Outcome Measures.—To determine whether there is a significant difference in the iris dilator muscle or stromal thickness in those patients receiving tamsulosin treatment compared with age-matched controls.

Results.—The mean iris dilator muscle thickness in the tamsulosin-treated group (6.53 ± 1.99 μm) was significantly thinner compared with that of the control group (8.50 ± 1.61 μm) ($P=0.006$). There was no difference in iris stromal thickness between the 2 groups ($P=0.268$). There was no direct relationship between duration of tamsulosin use and iris dilator muscle or stromal thickness. Statistical significance was maintained when the iris dilator muscle thickness was compared between the groups using history of diabetes and cataract extraction as separate variables. No difference was noted when comparing the iris stromal thickness using diabetes as a separate variable. However, stromal thickness was significantly different between the groups in pseudophakic eyes ($P=0.005$).

Conclusions.—According to histologic examination of cadaver eyes, patients receiving tamsulosin treatment exhibited decreased iris dilator muscle thickness compared with control patients. There was no difference noted in the iris stromal thickness within the groups. We believe this

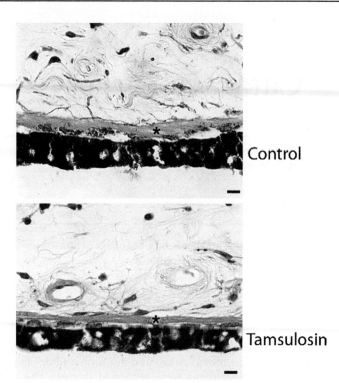

FIGURE 4.—Photomicrographs show representative iris samples from a control (*top*) and a tamsulosin subject (*bottom*) under ×600 magnification (hematoxylin and eosin). The average dilator smooth muscle (*) thickness was 8.5 μm for the control subject and 6.5 μm for the tamsulosin subject. Magnification bar = 10 μm. (Reprinted from Santaella RM, Destafeno JJ, Stinnett SS, et al. The effect of α_1-adrenergic receptor antagonist tamsulosin (Flomax) on iris dilator smooth muscle anatomy. *Ophthalmology.* 2010;117:1743-1749, Copyright 2010, with permission from the American Academy of Ophthalmology.)

finding may shed light on the pathophysiology of intraoperative floppy iris syndrome. Further studies need to be performed to assess the significance of this histologic finding (Fig 4).

▶ Starting with the ground-breaking reports by Chang and Campbell in 2005,[1] cataract surgeons have become aware of the association of intraoperative floppy iris syndrome (IFIS) with use of the oral medication tamsulosin (Flomax). Clinically, IFIS can occur with varying severity in a dose-independent fashion. Significantly, cessation of tamsulosin prior to cataract surgery does not affect the occurrence or severity of IFIS.

This study provides an anatomical explanation for these clinical observations. The authors found histopathologic thinning of the iris dilator muscle post-mortem in eyes of patients who had taken Flomax (Fig 4). This finding supports the theory that long-term or irreversible α_{1A} receptor blockade by Flomax results in disuse atrophy of iris smooth muscle. Iris dilator muscle atrophy leads to loss of iris rigidity, resulting in the characteristic triad of IFIS: flaccid iris stroma, tendency for prolapse through incisions during surgery, and progressive miosis. Difficulty completing cataract surgery safely and increased risk for intraoperative complications such as vitreous loss are well known in cases of IFIS.

This study should help cataract surgeons understand the frustrating problem of IFIS and how best to prevent it or minimize complications when it does occur.

M. F. Pyfer, MD

Reference

1. Chang DF, Campbell JR. Intraoperative floppy iris syndrome associated with tamsulosin. *J Cataract Refract Surg.* 2005;31:664-673.

Prevalence and Predictors of Ocular Complications Associated with Cataract Surgery in United States Veterans
Greenberg PB, Tseng VL, Wu W-C, et al (VA Med Ctr, Providence, RI; et al)
Ophthalmology 118:507-514, 2011

Purpose.—To investigate the prevalence and predictors of intraoperative and 90-day postoperative ocular complications associated with cataract surgery performed in the United States Veterans Health Administration (VHA) system.

Design.—Retrospective cohort study.

Participants.—Forty-five thousand eighty-two veterans who underwent cataract surgery in the VHA.

Methods.—The National Patient Care Database was used to identify all VHA patients who underwent outpatient extracapsular cataract surgery and who underwent only 1 cataract surgery within 90 days of the index surgery between October 1, 2005, and September 30, 2007. Data collected include demographics, preoperative systemic and ocular comorbidities, intraoperative complications, and 90-day postoperative complications. Adjusted odds ratios (ORs) of factors predictive of complications were calculated using logistic regression modeling.

Main Outcome Measures.—Intraoperative and postoperative ocular complications within 90 days of cataract surgery.

Results.—During the study period, 53 786 veterans underwent cataract surgery; 45 082 met inclusion criteria. Common preoperative systemic and ocular comorbidities included diabetes mellitus (40.6%), chronic pulmonary disease (21.2%), age-related macular degeneration (14.4%), and diabetes with ophthalmic manifestations (14.0%). The most common ocular complications were posterior capsular tear, anterior vitrectomy, or both during surgery (3.5%) and posterior capsular opacification after surgery (4.2%). Predictors of complications included: black race (OR, 1.38; 95% confidence interval [CI], 1.28—1.50), divorced status (OR, 1.10; 95% CI, 1.03—1.18), never married (OR, 1.26; 95% CI, 1.14—1.38), diabetes with ophthalmic manifestations (OR, 1.33; 95% CI, 1.23—1.43), traumatic cataract (OR,

1.80; 95% CI, 1.40—2.31), previous ocular surgery (OR, 1.29; 95% CI, 1.02—1.63), and older age.

Conclusions.—In a cohort of United States veterans with a high preoperative disease burden, selected demographic factors and ocular comorbidities were associated with greater risks of cataract surgery complications. Further large-scale studies are warranted to investigate cataract surgery outcomes for non-VHA United States patient populations.

▶ This is one of the largest population studies of cataract surgical outcomes in the United States ever published. It represents a paradigm shift in large surgical outcomes and comorbidity studies brought on by the advent of electronic medical records (EMR). The Veterans Health Administration uses the Vista EMR system since at least 2005. Data were collected from this system to examine incidence of intraoperative and postoperative complications of cataract surgery and their relationship to various comorbidity factors. When you read this article, it is important to view the supporting tables published only online, not in print. There you will find, for example, in Table 5 in the original article, that glaucoma is a risk factor for complications from cataract surgery, with a *P* value of .0061, but posterior polar cataract is not (*P* = .3410).

This study without EMR would require manual review of over 45 000 charts, a daunting proposition at best. Now, and increasingly so in the future, we will have relatively easy access to statistical data over large populations, so rare events such as postoperative endophthalmitis can finally be studied at least retrospectively in a straightforward manner. This is one reason that government mandates for EMR should be accompanied by uniform standards for data format and interconnection of different vendors' systems to allow simple automated epidemiologic data collection. Otherwise, there is relatively little public benefit to the nation as a whole from EMR use by private physicians.

M. F. Pyfer, MD

The Cataract National Dataset Electronic Multi-centre Audit of 55,567 Operations: Variation in Posterior Capsule Rupture Rates between Surgeons
Johnston RL, Taylor H, Smith R, et al (Cheltenham General Hosp, UK; Univ Hosps Bristol NHS Foundation Trust, UK; Stoke Mandeville Hosp, Aylesbury, UK; et al)
Eye 24:894-900, 2010

Aims.—To demonstrate variations in posterior capsule rupture (PCR) rate between surgeons of the same and different grades as a by-product of routine clinical care.

Method.—NHS departments using electronic medical record (EMR) systems to collect the Cataract National Dataset (CND) were invited to submit data. Data were remotely extracted, anonymised, assessed for conformity and completeness, and analysed for rates of PCR for individual surgeons within each of the three grades.

Results.—Data were extracted on 55 567 cataract operations performed at 12 NHS trusts by 406 surgeons between November 2001 and July 2006. Data on the grade of 404 of the 406 surgeons who contributed to the study were available for 55 515 cases (99.9%) and were used for this analysis. Variation in PCR rate between surgeons was highest for the most junior grade of surgeon and between those surgeons contributing relatively few cases to the data set. Variation in PCR was lowest among experienced surgeons contributing large numbers of cases to the data set.

Conclusions.—Considerable variation in PCR rate exists both between and within surgical grades. Routine electronic collection of the CND allows detailed analysis of variations in PCR rates between individual surgeons. To define acceptable limits for this benchmark complication of cataract surgery, further work is needed to adjust surgeons' outcomes for the case mix complexity.

▶ The collection of statistics purported to measure quality of care in medicine is controversial but likely inevitable. Statistical data on the incidence and outcomes of uncommon conditions over large populations should ultimately improve medical care and is much stronger evidence than anecdotal opinions of individual experts. This study, from the United Kingdom, is the first to use an electronic health record (EHR) system to extract data collected during clinical care to examine variation among surgeons in posterior capsule rupture rate during cataract surgery. Adoption of EHR in the United States is proceeding by government mandate and will certainly make this type of study much simpler.

Sometimes large population studies defy conventional wisdom and have a surprising finding, but not in this case. More experienced surgeons have a lower incidence of posterior capsule rupture during cataract surgery. No adjustment was made for surgical complexity or comorbid conditions, such as history of tamsulosin (Flomax) use, exfoliation syndrome, or cataract density.

M. F. Pyfer, MD

Age-Related Cataract in a Randomized Trial of Vitamins E and C in Men
Christen WG, Glynn RJ, Sesso HD, et al (Brigham and Women's Hosp and Harvard Med School, Boston, MA)
Arch Ophthalmol 128:1397-1405, 2010

Objective.—To test whether supplementation with alternate-day vitamin E or daily vitamin C affects the incidence of age-related cataract in a large cohort of men.

Methods.—In a randomized, double-masked, placebo-controlled trial, 11 545 apparently healthy US male physicians 50 years or older without a diagnosis of cataract at baseline were randomly assigned to receive 400 IU of vitamin E or placebo on alternate days and 500 mg of vitamin C or placebo daily.

Main Outcome Measure.—Incident cataract responsible for a reduction in best-corrected visual acuity to 20/30 or worse based on self-report confirmed by medical record review.

Application to Clinical Practice.—Long-term use of vitamin E and C supplements has no appreciable effect on cataract.

Results.—After 8 years of treatment and follow-up, 1174 incident cataracts were confirmed. There were 579 cataracts in the vitamin E−treated group and 595 in the vitamin E placebo group (hazard ratio, 0.99; 95% confidence interval, 0.88-1.11). For vitamin C, there were 593 cataracts in the treated group and 581 in the placebo group (hazard ratio, 1.02; 95% confidence interval, 0.91-1.14).

Conclusion.—Long-term alternate-day use of 400 IU of vitamin E and daily use of 500 mg of vitamin C had no notable beneficial or harmful effect on the risk of cataract.

Trial Registration.—clinicaltrials.gov Identifier: NCT00270647.

▶ When diagnosed with cataract, our patients frequently ask whether vitamin supplements can slow the progression and perhaps delay the need for surgery. This is understandable, given that we frequently recommend vitamins and good nutrition per the Age-Related Eye Disease Study (AREDS) trial for macular degeneration. This study followed up over 11 000 healthy male physicians aged 50 years or more who started without cataracts. After 8 years, there was no benefit of vitamin C or vitamin E supplements with regard to development of cataract. This result is consistent with other published trials, including AREDS, that found minimal to no benefit for these 2 antioxidant vitamins on cataract. An interesting statistic from this article is the overall cumulative incidence of visually significant cataract (20/30 or worse), which was about 10% over 8 years across all groups (Fig 3 in the original article).

M. F. Pyfer, MD

Visual Acuity Outcomes after Cataract Surgery in Patients with Age-Related Macular Degeneration: Age-Related Eye Disease Study Report No. 27
Forooghian F, for the AREDS Research Group (Natl Eye Inst/Natl Insts of Health, Bethesda, MD; et al)
Ophthalmology 116:2093-2100, 2009

Objective.—To evaluate visual acuity outcomes after cataract surgery in patients with varying degrees of age-related macular degeneration (AMD).

Design.—Cohort study.

Participants.—A total of 4757 participants enrolled in the Age-Related Eye Disease Study (AREDS), a prospective, multicenter, epidemiological study of the clinical course of cataract and AMD and a randomized controlled trial of antioxidants and minerals.

Methods.—Standardized lens and fundus photographs, performed at baseline and annual visits, were graded by a centralized reading center using standardized protocols for severity of AMD and lens opacities. History of cataract surgery was obtained every 6 months. Analyses were conducted using multivariate logistic regression.

Main Outcome Measure.—The change in best-corrected visual acuity (BCVA) after cataract surgery compared with preoperative BCVA.

Results.—Visual acuity results were analyzed for 1939 eyes that had cataract surgery during AREDS. The mean time from cataract surgery to measurement of postoperative BCVA was 6.9 months. After adjustment for age at surgery, gender, type, and severity of cataract, the mean change in visual acuity at the next study visit after the cataract surgery was as follows: Eyes without AMD gained 8.4 letters of acuity ($P < 0.0001$), eyes with mild AMD gained 6.1 letters of visual acuity ($P < 0.0001$), eyes with moderate AMD gained 3.9 letters ($P < 0.0001$), and eyes with advanced AMD gained 1.9 letters ($P = 0.04$). The statistically significant gain in visual acuity after cataract surgery was maintained an average of 1.4 years after cataract surgery.

Conclusions.—On average, participants with varying severity of AMD benefited from cataract surgery with an increase in visual acuity

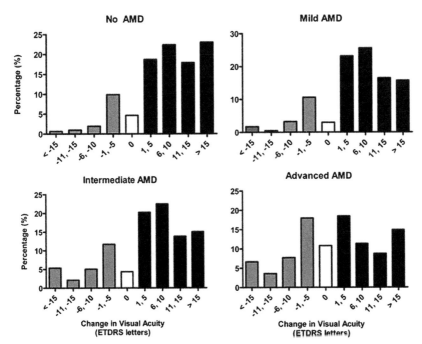

FIGURE 4.—Change in visual acuity after cataract surgery in patients with varying severity of AMD. Percentage of patients with gain or loss of letters on the logarithm of the minimal angle of resolution visual acuity chart is shown for eyes with no AMD, mild AMD, intermediate AMD, and advanced AMD. AMD = age-related macular degeneration; ETDRS = Early Treatment Diabetic Retinopathy Study. (Reprinted from Forooghian F, for the AREDS Research Group. Visual acuity outcomes after cataract surgery in patients with age-related macular degeneration: age-related eye disease study report no. 27. *Ophthalmology.* 2009;116:2093-2100, Copyright 2009, with permission from American Academy of Ophthalmology.)

postoperatively. This average gain in visual acuity persisted for at least 18 months (Fig 4).

▶ This report from the landmark Age-Related Eye Disease Study project represents the largest published series of patients with age-related macular degeneration (AMD) undergoing cataract surgery. Several recent epidemiologic studies have suggested a risk for progression of AMD with resultant decline in vision after cataract surgery. Some cataract surgeons and retinal specialists advise a conservative approach toward cataract treatment in patients with AMD in light of these earlier publications.

This large case series indicates a gain in visual acuity after cataract surgery for patients with all grades of AMD. The largest increase in vision was associated with milder AMD and more advanced cataract, as might be expected (Fig.4). In fact, cataract extraction in AMD patients resulted in a gain of between 2 and 16 Early Treatment Diabetic Retinopathy Study chart letters, similar to the average vision improvement reported for patients with wet AMD treated with ranibizumab (Lucentis) in the Minimally Classic/Occult Trial of the Anti-VEGF Antibody Ranibizumab in the Treatment of Neovascular AMD, Anti-VEGF Antibody for the Treatment of Predominantly Classic Choroidal Neovascularization in Age-Related Macular Degeneration, and Prospective OCT Imaging of Patients with Neovascular AMD Treated with intraOcular Ranibizumab studies. This result should reassure physicians and their patients with coexisting cataract and AMD when considering cataract surgery.

M. F. Pyfer, MD

Evaluation of Axial Length Measurement of the Eye Using Partial Coherence Interferometry and Ultrasound in Cases of Macular Disease

Kojima T, Tamaoki A, Yoshida N, et al (Social Insurance Chukyo Hosp, Aichi, Japan; et al)
Ophthalmology 117:1750-1754, 2010

Purpose.—The present study evaluated the accuracy of using partial coherence interferometry (PCI) and ultrasound (US) to measure axial length in eyes with macular disease, the nature of the double peak (DP) in PCI measurements, and the applicability of intraocular lens (IOL) power calculation.

Design.—Retrospective noncomparative case series.

Participants.—We studied 132 eyes with macular edema, epiretinal membrane, and macular hole in 132 patients who underwent combined cataract and vitrectomy surgery.

Methods.—Axial length was measured using PCI and US. If a DP was observed in the PCI measurement, the posterior peak was used for the IOL calculation. The central retinal thickness (CRT) was measured using optical coherence tomography.

Main Outcome Measures.—Measurements were made of the frequency of DP observation in PCI measurement and the postoperative refractive errors when either PCI or US measurements were applied.

Results.—A DP was observed in 25 (18.7%) of 132 eyes in the axial length measurement using PCI. There was a significant correlation between the interpeak distance and the CRT ($P<0.001$, $r^2=0.3869$). The 6-month postoperative refractive errors in the DP and single peak (SP) groups were predicted correctly within ± 0.5 diopters in 56.0% (DP) and 61.7% (SP) of the cases and within ± 1.0 diopters in 92.0% (DP) and 92.2% (SP) of the cases. The accuracy of the axial length measurement was similar between PCI and US.

Conclusions.—Our results suggest that the longer axial length of the DP observed in PCI represents retinal pigment epithelium. If a DP was observed in PCI measurement, application of the longer peak for the IOL calculation resulted in a refractive error similar to that in the SP group (Fig 1).

▶ Cataract and retinal disease frequently coexist, and cataract surgeons are often confronted with patients who will require either combined or consecutive cataract extraction and vitrectomy. Partial coherence interferometry typically using the IOLMaster device (Carl Zeiss, Heidelberg, Germany) has become the method of choice for accurate preoperative axial length (AL) measurement. Occasionally, a double peak is observed in patients with thickness altering

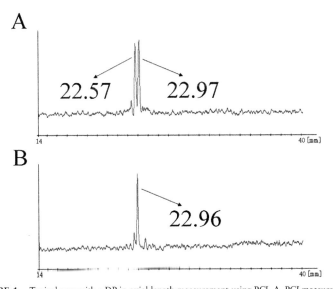

FIGURE 1.—Typical case with a DP in axial length measurement using PCI. A, PCI measurement data before vitrectomy for a case of epiretinal membrane. B, PCI measurement after vitrectomy. The DP disappeared. DP = double peak; PCI = partial coherence interferometry. (Reprinted from Kojima T, Tamaoki A, Yoshida N, et al. Evaluation of axial length measurement of the eye using partial coherence interferometry and ultrasound in cases of macular disease. *Ophthalmology.* 2010;117:1750-1754, with permission from the American Academy of Ophthalmology.)

macular pathology such as epiretinal membrane, macular edema, and macular hole, presumably because of an extra reflective surface anterior to the retinal pigment epithelium (Fig 1). The IOLMaster software will choose the peak with greater signal strength, which may cause an error in AL determination.

In this retrospective case series, the authors found a double peak in about 20% of eyes with macular pathology. The best refractive outcome was achieved when the posterior peak was used to determine AL.

The Zeiss IOLMaster software allows the user to select the anterior or posterior peak to use for calculations when a double peak occurs. This study supports always selecting the posterior peak for greatest accuracy in cases with altered central retinal thickness because of macular pucker, edema, or hole.

M. F. Pyfer, MD

Efficacy of bromfenac sodium ophthalmic solution in preventing cystoid macular oedema after cataract surgery in patients with diabetes
Endo N, Kato S, Haruyama K, et al (Tokyo Women's Med Univ, Japan; Univ of Tokyo School of Medicine, Japan)
Acta Ophthalmol 88:896-900, 2010

Purpose.—To compare the efficacy of bromfenac sodium ophthalmic solution (BF) and a steroidal solution (ST) administered prophylactically against cystoid macular oedema and anterior-chamber inflammation after phacoemulsification and intraocular lens implantation and to assess macular thickness changes using optical coherence tomography (OCT).

Methods.—In this prospective study, 62 eyes of 62 patients were randomized to either the BF group ($n = 31$) or the ST group ($n = 31$). The average perifoveal thickness (AFT) was measured by OCT preoperatively, and 1 day and 1, 2, 4 and 6 weeks postoperatively. The best-corrected visual acuity, intraocular pressure and flare in the anterior chamber were recorded at each visit. The same method was used to compare patients with non-proliferative diabetic retinopathy (NPDR) in the BF ($n = 16$) and ST ($n = 11$) groups.

Results.—In the analysis of all patients, flare in the anterior chamber was significantly ($p = 0.007$) lower in the BF group 2 weeks postoperatively. In patients with NPDR, the anterior chamber flare values were significantly lower in the BF group at 4 weeks ($p = 0.0009$) and 6 weeks ($p = 0.005$). The AFT values were significantly lower in the BF group at 4 weeks ($p < 0.0001$) and 6 weeks ($p < 0.0001$). No adverse events occurred in either group.

Conclusion.—BF suppressed anterior chamber inflammation and increasing retinal thickening after cataract surgery in patients with NPDR.

▶ This report describes a randomized trial that could have been an important practical advance in guiding clinical decision making for cataract surgeons except for a peculiar design flaw. The authors chose to compare the effects of a topical nonsteroidal agent (nonsteroidal anti-inflammatory drug [NSAID]), bromfenac, with the effects of topical steroid treatment after cataract surgery for 6 weeks. The authors found a clear benefit to treatment with the NSAID in terms of aqueous flare and a trend towards a benefit in terms of reducing macular edema. This was true for all diabetic patients, including those with preexisting retinopathy. The problem is that the protocol required switching all steroid-treated patients from betamethasone to fluorometholone (FML) at week 1. The authors were concerned about the potential for steroid-related side effects if use was to be continued for 6 weeks. While this concern is understandable, FML is a very weak steroid with limited intraocular penetration, and it likely has little if any effect on anterior segment inflammation and even less effect on macular pathology. This choice renders this group of patients as something of a control group with no meaningful treatment beyond week 1. Given that, we can still draw meaningful conclusions. Bromfenac does appear to have an effect on reduction of macular edema in these high-risk patients (ie, diabetic patients). The drug is well tolerated, and routine off-label use for several weeks after cataract surgery is reasonable, if still not definitively proven. Whether concomitant use of or substitution with a stronger topical steroid is preferable remains unknown.

J. F. Vander, MD

Outcomes of Corneal Spherical Aberration-guided Cataract Surgery Measured by the OPD-Scan

Solomon JD (Solomon Eye Physicians & Surgeons, Bowie, MD)
J Refract Surg 26:863-869, 2010

Purpose.—To determine based on preoperative corneal spherical aberration, the practicality of targeting zero total ocular postoperative spherical aberration when selecting an aspheric intraocular lens (IOL).

Methods.—Consecutive cataract patients were selected to receive an aspheric IOL based on corneal spherical aberration. A target of zero postoperative total spherical aberration $Z(4,0)$ was calculated. One of three IOLs was chosen, based on the corneal spherical aberration $Z(4,0)$ measurement at the 6-mm optical zone. The IOL was selected based on the summation of the corneal spherical aberration and the aspheric value of the prolate optic. The intention was an absolute value of zero total spherical aberration. Statistical analysis of the postoperative total ocular wavefront profile was performed to assess the accuracy of aspheric IOL selection.

Results.—Forty eyes of 40 patients were available for postoperative assessment. The Tecnis Z9003 (Abbott Medical Optics) was implanted in 25 eyes with a preoperative corneal spherical aberration of +0.311 ± 0.054 μm, the AcrySof IQ (Alcon Laboratories Inc) in 13 eyes (+0.188 ± 0.034 μm), and the SofPort-Advanced Optic with Violet Shield (Bausch & Lomb) was implanted in 2 eyes (+0.0915 μm). Total postoperative ocular spherical aberration for the entire group measured + 0.019 ± 0.051 μm (Tecnis: +0.024 ± 0.058 μm; AcrySof IQ: +0.010 ± 0.035 μm; and SofPort AOV: +0.037 μm).

Mean absolute predictive error, for the entire group, measured +0.025 ± 0.020 μm.

Conclusions.—Skiascopy-derived total wavefront measurement of spherical aberration is a reproducible method of aspheric IOL selection and permits more precise control of total ocular spherical aberration.

▶ This study examined the feasibility of targeting zero total ocular spherical aberration (SA) after cataract surgery by using 1 of 3 currently available aspheric intraocular lenses (IOLs) custom matched to the calculated SA of the patient's cornea preoperatively. These 3 lenses are Abbott Medical Optics Tecnis, Alcon AcrySof IQ, and Bausch & Lomb (B&L) Advanced Optic. These lenses are made with negative SA (Tecnis and AcrySof IQ) or zero SA (B&L) to balance the natural positive SA of the cornea. The goal of near-zero total ocular SA was achieved for all eyes with less than 0.35 μm of corneal SA (Fig 2 in the original article). The author makes no attempt to assess the effect of near-zero SA on the patients' visual acuity or contrast sensitivity, however. Customized IOLs to optimize not only low-order aberrations (the well-known sphere and cylinder power correction) but also high-order aberrations, such as coma, trefoil, and SA, may be on the horizon in the future. This capability to reduce ocular higher order aberrations is already in common use in wavefront-guided excimer laser vision correction.

M. F Pyfer, MD

Accuracy of Intraocular Lens Calculations Using the IOLMaster in Eyes with Long Axial Length and a Comparison of Various Formulas
Bang S, Edell E, Yu Q, et al (The Johns Hopkins Univ, Baltimore, MD)
Ophthalmology 118:503-506, 2011

Purpose.—To evaluate the relationship between eyes with long axial length (AL) and postoperative refractive errors as predicted by various commonly used intraocular lens (IOL) formulas using the Zeiss IOLMaster (Carl Zeiss Meditec, Jena, Germany).

Design.—Retrospective chart review.

Participants.—A total of 53 eyes of 36 patients with an AL of more than 27 mm who underwent uncomplicated cataract extraction with IOL implantation.

Methods.—Data were obtained from patient charts and the IOLMaster.

Main Outcome Measures.—The main parameters assessed were AL, preoperative best-corrected visual acuity (BCVA), postoperative BCVA, and mean absolute error (actual postoperative spherical equivalent minus predicted postoperative spherical equivalent). Mean absolute error was calculated using predicted spherical equivalents obtained from the Holladay 1, Holladay 2, SRK/T, Hoffer Q, and Haigis formulas.

Results.—The Haigis formula was found to be the most accurate in predicting postoperative refractive error in long eyes. The SRK/T formula

TABLE 1.—Overall Mean Absolute Error* by Formula

Formula	Mean	Standard Deviation	Lower 95% Confidence Interval	Upper 95% Confidence Interval	Minimum	Maximum
Holladay1	0.96	0.63	0.78	1.14	−0.05	2.08
Holladay 2	0.81	0.81	0.58	1.04	−0.80	2.15
SRK/T	0.62	0.77	0.40	0.84	−0.52	2.22
Hoffer Q	1.02	0.88	0.77	1.26	−0.70	2.45
Haigis	0.52	0.63	0.34	0.70	−0.51	2.12

*Overall mean absolute error = (predicted spherical equivalent−actual postoperative spherical equivalent).

was the second most accurate, followed by the Holladay 2, then the Holladay 1, then the Hoffer Q. All formulas predicted a more myopic outcome than was actually achieved.

Conclusions.—These results suggest using the Haigis, SRK/T, or Holladay 2 formulas for very long eyes. It is also advisable to aim for a more myopic result than is intended (Table 1).

▶ Eyes with long axial length are challenging to measure and can be more difficult to achieve a targeted refractive outcome after cataract surgery. This is because of uncertainty in axial length measurement, variability in final intraocular lens (IOL) position, and inaccuracy of predictive formulas for unusually long (and also short) eyes. Partial coherence optical measurement of axial length, as used in the IOLMaster (Carl Zeiss, Inc) instrument, has improved the accuracy of axial length measurement of long eyes but does not reduce the other sources of error.

This study found that the Haigis and SRK/T formulas gave the most accurate results for eyes greater than 27 mm long (Table 1). The authors do not specify if their Haigis formula A constants were optimized with surgeon-specific outcomes. This is an important detail because in previous studies, the nonoptimized Haigis formula was somewhat inferior to SRK/T and Holladay 2.[1]

The authors found that all of the formulas yielded a more hyperopic outcome than predicted, so they recommend a target of mild myopia in longer eyes to avoid hyperopic surprise. This phenomenon is well known to most cataract surgeons and agrees with prior studies,[2] so their advice is prudent.

M. F. Pyfer, MD

References

1. Haigis W. Intraocular lens calculation in extreme myopia. *J Cataract Refract Surg.* 2009;35:906-912.
2. Wang JK, Hu CY, Chang SW. Intraocular lens power calculation using the IOL Master and various formulas in eyes with long axial length. *J Cataract Refract Surg.* 2008;34:262-267.

Comparison of visual performance with blue light-filtering and ultraviolet light-filtering intraocular lenses

Neumaier-Ammerer B, Felke S, Hagen S, et al (Rudolf Foundation Clinic Vienna, Austria; et al)
J Cataract Refract Surg 36:2073-2079, 2010

Purpose.—To compare the contrast sensitivity, glare, color perception, and visual acuity at different light intensities with yellow-tinted and clear intraocular lenses (IOLs) by different manufacturers.

Setting.—Ludwig Boltzmann Institute of Retinology and Biomicroscopic Laser-Surgery, Department of Ophthalmology, Rudolf Foundation Clinic, Vienna, Austria.

Design.—Comparative case series.

Methods.—Eyes were randomized to 1 of the following IOLs: AF-1 (UY) (yellow tinted), AcrySof SN60AT (yellow tinted), AF-1 (UV) (clear), or AcrySof SA60AT (clear). One week and 2 months postoperatively, monocular contrast sensitivity function and color discrimination were tested and the corrected distance and near visual acuities were evaluated. All tests were performed under different light intensities (10 to 1000 lux).

Results.—Of the 80 patients enrolled, 76 completed the study; there were 37 eyes in the yellow-tinted IOL group and 39 in the clear IOL group. There were no significant differences between yellow-tinted IOLs and clear IOLs except in color vision under mesopic conditions (10 lux). Patients with a yellow-tinted IOL made significantly more mistakes in the blue-light spectrum than patients with clear IOLs ($P = .00015$). There was no significant difference under photopic conditions (1000 lux).

Conclusions.—The yellow-tinted IOLs were equivalent to the clear IOLs in postoperative contrast sensitivity, visual acuity, and color perception under photopic conditions. Patients with yellow-tinted IOLs made statistically significantly more mistakes in the blue range under dim light than patients with clear IOLs (Table 3).

▶ Intraocular lenses (IOLs) containing yellow chromophore have been well accepted by cataract surgeons both in the United States and worldwide, and millions of these IOLs have been implanted in patients since their introduction over 8 years ago. Theoretically, blue-blocking (yellow-tinted) IOLs may help protect the macula from oxidative free radical damage induced by high-energy blue light exposure. There is no clear consensus on the visual effects of blue-blocking IOLs, although clinically it is clear to most surgeons that these lenses perform well. Some authors have postulated that because blue light is important for stimulation of melatonin production and maintenance of circadian rhythm in humans, yellow IOLs may result in sleep disturbance.[1]

This study examined contrast sensitivity and color perception in photopic and mesopic conditions, comparing patients with yellow-tinted and clear IOLs. There was a statistically significant difference in blue color perception for the yellow IOL group only under mesopic conditions (Table 3). No difference in acuity, contrast sensitivity, or photopic color perception was found in this

TABLE 3.—Mistakes in the Blue Light Spectrum of the Hue Test 8 Weeks Postoperatively Under Different Lighting Intensities

	Yellow IOL		Untinted IOL		Both Yellow IOLs (n = 37)	Both Clear IOLs (n = 39)	P Value*	
Lighting	Hoya (n = 19)	Alcon (n = 18)	Hoya (n = 20)	Alcon (n = 19)			Yellow Vs Untinted	Between Yellow IOLs
1000 lux	0.72 ± 0.89	1.12 ± 1.32	0.79 ± 1.03	0.89 ± 1.10	0.91 ± 2.20	0.84 ± 1.05	.8081	.4577
10 lux	3.11 ± 1.97	3.82 ± 2.43	1.84 ± 1.74	2.16 ± 1.57	3.46 ± 2.20	2.00 ± 1.64	.0015	.4678

IOL = intraocular lers.
*Mann-Whitney *U* test.

study when comparing yellow-tinted IOLs with their clear versions by the same manufacturer. This should reassure surgeons who implant these yellow lenses that the benefit of macular photoprotection does not come at the expense of compromised visual perception.

M. F. Pyfer, MD

Reference

1. Mainster MA. Violet and blue light blocking intraocular lenses: photoprotection versus photoreception. *Br J Ophthalmol.* 2006;90:784-792.

Correction of Astigmatism During Cataract Surgery: Toric Intraocular Lens Compared to Peripheral Corneal Relaxing Incisions
Poll JT, Wang L, Koch DD, et al (Baylor College of Medicine, Houston, TX)
J Refract Surg 27:165-171, 2011

Purpose.—To compare the efficacy of astigmatic correction achieved at the time of cataract surgery using toric intraocular lens (IOL) implantation versus peripheral corneal relaxing incisions.

Methods.—A retrospective review assessed the outcomes of phacoemulsification cataract surgery performed between January 2006 and January 2008 by a single surgeon. Patients receiving a toric IOL (toric IOL group) or peripheral corneal relaxing incisions (relaxing incisions group) were included in the study. Main outcome variables included postoperative uncorrected distance visual acuity (UDVA) and manifest refractive cylinder. Each treatment modality was stratified by amount of preoperative keratometric astigmatism into three groups (low, moderate, and high astigmatism) for comparative analysis.

Results.—A total of 192 eyes were included in the study; 77 received a toric IOL and 115 received peripheral corneal relaxing incisions. Preoperative data were not significantly different between the two groups except regarding keratometric astigmatism, which was higher in the toric IOL group ($P<.05$). Average postoperative astigmatism was 0.42 diopters (D) and 0.46 D in the toric and relaxing incisions groups, respectively. In subgroup analysis, no statistical significance separated the two treatment options in terms of amount of surgically induced astigmatism or residual astigmatism. Eyes with astigmatism $\geq$2.26 D were more likely to achieve 20/40 UDVA from a toric IOL.

Conclusions.—Toric IOL implantation and peripheral corneal relaxing incisions yielded similar results regarding surgical correction of astigmatism at the time of phacoemulsification cataract surgery. Both treatment modalities achieved comparable results with mild-to-moderate astigmatism. Higher degrees of astigmatism favor use of a toric IOL.

▶ Refractive-oriented cataract surgeons now have in their armamentarium at least 3 options for correction of astigmatism along with cataract surgery.

These options are toric intraocular lenses (IOLs, typically Alcon AcrySof toric), intraoperative and/or postoperative limbal relaxing incisions, and postoperative excimer laser corneal surgery. An advantage of postoperative excimer laser ablation (sometimes called the corneal bioptic procedure) is that any residual spherical error can be corrected at the same time as the astigmatism. Disadvantages of the bioptic technique include the need for 2 separate procedures and higher cost.

This article compares the first 2 techniques, toric IOL placement versus limbal/peripheral corneal relaxing incisions (PCRIs) in treating low-to-moderate corneal astigmatism simultaneously with cataract surgery. The authors found both methods effective, with a slight edge in accuracy for the toric IOL (Fig 5 in the original article). The procedures were performed by a single surgeon using an optimized nomogram for the PCRIs. One significant deficiency of this study is that results were assessed at 1 month. It is well known that limbal/PCRIs may continue to drift or decline in effect, while the cornea heals beyond 1 month. While it presents useful information, the study would be more robust if data at 1 year was included.

The authors' final recommendation for the management of patients with significant astigmatism is as follows:

"1) Eyes with approximately 1.00 D of cylinder or those eyes receiving a multifocal or accommodating IOL typically receive peripheral corneal relaxing incisions; 2) eyes in the 1.00- to 1.50-D range may receive either treatment modality depending on other factors that include symmetry of astigmatism, affordability, corneal status and need for negative asphericity in the IOL; 3) eyes with 1.50 to 3.00 D most often receive a toric IOL; and 4) eyes with > 3.00 D are managed by implanting a toric IOL and performing peripheral corneal relaxing incisions at the time of surgery or a few weeks postoperatively." Based on current technology, this is a useful algorithm that should serve most refractive cataract surgeons and their patients well.

M. F. Pyfer, MD

Visual function and patient satisfaction: Comparison between bilateral diffractive multifocal intraocular lenses and monovision pseudophakia

Zhang F, Sugar A, Jacobsen G, et al (Henry Ford Health System, Taylor, MI; Univ of Michigan, Ann Arbor; Henry Ford Health System, Detroit, MI)
J Cataract Refract Surg 37:446-453, 2011

Purpose.—To compare visual function and patient satisfaction in patients with bilateral diffractive multifocal intraocular lenses (IOLs) and patients with monofocal IOL monovision.

Setting.—Department of Ophthalmology, Henry Ford Health System, Detroit, Michigan, USA.

Design.—Cohort study.

Methods.—This study comprised consecutive bilateral cataract patients having implantation of AcrySof ReSTOR SN60D3 multifocal IOLs or AcrySof SN60WF IOLs as monovision between July 2007 and June

2009. Parameters analyzed 3 months postoperatively included binocular uncorrected distance, intermediate, and near visual acuities; stereo vision; spectacle independence; subjective visual symptoms; and patient satisfaction. Patients were administered the Visual Function Questionnaire-25 preoperatively and postoperatively.

Results.—The multifocal IOL group comprised 21 patients and the monovision group, 22 patients. Although bilateral uncorrected distance vision and near vision were slightly better in the multifocal IOL group than in the monovision group, there was no statistically significant difference between the 2 groups. The monovision group had better intermediate vision than the multifocal IOL group and had less difficulty using computers without glasses; the differences between the 2 groups were statistically significant. Patients with monovision had a slightly higher overall satisfaction score, significantly fewer complaints, and less out-of-pocket cost.

Conclusions.—Pseudophakic monovision achieved distance vision and near vision that were comparable to those with bilateral multifocal IOLs without the inherent risk for disturbing visual symptoms associated with multifocal IOLs. Monovision patients also had significantly better intermediate vision and less difficulty using computers without glasses.

▶ This is a well-organized compelling study comparing a small group of patients who received bilateral AcrySof ReSTOR multifocal intraocular lenses (IOLs) against another group who had planned monovision with the aspheric monofocal AcrySof, both with optimal correction of astigmatism using limbal relaxing incisions when needed. When questioned about visual symptoms such as glare, halos, or difficulty driving in low light or low contrast situations, the monovision patients overall had slightly greater satisfaction with vision. Multifocal patients performed better on stereo testing, but the authors point out that when stereo vision is needed or binocular distance vision is required, a simple pair of single vision glasses will work for the monovision patients. Visual symptoms such as glare and halos, as well as decreased contrast, in patients with multifocal lens are generally not improved with spectacle correction unless significant refractive error remains. Monovision patients also had greater satisfaction with intermediate distance visual tasks such as computer use.

Satisfaction survey questions were asked, and these were about equal between the 2 groups, and no IOL exchanges were required because of intolerance of visual side effects.

One significant limitation of this study is that the first-generation ReSTOR lens was tested. Presently, it is available in an aspheric version and with 3.00 D add rather than 4.00 D as was tested in this study. This newest multifocal IOL should have better intermediate vision performance and perhaps improved contrast sensitivity because of asphericity. I would encourage the authors to repeat their study using the latest multifocal lens design.

M. F. Pyfer, MD

Straylight measurements in pseudophakic eyes with natural and dilated pupils: One-year follow-up

van Gaalen KW, Koopmans SA, Hooymans JMM, et al (Univ of Groningen, The Netherlands)
J Cataract Refract Surg 36:923-928, 2010

Purpose.—To compare the amount of straylight in natural pupils and dilated pupils in pseudophakic eyes 6 weeks and 1 year after cataract extraction.

Setting.—Laboratory of Experimental Ophthalmology, University Medical Center Groningen, University of Groningen, Groningen, The Netherlands.

Methods.—This study evaluated patients with bilateral age-related cataract who had cataract surgery with implantation of an aspheric Tecnis ZA9003 or spherical Sensar AR40e intraocular lens (IOL). Straylight measurements were performed with a C-Quant straylight meter 6 weeks after surgery (with natural pupils) and 1 year after surgery (with natural and dilated pupils) in a randomly chosen eye. Retroillumination photographs of dilated pupils were taken to document posterior capsule opacification. The main outcome variable for straylight measurements was the logarithmic straylight parameter, log(s).

Results.—Twenty-two patients were evaluated. There was a statistically significant decrease in straylight in a natural pupil between 6 weeks (mean 1.44 log[s]) and 1 year (mean 1.30 log[s]) postoperatively ($P = .012$). The straylight parameter was greater after dilation (mean 1.48 log[s]) than with a natural pupil (1.29 log[s]) at 1 year ($P = .012$). This difference was greater when more anterior capsule was visible in the pupillary area ($P = .031$).

Conclusions.—Straylight decreased significantly in the first year after cataract surgery. Furthermore, it increased with increasing pupil size, which was associated with a capsulorhexis smaller than the pupil. This indicates the capsulorhexis should be as large as possible to prevent straylight, especially under low-luminance conditions when the pupil is large.

▶ Ocular straylight measurements using the C-Quant straylight meter (Oculus Instruments) are a valid method for quantifying glare and halo-like visual phenomena in patients. This study examined pseudophakes with standard monofocal intraocular lenses and without other ocular pathology preoperatively and at 6 weeks and 1 year postoperatively. The findings show that straylight decreases after cataract surgery, not surprisingly. Also, there is a further decrease between 6 weeks and 1 year after surgery, possibly because of resolution of subclinical corneal or macular edema. Finally, straylight in pseudophakic eyes when the pupil is dilated is directly proportional to the amount of anterior capsule visible within the pupil. This result indicates that a small capsulorhexis or progressive anterior capsule phimosis postoperatively may contribute to nighttime glare symptoms that some patients notice after cataract surgery. This study did not attempt to correlate subjective complaints with the straylight measurements. This result also lends credence to recent reports by Masket et al[1] relating negative dysphotopsia symptoms in pseudophakes to excess anterior capsule overlap of the optic.

M. F. Pyfer, MD

Reference

1. Masket S, Fram NR. Pseudophakic negative dysphotopsia: Surgical management and new theory of etiology. *J Cataract Refract Surg.* 2011;37(7):1199-1207.

Ablation of lens epithelial cells with a laser photolysis system: Histopathology, ultrastructure, and immunochemistry
Mamalis N, Grossniklaus HE, Waring GO III, et al (Univ of Utah, Salt Lake City; Emory Univ, Atlanta, GA; et al)
J Cataract Refract Surg 36:1003-1010, 2010

Purpose.—To evaluate efficacy of a neodymium:YAG (Nd:YAG) laser photolysis system in removing lens epithelial cells (LECs) and characterize the effect of the laser on laminin and fibronectin involved in LEC adhesion and migration.

Methods. Cadaver eyes were evaluated using the Miyake technique. The lenses were removed with phacoemulsification. The modified Nd:YAG laser was used to clean the LECs from the capsule. Only the fornix was cleaned in some eyes and the anterior subcapsular area in other eyes. Some areas were not treated and acted as controls. Standard irrigation/aspiration (I/A) removal of LECs was performed in additional eyes. The eyes were analyzed using light microscopy and immunohistochemical staining.

Results.—Histopathologic evaluation showed that the laser removed the LECs from the anterior lens capsule and from the fornix. Immunohistochemical staining showed fibronectin and laminin staining in the untreated areas that was absent in the treated areas. Standard I/A removal of the LECs showed absence of cells but persistent laminin and fibronectin. Electron microscopy showed epithelial cells in untreated areas with an absence of the LECs and debris in treated areas.

Conclusions.—The laser photolysis system removed LECs from the anterior lens capsule and capsule fornix. Along with the cells, laminin, fibronectin, and cell debris remained in the untreated areas but were removed by the treatment. This treatment may be useful in preventing posterior capsule opacification (Fig 1).

▶ This article describes the laboratory study of a neodymium yttrium aluminum garnet (Nd:YAG) laser system used to remove the lens epithelial cells (LECs) and cell adhesion molecules (CAMs) within the capsular bag after phacoemulsification. It should be read in tandem with the clinical study of the same device.[1] Human cadaver eyes were treated (Fig 1) and then examined in the histopathology lab to determine the effectiveness of the technique. Comparison with standard irrigation/aspiration (I/A) removal of LECs was also made. The

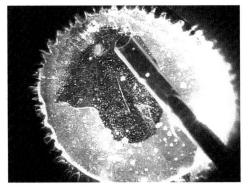

FIGURE 1.—Removal of LECs from a human cadaver eye using the Miyake technique. (Reprinted from Mamalis N, Grossniklaus HE, Waring GO III, et al. Ablation of lens epithelial cells with a laser photolysis system: histopathology, ultrastructure, and immunochemistry. *J Cataract Refract Surg.* 2010;36:1003-1010, Copyright 2010, with permission from ASCRS and ESCRS.)

Nd:YAG laser was effective in removing all cellular material, debris, and CAMs, without damaging the underlying capsule, whereas I/A left some cells, debris, and most of the CAMs behind. If this technique can be performed efficiently through a sub-3-mm temporal clear corneal incision, which has yet to be demonstrated in significant numbers of patients, then it looks promising for prevention of postcataract surgical capsular fibrosis and opacification. This is especially important for optimal performance of accommodating and multifocal intraocular lenses.

M. F. Pyfer, MD

Reference

1. Wehner W, Waring GO 3rd, Mamalis N, Walker R, Thyzel R. Prevention of lens capsule opacification with ARC neodymium:YAG laser photolysis after phacoemulsification. *J Cataract Refract Surg.* 2010;36:881-884.

Prevention of lens capsule opacification with ARC neodymium:YAG laser photolysis after phacoemulsification
Wehner W, Waring GO III, Mamalis N, et al (Maximilian Eye Clinic, Nuremberg, Germany; Eye 1st Vision and Laser, Atlanta, GA; Univ of Utah, Salt Lake City; et al)
J Cataract Refract Surg 36:881-884, 2010

We describe a technique that uses a neodymium:YAG (Nd:YAG) laser photolysis system to prevent lens capsule opacification. The photolysis instrument consists of a 1064 nm Nd:YAG laser transmitted along a fiber-optic cable into a handpiece containing an angulated titanium plate that the laser beam strikes, creating plasma and a shockwave that exits the handpiece through an aperture. Under direct visualization, the

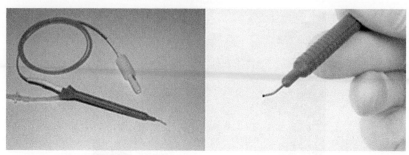

FIGURE 1.—The laser photolysis handpiece. *Left*: The green handpiece has an angled tip. The orange coiled fiber is the fiberoptic cable that relays the laser pulses. The white coupling device inserts into the laser console. The infusion fluid tubing is the clear tubing in the lower left of the picture. *Right*: The handpiece tip is 1.05 mm in diameter. For interpretation of the references to color in this figure legend, the reader is referred to web version of this article. (Reprinted from Journal of Cataract & Refractive Surgery. Wehner W, Waring GO III, Mamalis N, et al. Prevention of lens capsule opacification with ARC neodymium:YAG laser photolysis after phacoemulsification. *J Cataract Refract Surg*. 2010;36:881-884, Copyright 2010, with permission from ASCRS and ESCRS.)

shockwave is aimed at the inner surface of the anterior capsule, where it removes LECs and proteoglycan attachment molecules; the shockwave probably extends to the capsule fornix, destroying germinal epithelial cells. We report preliminary results in 12 eyes followed for approximately 2.5 years in which the treated nasal anterior capsule remained clear or with only slight opacity and the untreated temporal capsule developed moderate to severe opacification (Fig 1).

▶ Advanced intraocular lenses increasingly depend on a persistently clear capsular bag with minimal fibrosis and contracture for optimal performance. However, current literature cites posterior capsule opacification requiring YAG laser capsulotomy as the most frequent postoperative complication of modern phacoemulsification cataract surgery. This article and the study by Mamalis et al[1] describe the laboratory science and experimental surgical technique for an Nd:YAG laser photolysis instrument used to clean residual lens epithelial cells, debris, and cell adhesion substances from the internal capsular bag atraumatically. The device tested (Fig 1) is a modification of the Dodick laser photolysis system originally introduced for laser phacoemulsification 10 years ago but never marketed.[1] It creates a shock wave that disrupts cells and adherent molecules without damaging the capsular basement membrane or zonular apparatus. Other methods proposed for terminal capsular bag cleaning have relied on chemical or osmotic disruption, and are not practical, because a means for isolating the internal capsular bag from the rest of the eye has not been developed yet. The pilot study showed successful posterior capsule opacification prevention in the treated area of the capsule in 12 eyes for up to 2.5 years. This is an intriguing technique that could be used after routine phacoemulsification, especially with presbyopia-correcting multifocal or accommodating intraocular lenses.

M. F. Pyfer, MD

Reference

1. Mamalis N, Grossniklaus HE, Waring GO 3rd, et al. Ablation of lens epithelial cells with a laser photolysis system: Histopathology, ultrastructure, and immunochemistry. *J Cataract Refract Surg.* 2010;36:1003-1010.

Accelerated 20-year sunlight exposure simulation of a photochromic foldable intraocular lens in a rabbit model
Werner L, Abdel-Aziz S, Peck CC, et al (Univ of Utah, Salt Lake City; et al)
J Cataract Refract Surg 37:378-385, 2011

Purpose.—To assess the long-term biocompatibility and photochromic stability of a new photochromic hydrophobic acrylic intraocular lens (IOL) under extended ultraviolet (UV) light exposure.

Setting.—John A. Moran Eye Center, University of Utah, Salt Lake City, Utah, USA.

Design.—Experimental study.

Methods.—A Matrix Aurium photochromic IOL was implanted in right eyes and a Matrix Acrylic IOL without photochromic properties (n = 6) or a single-piece AcrySof Natural SN60AT IOL (n = 5) in left eyes of 11 New Zealand rabbits. The rabbits were exposed to a UV light source of 5 mW/cm^2 for 3 hours during every 8-hour period, equivalent to 9 hours a day, and followed for up to 12 months. The photochromic changes were evaluated during slitlamp examination by shining a penlight UV source in the right eye. After the rabbits were humanely killed and the eyes enucleated, study and control IOLs were explanted and evaluated in vitro on UV exposure and studied histopathologically.

Results.—The photochromic IOL was as biocompatible as the control IOLs after 12 months under conditions simulating at least 20 years of UV exposure. In vitro evaluation confirmed the retained optical properties, with photochromic changes observed within 7 seconds of UV exposure. The rabbit eyes had clinical and histopathological changes expected in this model with a 12-month follow-up.

Conclusions.—The new photochromic IOL turned yellow only on exposure to UV light. The photochromic changes were reversible, reproducible, and stable over time. The IOL was biocompatible with up to 12 months of accelerated UV exposure simulation (Fig 3).

▶ An intraocular lens (IOL) that reliably becomes tinted in bright light while remaining clear in dim light, much like currently available photochromic sunglasses, is an appealing concept. It would seem to represent the best of both worlds between a yellow (blue-blocking) IOL and an optically clear IOL. Well, this concept is now a reality, as this article demonstrates.

This study examined the performance of the new Matrix Aurium photochromic IOL in vivo using the albino rabbit model. This is a unique IOL developed by Medennium and currently available outside the United States in a 3-piece design.

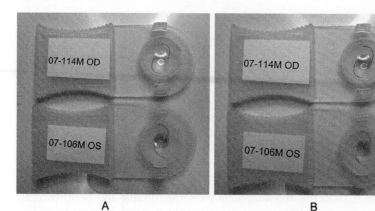

A   B

FIGURE 3.—Gross photographs of explanted study IOL (*top*) and control IOL 2 (*bottom*) before (A) and immediately after (B) exposure of the IOLs to an UV penlight for 7 seconds. (Reprinted from Werner L, Abdel-Aziz S, Peck CC, et al. Accelerated 20-year sunlight exposure simulation of a photochromic foldable intraocular lens in a rabbit model. *J Cataract Refract Surg.* 2011;37:378-385, Copyright 2011, with permission from ASCRS and ESCRS.)

It is a hydrophobic acrylic lens with a blue light absorption curve similar to the AcrySof Natural IOL (Alcon Laboratories, Inc) when exposed to ultraviolet (UV) light such as natural sunlight. Under these conditions, the optic of the IOL turns yellow in color and blue light is absorbed. In low UV illumination, such as indoors or at night, it behaves as a standard UV-filtering IOL with a clear optic.

The AcrySof Natural blue light—filtering IOL has gained wide acceptance in the United States, providing protection of the retina against short-wavelength light that may generate free radicals and cause oxidative photoreceptor damage possibly contributing to macular degeneration. However, blue light is important for maintenance of circadian rhythms in humans, and yellow filtration in low-light situations has been shown to decrease contrast sensitivity. Thus, the theoretical benefit of a yellow-tinted IOL is maximized when it is used only in bright light environments, so a photochromic IOL seems ideal as long as its properties are stable in the eye over the patient's lifetime. This study demonstrated no degradation of the Matrix Aurium photochromic IOL after accelerated 20-year equivalent of UV exposure in the rabbit eye (Fig 3).

In a prospective comparative clinical study of 15 patients in Mexico,[1] the Matrix Aurium IOL was randomly implanted in 1 eye and an Alcon AcrySof SN60WF (yellow aspheric IOL) in the other eye. The photochromic IOL outperformed the SN60WF under low-level illumination conditions (from 11 to 500 lux), and in other conditions there was no difference. Prior laboratory testing[2,3] also showed in vitro stability of the Matrix Aurium IOL after prolonged UV irradiation and to Nd:YAG laser exposure.

M. F. Pyfer, MD

References

1. Mendez D, Mendez A. First photochromic intraocular lens (matrix acrylic aurium)—two year clinical experience in humans. Presented at the Annual Meeting of the American Academy of Ophthalmology; November 2008; Atlanta, GA.

2. Werner L, Mamalis N, Wilcox C, Zhou S. In Vitro and in Vivo Studies for Evaluation of the Matrix Acrylic Aurium Photochromic Intraocular Lens. Presented at the XXV Congress of the European Society of Cataract and Refractive Surgeons; September 2007; Stockholm, Sweden.
3. Brubaker JW, Espandar L, Davis DK, Wilcox C, Mamalis N. Stability of a Novel Photochromic IOL After Simulated 20 Years in the Eye Using Nd: YAG Laser Exposure Test. Presented at the ASCRS Symposium on Cataract, IOL and Refractive Surgery; April 2008; Chicago, IL.

Evaluation of the Calhoun Vision UV Light Adjustable Lens Implanted Following Cataract Removal

Hengerer FH, Conrad-Hengerer I, Buchner SE, et al (Ruhr Univ Eye Clinic, Bochum, Germany)
J Refract Surg 26:716-721, 2010

Purpose.—To evaluate the effectiveness of a silicone intraocular lens (IOL) that can be adjusted following implantation using ultraviolet (UV) irradiation.

Methods.—Prospective clinical trial of 40 patients (40 eyes) with visually significant cataract. Participants underwent small-incision phacoemulsification followed by implantation of a light-adjustable, silicone IOL (Light Adjustable Lens [LAL], Calhoun Vision). All patients were required to wear UV-protective eyewear at all times, until final lock-in. Pre- and postoperative clinical parameters included distance visual acuity and manifest refraction.

Results.—At average 2 weeks postoperative (range: 10 to 21 days), patients were seen and refracted to determine type and magnitude of refractive error needing correction. All patients required an initial adjustment of the LAL, whereas 28 required a second UV treatment and none required a third adjustment. At 4 months postoperative, mean refraction was 0.04 ± 0.37 diopters (D) (range: -0.88 to 0.50 D), mean sphere was 0.24 ± 0.40 D (range: -0.50 to 0.75 D), and mean cylinder was 0.41 ± 0.25 D (range: 1.00 to 0.0 D). Eighty-one percent of eyes gained 2 or more lines of corrected distance visual acuity.

Conclusions.—The adjustment and lock-in procedures were well tolerated by patients. The Calhoun Vision LAL is a promising technology with the potential to eliminate postoperative refractive surprises of up to 2.00 D of refractive and cylindrical error following implantation.

▶ Since the first laboratory studies were published in 2003, the light-adjustable lens (LAL), developed by Calhoun Vision in Pasadena, CA, has made slow but steady progress toward clinical utility. A recent report[1] from the Codet Vision Institute in Tijuana, Mexico, demonstrates successful postimplantation adjustment of both spherical and toric refractive status in 5 patients. They achieved 20/25 or better uncorrected visual acuity with a stable postadjustment refraction for 9 months. This larger series of 40 patients at Ruhr University Eye Hospital in Germany included both spherical and toric adjustments of up to 2-dimensional.

They demonstrated stability and good visual acuity up to 4 months post–lock-in. Several earlier reports[2-4] present short-term results for the LAL undergoing myopic and hyperopic postimplantation adjustments.

This is an exciting technology that allows noninvasive postoperative adjustment of the refractive power of a silicone intraocular lens (IOL) implant. Limitations of the current design are that the power cannot be changed after lock-in and that exposure to UV light prior to adjustment and lock-in can cause unpredictable results and must be prevented.[5] Despite these limitations, this technology could be extended to provide customized correction for higher-order aberrations and even combined with accommodative or multifocal lens designs for both primary and secondary (piggy-back) IOL implantation to create a wide range of new applications for pseudophakic patients.

M. F. Pyfer, MD

References

1. Chayet A, Sandstedt C, Chang S, et al. Use of the light-adjustable lens to correct astigmatism after cataract surgery. *Br J Ophthalmol*. 2010;94:690-692.
2. Chayet A, Sandstedt CA, Chang SH, Rhee P, Tsuchiyama B, Schwartz D. Correction of residual hyperopia after cataract surgery using the light adjustable intraocular lens technology. *Am J Ophthalmol*. 2009;147:392-397.
3. von Mohrenfels CW, Salgado J, Khoramnia R, Maier M, Lohmann CP. Clinical results with the light adjustable intraocular lens after cataract surgery. *J Refract Surg*. 2010;26:314-320.
4. Chayet A, Sandstedt C, Chang S, et al. Correction of myopia after cataract surgery with a light-adjustable lens. *Ophthalmology*. 2009;116:1432-1435.
5. Hafezi F, Seiler T, Iseli HP. Light-adjustable lens complication [Letter]. *Ophthalmology*. 2010;117:848-848.e1.

Ab externo iris fixation of posterior chamber intraocular lens through small incision

Zandian M, Moghimi S, Fallah M, et al (Tehran Univ of Med Sciences, Iran; et al)
J Cataract Refract Surg 36:2032-2034, 2010

During secondary posterior chamber intraocular lens (PC IOL) implantation with iris fixation in the absence of capsule support, we implanted an acrylic 3-piece PC IOL through a small clear corneal incision with haptics secured in knots; there was no need for IOL capture. Sutures were placed appropriately in the iris tissue before the IOL was inserted, ensuring safety of the procedure and centration of the IOL (Fig 1).

▶ Fixation of a posterior chamber intraocular lens in the absence of capsular support can be challenging. A variety of techniques have been described, including scleral suture fixation and iris suture fixation. Iris-sutured intraocular lenses (IOLs) avoid the problem of suture or knot erosion to the external ocular surface and at least theoretically have a lower risk for late-onset endophthalmitis that may result from an exposed suture. Iris fixation has its own set of potential

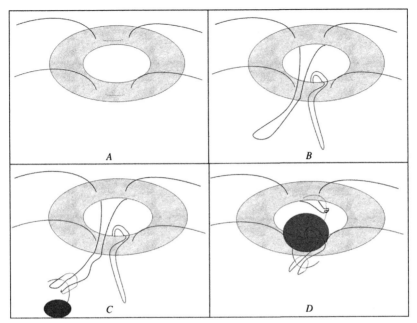

FIGURE 1.—*A*: Entering from the limbal region, polypropylene 10.0 sutures are passed through the peripheral iris with a 2.0 mm bite and exit the opposite limbus. *B*: Using a side-port stab incision opposite the main incision, the loops are grasped and pulled out through the main incision. *C*: A girth-hitch knot is used to secure the leading haptic at the optic—haptic junction. After the IOL is folded, it is placed under the iris. *D*: Another girthhitch knot is used to secure the trailing haptic in the subincisional loop, and the haptic is placed under the iris. (Reprinted from Zandian M, Moghimi S, Fallah M, et al. Ab externo iris fixation of posterior chamber intraocular lens through small incision. *J Cataract Refract Surg.* 2010;36: 2032-2034, Copyright 2010, with permission from ASCRS and ESCRS.)

problems, including pupil distortion, pigment dispersion, and chronic iris. Also, in all suture techniques, late failure of the suture or cheese-wiring through the tissue have been reported, resulting in potential subluxation of the IOL.

This article describes a novel technique for iris suture fixation of an IOL using an external knot. It avoids blind passes of the suture needle through the iris to capture the IOL haptic that are necessary in the standard iris fixation method. This should result in better centration of the iris-sutured IOL and less distortion of the pupil because of more accurate suture placement in the midperipheral iris. Fig 1 shows the essential elements of this straightforward technique for small-incision iris fixation of a foldable IOL.

M. F. Pyfer, MD

Use of a Microvascular Clip for Iris Fixation of an Intraocular Lens: A Laboratory Model

Tzu JH, Desai NR, Akpek EK (Johns Hopkins Hosp, Baltimore, MD)
Arch Ophthalmol 128:114-116, 2010

Here we present a potential novel surgical technique consisting of fixation of a posterior-chamber intraocular lens to the iris that may be used in the treatment of aphakia or the management of intraocular lens complications when capsular support has been compromised. The technique was performed in a laboratory model using cadaveric human eyes. A commercially available neurovascular clip was used to securely fasten the intraocular lens to the iris with minimal trauma. The use of a metal clip has the advantage of avoiding potential risks of suture fixation such as suture breakage. Also, this technique is easier than suturing and may potentially serve as another tool in a cornea surgeon's armamentarium.

▶ Hardware clips and staples for anchoring tissue as an alternative to sutures are commonly used in many surgical applications, but so far have not been developed for ophthalmic surgery. This article presents a titanium clip designed for neurovascular surgery, used experimentally in cadaver eyes to secure an intraocular lens to the posterior iris instead of sutures. Surgical speed and efficiency, as well as long-term durability, may benefit from the use of a clip like this. Ideally, it would be redesigned, specifically for ophthalmic use, with reduced bulk and reflectivity to make it less visible on the anterior iris surface (Figs 1-3 in the original article). Permanent easily-implantable tissue anchors for the eye represent an intriguing area ripe for new development in ophthalmic surgery.

M. F. Pyfer, MD

2 Refractive Surgery

One-Year Follow-up of Posterior Chamber Toric Phakic Intraocular Lens Implantation for Moderate to High Myopic Astigmatism
Kamiya K, Shimizu K, Aizawa D, et al (Univ of Kitasato School of Medicine, Kanagawa, Japan; et al)
Ophthalmology 117:2287-2294, 2010

Objective.—To assess the 1-year clinical outcomes of toric Visian Implantable Collamer Lens (ICL; STAAR Surgical, Nidau, Switzerland) implantation for moderate to high myopic astigmatism.

Design.—Prospective, observational case series.

Participants.—Fifty-six eyes of 32 consecutive patients, with spherical equivalent errors of −4.00 to −17.25 diopters (D) and cylindrical errors of −0.75 to −4.00 D, who underwent toric ICL implantation.

Methods.—Before and 1 week and 1, 3, 6, and 12 months after surgery, the safety, efficacy, predictability, stability, and adverse events of the surgery were assessed in eyes undergoing toric ICL implantation. Ocular higher-order aberrations (HOAs) and contrast sensitivity (CS) function also were evaluated before and 1 year after surgery.

Main Outcome Measures.—Uncorrected visual acuity (UCVA), best spectacle-corrected visual acuity (BSCVA), safety index, efficacy index, predictability, stability, adverse events, HOAs, and CS function.

Results.—The logarithm of the minimum angle of resolution (logMAR) UCVA and logMAR BSCVA were −0.11 (corresponding to Snellen equivalent 20/16) ± 0.12 and −0.19 (corresponding to 20/12.5) ± 0.08 1 year after surgery, respectively. The safety and efficacy indices were 1.17 ± 0.21 and 1.00 ± 0.29. At 1 year, 91% and 100% of the eyes were within 0.5 and 1.0 D, respectively, of the targeted correction. Manifest refraction changes of −0.07 ± 0.27 D occurred from 1 week to 1 year. For a 4-mm pupil, fourth-order aberrations were changed, not significantly, from 0.05 ± 0.02 μm before surgery to 0.06 ± 0.03 μm after surgery ($P = 0.38$, Wilcoxon signed-rank test). Similarly, for a 6-mm pupil, fourth-order aberrations were not significantly changed, merely from 0.20 ± 0.08 μm before surgery to 0.23 ± 0.11 μm after surgery ($P = 0.15$). The area under the log CS function was significantly increased from 1.41 ± 0.15 before surgery to 1.50 ± 0.13 after surgery ($P<0.001$). No vision-threatening complications occurred during the observation period.

Conclusions.—In the authors' experience, the toric ICL performed well in correcting moderate to high myopic astigmatism during a 1-year observation

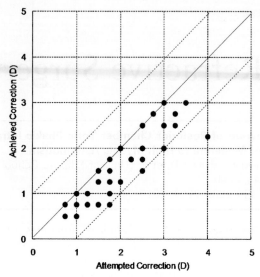

FIGURE 4.—Scatterplot showing attempted versus achieved correction (refractive cylinder) after toric Implantable Collamer Lens implantation. D = diopters. (Reprinted from Kamiya K, Shimizu K, Aizawa D, et al. One-year follow-up of posterior chamber toric phakic intraocular lens implantation for moderate to high myopic astigmatism. *Ophthalmology.* 2010;117:2287-2294, copyright © 2010, with permission from the American Academy of Ophthalmology.)

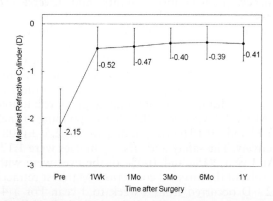

FIGURE 6.—Graph showing the time course of manifest refractive cylinder after toric Implantable Collamer Lens implantation. D = diopters; Y = year. (Reprinted from Kamiya K, Shimizu K, Aizawa D, et al. One-year follow-up of posterior chamber toric phakic intraocular lens implantation for moderate to high myopic astigmatism. *Ophthalmology.* 2010;117:2287-2294, copyright © 2010, with permission from the American Academy of Ophthalmology.)

period, suggesting its viability as a surgical option for the treatment of such eyes (Figs 4 and 6).

▶ Spherical implantable collamer lenses (ICLs) have been shown to be safe and effective in numerous studies, at least for several years. Cataracts and endothelial cell loss continue to be ongoing concerns. This study reported 1-year results of toric ICLs. These lenses are essentially identical to spherical ICLs, except the optic is designed to correct varying degrees of cylinder. They are not yet available in the United States. In addition to the expected issues of cataract and endothelial cell loss, toric ICLs have the additional concern of axis orientation. Axis misalignment can not only affect the refractive outcome and therefore the uncorrected visual acuity, but also potentially affect higher-order aberrations.

The overall results of toric ICL implantation at 1 year were quite good, comparable to spherical ICLs. There was, however, a statistically significant increase in total higher-order aberrations at both 4 and 6 mm pupil sizes ($P < .001$). Astigmatic correction was fairly good (Fig 4) and quite stable (Fig 6). Five eyes required ICL repositioning in the early postoperative period because of lens axis rotation that was greater than or equal to 10°. Four lenses were repositioned on postoperative day 1, and 1 lens was repositioned 1 week after surgery. Two additional eyes required ICL repositioning at a later date because of ocular trauma, totaling 7/56 (12.5%) requiring repositioning in the first year. Asymptomatic anterior subcapsular cataracts were noted in 5.4%. Mean endothelial cell loss was 2.9% at 1 year, which is better than reported for many other ICL series, but higher than the 0.6% yearly physiologic endothelial cell loss. ICLs certainly have a place in the refractive surgeon's arsenal. Hopefully, the toric ICL will be Food and Drug Administration approved in the near future to further expand our surgical options.

C. J. Rapuano, MD

Quality of Life in High Myopia before and after Implantable Collamer Lens Implantation
Ieong A, Hau SCH, Rubin GS, et al (Moorfields Eye Hosp, London, UK; UCL Inst of Ophthalmology, London, UK)
Ophthalmology 117:2295-2300, 2010

Purpose.—To examine changes in vision-related quality of life after implantable Collamer lens (ICL) implantation for the correction of myopia.

Design.—Prospective, interventional, consecutive case series.

Participants.—We included 34 consecutive patients (68% female; mean age, 37 years [range, 23–49]) with preoperative myopia (mean ± standard deviation [SD] refraction spherical equivalent, −11.0 ± 3.12).

Intervention.—Bilateral ICL implantation.

Main Outcome Measures.—Quality of life Impact of Refractive Correction (QIRC) score.

Results.—The median postoperative interval before questionnaire administration was 4 months (range, 3–7). The QIRC scores were significantly higher postoperatively (preoperative QIRC score [mean ± SD], 40.45 ± 4.83; postoperative QIRC score 53.79 ± 5.60; $P<0.001$), with significant improvements ($P<0.01$) for 14 of 19 items. Nineteen (58%) patients reported a worsening in night vision symptoms (mostly nonspecific glare

TABLE 2.—Quality of Life Impact of Refractive Correction (QIRC) Questionnaire Responses Before and After Bilateral Implantable Collamer Lens Implantation

QIRC Item	% N/A	Preoperatively	Postoperatively	P-Value (t-test)
1. Difficulty driving in glare conditions	3	47.87±12.49	45.06±12.62	**0.206**
2. Eyes feeling tired or strained	0	43.75±10.07	53.30±9.36	<0.001
3. Trouble using off the shelf sunglasses	3	42.67±14.64	56.71±0	<0.001
4. Trouble thinking about correction before traveling, sport, swimming	0	33.65±6.35	57.28±9.55	<0.001
5. Trouble not seeing on waking	0	30.24±5.05	58.41±5.30	<0.001
6. Trouble not seeing on beach, in pool	3	33.50±2.69	62.98±3.74	<0.001
7. Trouble with spectacles or contact lenses when doing gym or keep fit	55	38.32±14.64	N/A	N/A
8. Concern about initial cost of contact lenses or refractive surgery	0	40.98±10.23	52.90±12.23	<0.001
9. Concern about ongoing cost	0	41.09±12.21	49.72±9.71	**0.06**
10. Concern about increasing reliance on specs or contact lenses	3	41.80±11.76	58.64±10.89	<0.001
11. Concern about vision not being as good as it could be	0	35.60±4.45	54.23±12.32	<0.001
12. Concern over medical complications from refractive surgery or contact lens wear	0	40.86±11.27	48.58±10.44	**0.03**
13. Concern about eye protection from UV radiation	0	46.17±11.86	53.44±12.10	**0.07**
14. How much time you looked your best	0	41.25±12.42	54.04±14.35	<0.001
15. How much time you projected a positive image to others	3	45.58±12.82	57.09±15.56	<0.001
16. How much time have you felt complimented	3	42.45±8.95	54.13±14.40	<0.001
17. How much time you felt confident	0	44.69±13.58	55.47±14.13	0.01
18. How much time you felt happy	0	43.48±13.61	54.90±13.69	<0.001
19. How much time you felt able to do the things you want	0	36.55±15.7	49.32±14.10	<0.001
20. How much time you felt eager to try new things	0	36.28±14.32	45.27±14.97	0.01
Total QIRC scores		40.45±4.83	53.79±5.60	<0.001

The QIRC questionnaire items and Rasch-weighted response scores (mean±standard deviation [SD]) for implantable Collamer lens (ICL) recipients before and after surgery are summarized. Higher scores suggest better vision related quality of life. P-values for items with a significant change after surgery ($P \leq 0.01$) are highlighted in bold text. The percentage of patients not answering a given questionnaire item (%N/A) was particularly high for question 7, which 55% of patients felt they could not answer after surgery because they were no longer wearing any correction. This item was excluded from the analysis.

and halo or arc effects) after surgery, but overall levels of satisfaction were high; 88% were either satisfied or very satisfied with the results of surgery. No patients reported overall dissatisfaction. In free text responses, 11 patients (32%) described ICL implantation as life changing or wished that they had opted for the surgery sooner.

Conclusions.—Implantation of an ICL for myopia is associated with significant improvements in quality of life. Any dissatisfaction with the procedure largely relates to night vision symptoms, which are common in the early postoperative period (Table 2).

▶ Defining quality of life is a little like defining pornography, in that we all have a good idea what each is, but they are both difficult to define and therefore difficult to measure. Quality of life has been assessed in a variety of ways but most commonly by questionnaires, of which there are numerous validated ones. The authors of this study used one specifically designed to measure quality of life as related to refractive correction called the Quality of Life Impact of Refractive Correction questionnaire that involves answering 20 questions (Table 2).

Results of this study reveal that almost all measures of quality of life were highly statistically significantly better after implantable Collamer lens (ICL) surgery. One measure that wasn't better was difficulty driving in glare conditions, which was slightly worse after surgery. Specifically, 58% of patients felt that night vision symptoms were worse, 27% felt they were the same, and 15% felt they were improved after ICL implantation. Such symptoms tend to improve over time after surgery, and it wasn't reported whether there was a correlation of improved symptoms with greater follow-up time after surgery.

Worsening night vision symptoms after ICL surgery should be further investigated. Correlation to age, pupil size, ICL power, use of toric ICL, residual refractive error, and time since surgery are among the parameters that would be interesting to look at but would likely require many more patients than in this study.

C. J. Rapuano, MD

Refractive surgical correction of presbyopia with the AcuFocus small aperture corneal inlay: two-year follow up
Seyeddain O, Riha W, Hohensinn M, et al (Paracelsus Med Univ, Salzburg, Austria)
J Refract Surg 26:707-715, 2010

Purpose.—To evaluate the safety and efficacy of the AcuFocus Corneal Inlay 7000 (ACI 7000) implanted in emmetropic presbyopic patients for the improvement of near and intermediate vision over 2-year follow-up.

Methods.—This prospective, non-randomized, non-comparative study included 32 naturally emmetropic presbyopic patients. The intracorneal inlay was implanted in the non-dominant eye over the pupil by creating a superior-hinged flap with the IntraLase 60-kHz femtosecond laser (Abbott Medical Optics). Inlay centration was over the line of sight. Minimum postoperative follow-up was 24 months.

Results.—After mean follow-up of 24.2 ± 0.8 months (range: 24 to 26 months), 96.9% of patients read J3 or better in the implanted eye. Mean binocular uncorrected near visual acuity improved from J6 preoperatively to J1 after 24 months. Mean binocular uncorrected intermediate visual acuity (UIVA) was 20/20 at 1 month and remained 20/20 throughout 24-month follow-up, with 71.9% of eyes reaching UIVA of 20/20 or better. At 24 months, mean uncorrected distance visual acuity was 20/20 in the implanted eye and 20/16 binocularly. No inlay was explanted during the study. Two decentered inlays were recentered after 6 months because of in-sufficient increase in near and intermediate visual acuity. Both patients' near and intermediate visual acuity improved significantly after recentration.

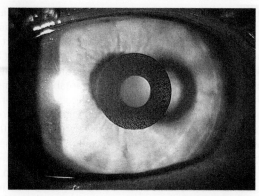

FIGURE 1.—AcuFocus Corneal Inlay 7000 in a patient eye. (Reprinted from Seyeddain O, Riha W, Hohensinn M, et al. Refractive surgical correction of presbyopia with the AcuFocus small aperture corneal inlay: two-year follow up. *J Refract Surg.* 2010;26:707-715, with permission from SLACK Incorporated.)

Conclusions.—The ACI 7000 seems to provide a safe and effective treatment for presbyopia over follow-up of 2 years.

▶ This is exciting new technology! While corneal inlays have been used for decades to correct refractive errors, none have been very successful for a variety of reasons. The only currently Food and Drug Administration (FDA)-approved corneal inlay is Intacs, which is hardly ever used for myopia (it is also FDA approved to treat mild to moderate contact lens—intolerant keratoconus, its primary indication these days).

The AcuFocus corneal inlay (ACI) is based on the small aperture optics concept, long used in photography, in which the depth of the field increases as the aperture size decreases. Through computer modeling, a central aperture size of 1.6 mm was determined to be the optimal size for the ACI to increase near and intermediate vision while minimally affecting distance vision.

The ACI is made of polyvinylidene fluoride material. It is 10-μm thick and 3.8 mm in diameter with a central opening of 1.6 mm. It is pigmented with nanoparticles of carbon to make it essentially opaque (Fig 1). Sixteen hundred small (25 μm in diameter) holes in the inlay allow nutrients to flow through it. The inlay is placed under a 170-μm thick laser-assisted in situ keratomileusis (LASIK) flap. Perfect centration is key given the small size of the inlay and the tiny central opening. It is placed only in the nondominant eye.

By 24 months, the visual results were remarkable. Mean uncorrected near vision improved from J6 to J2. Mean uncorrected intermediate vision improved from 20/40 to 20/25. Mean uncorrected distance vision remained essentially 20/20 in the implanted eye and was 20/16 binocularly. While this study only included emmetropic presbyopes, the authors note that the procedure can be safely performed in patients with hyperopic or myopic presbyopia undergoing LASIK as a combined procedure to correct the refractive error and presbyopia at the same time. I am really looking forward to this technology becoming available in the United States.

C. J. Rapuano, MD

Long-term comparison of corneal aberration changes after laser in situ keratomileusis: Mechanical microkeratome versus femtosecond laser flap creation

Muñoz G, Albarrán-Diego C, Ferrer-Blasco T, et al (Univ of Valencia, Spain)
J Cataract Refract Surg 36:1934-1944, 2010

Purpose.—To compute and compare visual acuity, refractive outcomes, and anterior corneal aberration changes after myopic laser in situ keratomileusis (LASIK) with flap creation by a mechanical microkeratome and by a femtosecond laser.

Setting.—Private practice refractive surgery center, Valencia, Spain.

Design.—Comparative case series.

Methods.—Patients were assigned to have LASIK flap creation with a mechanical microkeratome (Carriazo-Barraquer) or a femtosecond laser (IntraLase). The Visx S2 excimer laser was used for myopic ablation in all cases. Main outcome measures included uncorrected and corrected distance visual acuities and the defocus equivalent. Higher-order aberrations (HOAs) were computed from the anterior corneal surface measured with topography for 4.0 mm and 6.0 mm pupil diameters before and 48 months after surgery.

Results.—The study evaluated 50 patients (98 eyes). The root mean square of HOAs increased postoperatively by a factor of approximately 1.9 in both groups and with both pupil diameters. There were no statistically significant differences between the 2 groups in the increase in anterior corneal aberrations, mean postoperative visual acuity, or residual refraction. All visual and optical performance metrics remained stable throughout the 4-year follow-up. There were no complications with flap creation and no postoperative complications.

Conclusions.—The increase in anterior corneal aberrations after myopic LASIK was similar after mechanical microkeratome and femtosecond laser flap creation. Visual acuity, refraction, and the optical quality of the cornea after LASIK remained stable through 4 years postoperatively in both groups (Fig 7).

▶ Purported advantages of using the femtosecond laser versus a mechanical microkeratome to create laser in situ keratomileusis (LASIK) flaps include greater predictability of flap parameters (eg, thickness, size, and hinge width) but also less-induced corneal aberration, which should theoretically translate into better quality of vision.

The authors performed a prospective study randomizing patients to receive a LASIK flap with a mechanical microkeratome (Carriazo-Barraquer) or a femtosecond laser (IntraLase 15 kHz). Standard noncustom wavefront ablations were performed in all eyes. At 48 months, visual acuity results were essentially identical between the 2 groups. Changes in higher-order aberrations were also not statistically significantly different between the 2 groups, although there was a slightly greater increase in higher-order aberrations in the femtosecond laser

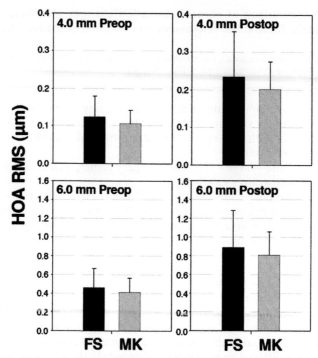

FIGURE 7.—Higher-order aberration RMS values (FS = femtosecond laser; HOA RMS = higher-order aberration root mean square; MK = microkeratome). (Reprinted from Muñoz G, Albarrán-Diego C, Ferrer-Blasco T, et al. Long-term comparison of corneal aberration changes after laser in situ keratomileusis: mechanical microkeratome versus femtosecond laser flap creation. *J Cataract Refract Surg.* 2010;36:1934-1944, copyright 2010, with permission from ASCRS and ESCRS.)

group than in the mechanical microkeratome group at both 4 and 6 mm pupil sizes (Fig 7).

Again, femtosecond laser LASIK flaps have some advantages over mechanical microkeratome flaps but less induced higher-order aberrations does not seem to be one of them. Having said that, perhaps newer generation, faster femtosecond lasers or using custom wavefront ablations might show different results.

C. J. Rapuano, MD

Influence of flap thickness on visual and refractive outcomes after laser in situ keratomileusis performed with a mechanical keratome

Bansal AS, Doherty T, Randleman JB, et al (Emory Eye Ctr and Emory Vision, Atlanta, GA)
J Cataract Refract Surg 36:810-813, 2010

Purpose.—To study the effect of flap thickness on visual acuity and refractive outcomes after laser in situ keratomileusis (LASIK) using 2 blade types with a mechanical microkeratome.

Setting.—Emory Vision, Atlanta, Georgia, USA.

Methods.—This retrospective analysis was of LASIK cases performed between January 2005 and June 2006 using an Amadeus I microkeratome and an ML7090 CLB blade (blade A) or a Surepass blade (blade B). Outcomes analyzed included flap thickness, uncorrected distance visual acuity (UDVA), corrected distance visual acuity (CDVA), manifest refraction spherical equivalent (MRSE), the enhancement rate, and surgical complications 3 months postoperatively.

Results.—Two hundred sixty-three eyes of 153 patients were analyzed; blade A was used in 158 eyes and blade B, in 105 eyes. The mean flap thickness was significantly thinner with blade A than with blade B (107 µm ± 12 [SD] versus 130 ± 20 µm) (*P*<.0001). There was no overall correlation with either blade between flap thickness and UDVA, CDVA, or MRSE (all *r*<0.2). At 3 months, there was no statistically significant difference in UDVA, CDVA, or MRSE between the 2 blade groups at 3 months (all *P* > .10), and there was no difference in the complication rates.

Conclusion.—Flap thickness did not affect visual or refractive outcomes with a mechanical microkeratome with either blade type.

▶ Thinner laser-assisted in situ keratomileusis (LASIK) flaps result in increased residual stromal bed thickness and presumably decreased risk of postoperative ectasia. However, thinner flaps also increase the risk of flap complications such as buttonholes and striae. The ideal flap thickness is still unknown. In this study, there was no difference in visual acuity, refraction, enhancement rate, or complication rate between thinner and thicker LASIK flaps.

This study reinforced the fact that the thickness plate number for a mechanical microkeratome is not the expected value of the flap thickness. And the same thickness plate can yield rather different results depending on the specific blade. In this study, 1 blade resulted in a mean flap thickness of 107 µm while another blade resulted in a mean flap thickness of 130 µm using the same thickness plate. The blade with the thinner flaps also had a tighter standard deviation at 12 µm compared with 20 µm. It might be valuable for surgeons to know what blade is being used in their cases and whether it is the same blade each time.

C. J. Rapuano, MD

Incidence of diffuse lamellar keratitis after LASIK with 15 KHz, 30 KHz, and 60 KHz femtosecond laser flap creation

Choe CH, Guss C, Musch DC, et al (Univ of Michigan, Ann Arbor)
J Cataract Refract Surg 36:1912-1918, 2010

Purpose.—To compare the incidence of diffuse lamellar keratitis (DLK) after laser in situ keratomileusis (LASIK) with flap creation using the 15 kHz (FS15), 30 kHz (FS30), or 60 kHz (FS60) femtosecond laser.

Setting.—University-based academic practice, Ann Arbor, Michigan, USA.

Design.—Retrospective comparative case series.

Methods.—Consecutive myopic LASIK cases performed between January 1, 2005, and June 1, 2007, using the IntraLase FS15, FS30, or FS60 femtosecond laser for flap creation were reviewed. Preoperative clinical characteristics, treatment parameters, and intraoperative and postoperative complications were recorded. Statistical comparisons were made using repeated measures analysis, analysis of variance, chi-square, and Fisher exact tests.

Results.—Five hundred twenty eyes of 274 patients were included in the study. One hundred seventy-six eyes (93 patients) were treated with the FS15 laser, 180 eyes (93 patients) with the FS30 laser, and 164 eyes (89 patients) with the FS60 laser. Seventeen eyes (10%) in the FS15 laser group, 24 eyes (13%) in the FS30 laser group, and 23 eyes (14%) in the FS60 laser group developed DLK. There was no statistically significant difference in the incidence of DLK between the 3 groups ($P = .68$).

Conclusion.—There was no significant difference in the incidence of DLK between the FS15, FS30, and FS60 groups (Table 6).

▶ Diffuse lamellar keratitis (DLK) is a known complication of laser in situ keratomileusis (LASIK). Its exact cause is unknown. A variety of studies have proposed numerous causes including bacterial endotoxins, debris produced during autoclaving, microkeratome cleaning materials, epithelial defects, and others. Over the years, diligent efforts have been made to reduce the incidence of DLK. In fact, for mechanical microkeratomes, the incidence is quite low, generally reported to be less than 5%. However, for femtosecond laser LASIK, the incidence of DLK is much higher, often quoted to be 10% to 15%. The hypothesis is that femtosecond laser energy is causing DLK. When surgeons decreased their laser energy power (often as they gained more experience), they seemed to get less DLK. As femtosecond laser technology has evolved, faster lasers have become available, allowing less energy to be used per laser pulse, theoretically decreasing the risk of DLK.

The authors retrospectively compared the incidence of DLK using a 15 kHz, 30 kHz, and 60 kHz IntraLase femtosecond laser for LASIK. They found no

---

TABLE 6.—Diffuse Lamellar Keratitis by Flap Thickness

Group	<120 μm No DLK/Total (%)	≥120 μm No DLK/Total (%)	P Value*	OR (CI)	P Value**
FS15	3/26 (11.5)	14/150 (9.3)	.721	1.17 (0.30, 4.50)	.821
FS30	11/37 (29.7)	13/143 (9.1)	.001	4.69 (1.38, 15.97)	.014
FS60	6/34 (17.7)	17/130 (13.1)	.494	1.39 (0.53, 3.67)	.508
Total	20/97 (20.6)	44/423 (10.4)	.006	2.13 (1.10, 4.12)	.025

CI = confidence interval; DLK = diffuse lamellar keratitis; FS15 = 15 kHz femtosecond laser; FS30 = 30 kHz femtosecond laser; FS60 = 60 kHz femtosecond laser; OR = odds ratio.
*Calculated by chi-square or Fisher test.
**Calculated by logistic regression (GEE) model.

difference in the incidence of DLK (approximately 12%) between the 3 lasers. Interestingly, they found that eyes that developed DLK had slightly thinner flaps on average than eyes that did not develop DLK, although the differences were small. To look at it another way, they divided the eyes into flaps greater than or less than 120 μm. Eyes with flaps less than 120 μm had statistically significantly greater risk of DLK ($P = .02$) (Table 6).

Thinner flaps have the advantage of greater residual stromal bed thickness, but the increased DLK may be a disadvantage. Some of the results of this study may be confounded. The surgeons aimed for and achieved thinner flaps with the faster lasers, so the expected decrease in the DLK due to less energy per pulse in the faster lasers may have been overshadowed by an increase in DLK due to thinner flaps.

C. J. Rapuano, MD

Infectious Keratitis in 204 586 LASIK Procedures

Llovet F, de Rojas V, Interlandi E, et al (Instituto Oftalmológico Europeo, Spain)
Ophthalmology 117:232-238, 2010

Purpose.—To investigate the incidence, culture results, risk factors, and visual outcomes of infectious keratitis after LASIK, and examine treatment strategies.

Design.—Retrospective study.

Participants.—We included 107 613 patients who underwent LASIK at Clínica Baviera (Instituto Oftalmológico Europeo, Spain) from September 2002 to May 2008.

Methods.—The medical records of post-LASIK patients (204 586 eyes) were reviewed to identify cases of infectious keratitis. Incidence, risk factors, clinical course, days to diagnosis, medical and surgical treatment, and final visual outcomes were recorded.

Main Outcome Measures.—Incidence of post-LASIK infectious keratitis, culture results, response to treatment, and visual outcome.

Results.—Post-LASIK infectious keratitis was diagnosed in 72 eyes from 63 patients. Onset of infection was early (within 7 days after surgery) in 62.5% of cases. Cultures were positive in 21 of 54 cases in which samples were taken. The most frequently isolated microorganism was *Staphylococcus epidermidis* (9 cases). Immediate flap lifting and irrigation with antibiotics was performed in 54 eyes; late flap lifting was subsequently required in 10 out of 18 cases initially treated with topical antibiotics alone. One case required flap amputation owing to flap necrosis. Final best spectacle-corrected visual acuity (BSCVA) was ≥20/20 in 38 cases (52.7%) and ≥20/40 in 67 cases (93.05%); final BSCVA was <20/40 in 5 cases (6.94%).

Conclusions.—The incidence of post-LASIK infectious keratitis was 0.035% per procedure. Infectious keratitis after LASIK is a potentially vision-threatening complication. The appearance of infections in asymptomatic patients highlights the need for a proper schedule of follow-up

appointments. Prompt and aggressive management of this LASIK complication with early flap lifting, scraping, culture, and irrigation with antibiotics
is strongly recommended. Proper management can result in preserving
useful vision.

▶ The authors report the largest series I know of regarding infectious keratitis
after laser in situ keratomileusis (LASIK). Data are from a large private practice
institute with 19 centers throughout Spain, making postoperative visits (which
are free of charge) readily available, leading the authors to believe they have
captured most, if not all, postoperative information.

The good news is that the infection rate after LASIK is low, 0.035%. More
good news is that over 50% of eyes that developed infection had 20/20 or
better best spectacle-corrected vision and 93% had better than or equal to
20/40 best spectacle-corrected vision once the infection resolved. Doctors
(and patients) need to be vigilant about preventing infections. Promptly
managing eyes with suspected infectious keratitis after LASIK is critical. Immediate flap lifting and antibiotics (as were done in 75% of eyes in this series),
ideally with scraping for smears and cultures, should be considered. Aggressive
antibiotics and close follow-up are warranted.

C. J. Rapuano, MD

Incidence of epithelial ingrowth in primary and retreatment laser in situ keratomileusis

Caster AI, Friess DW, Schwendeman FJ (Private Practices, Beverly Hills, CA;
Private Practices, West Chester, PA; Private Practices, Overland Park, KS)
J Cataract Refract Surg 36:97-101, 2010

Purpose.—To analyze the risk for clinically significant epithelial ingrowth
after primary laser in situ keratomileusis (LASIK) and flap-lift retreatment
LASIK.

Setting.—Private practice, Beverly Hills, California, USA.

Methods.—All cases of primary and flap-lift retreatment LASIK performed by the same surgeon in a single surgical center between January
2004 and June 2007 were retrospectively reviewed. Cases that subsequently
developed clinically significant epithelial ingrowth, defined as epithelial
ingrowth impeding on the visual axis and negatively affecting uncorrected
or corrected distance visual acuity, were identified and analyzed.

Results.—Clinically significant epithelial ingrowth occurred in none of
the 3866 primary LASIK cases and in 15 (2.3%) of the 646 flap-lift retreatment cases (P<.0001). Clinically significant ingrowth was more frequent
when flap-lift retreatment was performed 3 or more years after primary
LASIK (7.7% versus 1.0%) (P =.0001). Patient age and sex did not have
a statistically significant effect on the epithelial ingrowth rate. There was
a nonsignificant trend toward increased epithelial ingrowth after flap-lift
retreatment of Automated Corneal Shaper (ACS) microkeratome flaps.

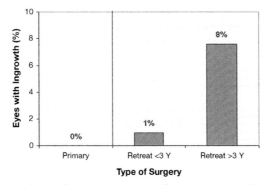

FIGURE 1.—Ingrowth rate after retreatment versus after primary surgery (Retreat = retreatment). (Reprinted from Caster AI, Friess DW, Schwendeman FJ. Incidence of epithelial ingrowth in primary and retreatment laser in situ keratomileusis. *J Cataract Refract Surg.* 2010;36:97-101, with permission from ASCRS and ESCRS.)

Conclusion.—Flap-lift retreatment performed 3 or more years after primary LASIK led to a higher risk of clinically significant epithelial ingrowth than primary LASIK or earlier flap-lift retreatment (Fig 1).

▶ Epithelial ingrowth after primary laser in situ keratomileusis (LASIK) is uncommon to rare. Interestingly, these authors found it nonexistent in 3866 eyes. They did find it in 15 (2.3%) of 646 flap-lift enhancement eyes (*P* < .0001). It was more common (7%) in eyes 3 or more years after the primary LASIK procedure than earlier (1%) (*P* = .0001) (Fig 1). Although all 15 eyes had the epithelial ingrowth removed, follow-up was available for 13 eyes. Twelve eyes had no recurrence of the ingrowth after treatment, whereas 1 eye required a second removal. No sutures, tissue glue, or alcohol was used in any of the epithelial ingrowth removal procedures.

This is one of the best series looking at the incidence of epithelial ingrowth after primary LASIK and flap-lift enhancement. Although there were no cases with epithelial ingrowth after primary LASIK, such cases certainly can be seen. Also, although all but one of the eyes with epithelial ingrowth were treated successfully with one procedure, recalcitrant epithelial ingrowth requiring more aggressive management can also occur.[1]

C. J. Rapuano, MD

Reference

1. Rapuano CJ. Management of epithelial ingrowth after laser in situ keratomileusis on a tertiary care cornea service. *Cornea.* 2010;29:307-313.

Management of Epithelial Ingrowth After Laser In Situ Keratomileusis on a Tertiary Care Cornea Service

Rapuano CJ (Jefferson Med College of Thomas Jefferson Univ, Philadelphia, PA)
Cornea 29:307-313, 2010

Purpose.—To review the management of epithelial ingrowth after laser in situ keratomileusis (LASIK) on the Wills Eye Institute Cornea Service from 1996 through 2007.

Methods.—Data of all patients referred to the Wills Eye Cornea Service after having undergone LASIK were reviewed. Charts of all patients with the diagnosis of epithelial ingrowth were analyzed. Data included patient demographics, previous ocular history, visual acuity, size and location of the ingrowth, and management. Additional data on eyes that underwent removal of the ingrowth at Wills were obtained.

Results.—Three hundred five patients (153 female and 152 male, mean age: 44.7 years) were referred for eye problems after LASIK during the study period. Epithelial ingrowth was confirmed in 46 patients (15%) (19 female and 27 male, mean age: 47.4 years) involving 55 eyes (27 right and 28 left). Patients with epithelial ingrowth were seen at a mean of 26 months after LASIK (range: 0.5—108 months). Twenty-four eyes had undergone previous enhancements, 2 twice. Fourteen eyes had undergone previous removal of epithelial ingrowth, 8 more than once (range: 2—8). In 35 eyes, simple observation was recommended. In 7 eyes, epithelial removal was recommended to the referring physician. Thirteen eyes underwent flap lift and epithelial removal at Wills Eye; 9 included flap suturing. One eye required repeat treatment with flap suturing and fibrin glue, after which no recurrence was found. In the other 12 eyes, there was no recurrence in 9, small recurrences in 2, and a large recurrence in 1 eye (mean follow-up: 16 months).

Conclusions.—Epithelial ingrowth after LASIK is not rare in our referral practice. Mild ingrowth can be observed, whereas significant ingrowth can respond well to removal with a low chance of significant recurrence (Tables 1 and 2).

▶ As a tertiary care cornea specialist who also performs laser in situ keratomileusis (LASIK), I seem to be preferentially referred patients with problems after refractive surgery. When I looked at our data, 15% of eyes referred for problems after LASIK over a 12-year period had some degree of epithelial ingrowth. Most were mild, not causing problems and not requiring treatment. I removed the ingrowth in 13 eyes, 10 of which had a history of flap lift enhancement, refloating, trauma, or a buttonhole. Another one had undergone cataract surgery after LASIK. Only 2 had no corneal issues after their primary LASIK procedure (see Table 1). In 9 eyes, I secured the flap with sutures. One eye required a repeat treatment with good results. Most of the others had minimal to no recurrent epithelial ingrowth (see Table 2).

TABLE 1.—Patients Treated With Epithelial Ingrowth Removal at Wills Eye

Patient Number	Sex	Age (yr)	First Seen	Eye	Months Since LASIK	Enhancement, Flap Repositioning, Trauma	Previous Epithelial Ingrowth Removal	UCVA	BCVA	Length of Ingrowth (mm)
1	F	39	January 21, 1998	L	10	Enhancement, October 1, 1997	No	20/30	20/30	1.5
2	M	46	September 10, 2002	L	5	Trauma, September 02, from a stick, explored, flap lifted, September 9, 2002	No	CF	CF	3
3	F	52	November 22, 2002	L	23	Trauma, September 6, 2002, dislodged flap from a stone from a lawn mower	No	20/50	20/50	3
4	F	49	February 21, 2003	R	1	Repositioned, February 1, 2003	3X, last with Tisseel	20/400	20/400	3
5	M	45	June 27, 2003	L	4	Partial flap, buttonhole, no laser treatment performed	2X	20/80	20/80	2
6	M	34	July 25, 2003	L	38	Enhancement, July 17, 2001	8X	20/40	20/25	2.5
7	M	46	March 3, 2004	R	1	Postoperative day 1 floated for striae	No	20/30	20/30	1.4
8	M	40	April 23, 2004	R	34	Trauma from an elbow, July 2001	1X	20/100	20/40	2.2
9	M	68	October 7, 2005	R	30	Cataract and lens implant surgery, February 2005	3X	CF	CF	3
10	F	48	January 24, 2007	R	16	Enhancement, April 20, 2006	No	20/30	20/30	1.4; 1.8
11	F	54	March 28, 2007	L	5	—	No	20/300	20/200	2.9
12	M	50	May 25, 2007	R	39	—	4X, last with MMC	20/80	20/50	5
13	F	62	September 17, 2007	L	12	Enhancement, September 11, 2007, caused DLK, epithelial defect	No	20/200	20/200	2

Patient Number	Width of Ingrowth (mm)	Location	Scraped	Sutured? (No. Sutures)	BSCL?	Additional Surgery	FU After Scrape (Mo)	Recurrent Ingrowth	Final UCVA	Final BCVA
1	3	Peripheral	January 13, 1998	No	No	—	1.25	No	20/40	20/40
2	3	Central	May 19, 2004	No	No	—	36	1 × 1.5 mm	20/40	20/40
3	3	Central	December 5, 2002	No	Yes	—	44	No	20/30	20/30
4	360 degrees	Peripheral	February 26, 2003	Yes (11)	No	—	0.75	1 × 3 mm	CF	CF
5	6	Peripheral	July 14, 2003	Yes (5)	Yes	—	52	Trace, edge	20/50	20/20 (RGPCL)
6	220 degrees	Peripheral	September 4, 2003	Yes (11)	No		10	1.5 × 2.5 mm	20/25	20/20
7	1.2	Central	July 22, 2004	No	Yes		40	No	20/20	20/20
8	4	Peripheral	May 13, 2004	Yes (7)	Yes		2	No	20/60	20/60

(Continued)

TABLE 1. (continued)

Patient Number	Width of Ingrowth (mm)	Location	Scraped	Sutured? (No. Sutures)	BSCL?	Additional Surgery	FU After Scrape (Mo)	Recurrent Ingrowth	Final UCVA	Final BCVA
9	6	Peripheral	October 7, 2005	Yes (10)	No	Scrape, 9 sutures, Tisseel October 20, 2005	5	No, small melt	20/80	20/50 (RGPCL)
10	1.3; 4.0	Peripheral	April 19, 2007	Yes (11)	No	—	4.5	No	20/50	20/25
11	7	Peripheral	October 15, 2007	Yes (13)	No	—	3.5	No	CF	20/400
12	4	Central	June 13, 2007	Yes (17)	No	—	9	No	20/20	20/20
13	4	Peripheral	September 26, 2007	Yes (14)	No	—	6.5	No	20/40	20/40

BCVA, best-corrected visual acuity; BSCL, bandage soft contact lens; FU, follow-up; L, left; R, right; RGPCL, rigid gas permeable contact lens; UCVA, uncorrected visual acuity.

TABLE 2.—Gain or Loss of Best-Corrected Snellen Visual Acuity

Loss of 2 lines	1 eyes
Loss of 1 line	3 eyes
Gain of 1 line	2 eyes
Gain of 2 lines	2 eyes
Gain of 4 lines	1 eye
Gain of 6 lines	1 eye
Gain of 7 lines	2 eye
Gain of 8 lines	1 eye

Epithelial ingrowth[1] can be successfully treated without flap suturing. The rationale for suturing is that the sutures tightly close the wound during the initial healing phase while the epithelium is growing to cover the edge of the flap. Without sutures, the wound often appears slightly gaped, allowing epithelium to enter the interface. Additionally, in some eyes with epithelial ingrowth, the edge of the flap has melted, decreasing its ability to seal quickly after the ingrowth has been removed. I think it is reasonable to try epithelial ingrowth removal without sutures initially, as it is a relatively straightforward procedure. However, in cases of multiple recurrences of epithelial ingrowth or if the edge of the flap doesn't appear to be sealing well, suturing or fibrin glue should be considered.

C. J. Rapuano, MD

Reference

1. Caster AI, Friess DW, Schwendeman FJ. Incidence of epithelial ingrowth in primary and retreatment laser in situ keratomileusis. *J Cataract Refract Surg.* 2010;36:97-101.

Straylight measurements before and after removal of epithelial ingrowth
Lapid-Gortzak R, van der Meulen I, van der Linden JW, et al (Univ of Amsterdam, the Netherlands; et al)
J Cataract Refract Surg 35:1829-1832, 2009

In 3 eyes with epithelial ingrowth after laser in situ keratomileusis, straylight was measured before and after the ingrowth was removed. In 2 eyes of 1 patient, epithelial ingrowth reached the pupillary axis. Straylight decreased (improved) significantly after ingrowth removal: a 3.6-fold decrease in the right eye and a 10-fold decrease in the left eye. The uncorrected distance visual acuity (UDVA) improved from 0.25 (20/80) in both eyes to 1.0 (20/20) and 0.8 (20/25), respectively. In 1 eye of another patient, from which epithelial ingrowth was removed to prevent flap melting and distortion, the pupillary opening was not obscured and no significant change in straylight was found. The UDVA improved from 0.32 (20/60) to 1.0 (20/20) after the ingrowth was removed. An increase in straylight can be a significant complication of epithelial ingrowth. After the interlamellar space is cleared, the improvement in straylight is several factors larger than the gain in UDVA.

▶ The authors write, "straylight is a functional measure of the effect of light spreading over the retina; the term is used...to define disability glare." This sounds like something very worthwhile to measure after refractive surgery, where glare is not an uncommon complaint. Interestingly the authors found that straylight values were statistically significantly better in over half of the eyes postoperatively in the laser in situ keratomileusis and laser epithelial keratomileusis groups. The *big* missing part of this study is that the authors did not attempt to correlate straylight measurement values and patients' symptoms or lack thereof. Since I am not an optical engineer, I must take it on faith that the Cataract Quantifier straylight meter used in this study actually measures straylight. But if the values don't correlate with a patient's symptoms, I can't see how helpful this measurement can be for me. That study needs to be done next.

C. J. Rapuano, MD

Subbasal Nerve Density and Corneal Sensitivity After Laser In Situ Keratomileusis: Femtosecond Laser vs Mechanical Microkeratome

Patel SV, McLaren JW, Kittleson KM, et al (Mayo Clinic, Rochester, MN)
Arch Ophthalmol 128:1413-1419, 2010

Objective.—To compare changes in subbasal nerve density and corneal sensitivity after laser in situ keratomileusis (LASIK) with the flap created by a femtosecond laser (bladeless) vs a mechanical microkeratome.

Design.—In a randomized paired-eye study, 21 patients received myopic LASIK with the flap created by a femtosecond laser in one eye and by a mechanical microkeratome in the fellow eye. Eyes were examined before and at 1, 3, 6, 12, and 36 months after LASIK. Central subbasal nerve density was measured by using confocal microscopy. Corneal mechanical sensitivity was measured by using a gas esthesiometer and was expressed as the ratio of mechanical threshold in eyes that received LASIK to mechanical threshold in concurrent control eyes.

Results.—Subbasal nerve density and corneal sensitivity did not differ between methods of flap creation at any examination. Mean (SD) nerve density was decreased at 1 month (bladeless, 974 [2453] $\mu m/mm^2$; microkeratome, 1308 [2881] $\mu m/mm^2$) compared with the preoperative examination (bladeless, 10 883 [5083] $\mu m/mm^2$, $P < .001$; microkeratome, 12 464 [6683] $\mu m/mm^2$, $P < .001$) and remained decreased through 12 months ($P < .001$). Mechanical threshold ratios did not differ from that at the preoperative examination through 36 months for either LASIK treatment; when all LASIK eyes were combined, the mechanical threshold ratio was transiently higher (decreased sensitivity) at 1 month (1.29 [0.85]) compared with the preoperative examination (0.89 [0.73], $P = .05$).

Conclusions.—The planar configuration of the femtosecond laser flaps is not associated with faster reinnervation compared with the microkeratome flaps. The prolonged decrease in subbasal nerve density after LASIK is not accompanied by a prolonged decrease in corneal sensitivity.

Trial Registration.—clinicaltrials.gov Identifier NCT00350246.

▶ It is well established that corneal nerves are severed and then ablated during a laser in situ keratomileusis (LASIK) procedure. Many studies also demonstrate a decrease in corneal sensation for weeks to many months after LASIK, presumably because of nerve damage inherent in the procedure. It was hypothesized that the different shape of the LASIK flap created with the femtosecond laser (ie, a planar flap with a steep entry wound) would allow improved realignment of the flap and promote faster and better corneal reinnervation.

The authors report a randomized paired-eye study where one eye received a femtosecond laser LASIK flap and the fellow received a mechanical microkeratome LASIK flap. All flaps had superior hinges. While the intended thickness of the femtosecond laser flap was 120 μm, at 1 month postoperation, the mean thickness was 143 μm. Similarly, while a 180-μm thickness plate of the microkeratome was used, at 1 month postoperation, the mean flap thickness was 138 μm, essentially the same as the femtosecond laser flaps.

They found statistically significant decreases in subbasal nerve density at 1 through 12 months postoperation and nonstatistically significant decreases at 36 months postoperation (Fig 1 in the original article). However, there was no difference in nerve density between the femtosecond laser flaps and the mechanical microkeratome flaps. While femtosecond laser LASIK flaps have certain advantages over mechanical microkeratome flaps, faster and better corneal reinnervation does not appear to be one of them.

C. J. Rapuano, MD

Upper and Lower Tear Menisci After Laser In Situ Keratomileusis
Tao A, Shen M, Wang J, et al (Wenzhou Med College, Zhejiang, China; Univ of Miami, FL)
Eye Contact Lens 36:81-85, 2010

Objectives.—To determine upper and lower tear menisci using optical coherence tomography (OCT) in volunteers after laser in situ keratomileusis (LASIK) for myopia.

Methods.—Thirty-five eyes of 35 nonsurgical volunteers were evaluated. Twenty-eight eyes of 28 volunteers who underwent LASIK served as the study group. The height, area, and volume of the upper and lower tear menisci were obtained in the study group, using OCT before surgery, 1 week, 1 month, and 20 months after surgery. At each visit, Schirmer test (type I, without anesthesia), tear break-up time, and corneal fluorescein staining score were evaluated. OCT imaging was conducted in the nonsurgical group with the same settings.

TABLE 1.—*Tear* Menisci Variables in the Nonsurgical Group ($n = 35$) and the Surgery Group ($n = 28$)

	Nonsurgical Group	Preoperative	1-wk Postoperative	1-mo Postoperative
UTMH (μm)	209 ± 39^a	163 ± 28	146 ± 24^a	153 ± 22
UTMA (μm²)	$14,153 \pm 4,405$	$13,144 \pm 3,169$	$10,711 \pm 2,148^a$	$10,922 \pm 2,292^a$
UTMV (μL)	0.48 ± 0.15	0.44 ± 0.11	0.36 ± 0.07^a	0.37 ± 0.08^a
LTMH (μm)	240 ± 53^a	205 ± 32	179 ± 29^a	180 ± 23^a
LTMA (μm²)	$20,054 \pm 6,700^a$	$15,669 \pm 4,246$	$12,049 \pm 3,145^a$	$12,832 \pm 2,952^a$
LTMV (μL)	0.69 ± 0.23^a	0.54 ± 0.15	0.41 ± 0.11^a	0.44 ± 0.10^a

[a]$P < 0.05$ compared with the preoperative value.

Results.—The lower tear meniscus volume at baseline were significantly smaller in the study group compared with the nonsurgical group (t test, $P < 0.01$). The upper tear meniscus volume decreased from 0.44 ± 0.11 μL to 0.37 ± 0.08 μL at 1 month after surgery ($P < 0.05$). The lower tear meniscus volume (0.54 ± 0.15 μL) reduced to 0.44 ± 0.10 μL at 1 month after surgery (posthoc, $P < 0.05$). For the subgroup analysis, tear menisci, Schirmer test, and tear break-up time after LASIK decreased during the first 1 month ($P < 0.05$) and recovered by 20 months after surgery (t test, $P > 0.05$).

Conclusions.—The upper and lower tear menisci decreased up to 1 month after LASIK and recovered by 20 months. OCT is a useful tool for evaluating the tear system in a noninvasive manner (Table 1).

▶ Studying dry eye disease is difficult for a number of reasons. One reason is that we do not have a test that correlates highly with the condition. Currently, we use a combination of history; symptoms; signs; Schirmer tests; tear break-up time; and fluorescein, rose bengal, and lissamine green testings, all of which have their limitations, including the fact that most are somewhat invasive. The measurement of the tear meniscus by optical coherence tomography (OCT) has several advantages, including being completely noninvasive and objective, and has numerous potential parameters, such as tear meniscus height or volume, that can be evaluated. Having said that, it still requires validation as an accurate and reproducible test for dry eye disease.

The results of this study are interesting. The preoperative tear meniscus measurements were statistically significantly smaller in the laser-assisted in-situ keratomileusis (LASIK) eye group than in normal controls, possibly because patients with dry eye are more likely to be contact lens intolerant and therefore more interested in refractive surgery. The authors did not detail the refractive error or contact lens status of the control eyes, but perhaps contact lens use itself may affect the tear meniscus.

All the tear meniscus measurements were decreased 1 week and 1 month after LASIK (Table 1). Eleven of the 28 patients who underwent LASIK were also followed up at 20 months postoperatively, and most, but not all, of the tear meniscus measurements had recovered to preoperative levels. It will be very helpful if further studies validate OCT measurements as a diagnostic test for dry eye disease, not only for refractive surgery screening purposes but for the general management of dry eyes.

C. J. Rapuano, MD

Visual outcomes after wavefront-guided photorefractive keratectomy and wavefront-guided laser in situ keratomileusis: Prospective comparison
Moshirfar M, Schliesser JA, Chang JC, et al (John A. Moran Eye Ctr, Salt Lake City, UT; Univ of Utah School of Medicine, Salt Lake City; et al)
J Cataract Refract Surg 36:1336-1343, 2010

Purpose.—To compare visual outcomes between wavefront-guided photorefractive keratectomy (PRK) and wavefront-guided laser in situ keratomileusis (LASIK).

Setting.—Academic center, Salt Lake City, Utah, USA.

Methods.—In this randomized prospective study, myopic eyes were treated with wavefront-guided PRK and or wavefront-guided LASIK using a Visx Star S4 CustomVue platform with iris registration. Primary outcome measures were uncorrected (UDVA) and corrected (CDVA) distance visual acuities and manifest refraction. Secondary outcome measures were higher-order aberrations (HOAs) and contrast sensitivity.

Results.—The PRK group comprised 101 eyes and the LASIK group, 102 eyes. At 6 months, the mean UDVA was −0.03 logMAR ± 0.10 [SD] (20/19) and 0.07 ± 0.09 logMAR (20/24), respectively ($P = .544$). In both groups, 75% eyes achieved a UDVA of 20/20 or better ($P = .923$); 77% of eyes in the PRK group and 88% in the LASIK group were within ±0.50 diopter of emmetropia ($P = .760$). There was no statistically significant difference between groups in contrast sensitivity at 3, 6, 12, or 18 cycles per degree. The mean postoperative HOA root mean square was 0.45 ± 0.13 μm in the PRK group and 0.59 ± 0.22 μm in the LASIK group ($P = .012$), representing an increase factor of 1.22 and 1.74, respectively.

Conclusions.—Wavefront-guided PRK and wavefront-guided LASIK had similar efficacy, predictability, safety, and contrast sensitivity; however, wavefront-guided PRK induced statistically fewer HOAs than wavefront-guided LASIK at 6 months (Fig 7).

▶ The authors compared custom wavefront photorefractive keratectomy (PRK) (20% ethanol for 35 seconds to remove the epithelium) with custom wavefront laser-assisted in-situ keratomileusis (LASIK) (flap made with a 60-kHz Intra-Lase femtosecond laser) using the VISX S4 excimer laser. Successful iris registration was required for inclusion in the study. Patients were randomized, and the 2 groups were equivalent preoperatively.

Three-month and 6-month results were fairly similar between the 2 groups. At 3 months, 80% of eyes in both groups had 20/20 or better uncorrected vision and 26% to 27% of both groups had 20/15 or better uncorrected vision. At 6 months (approximately 60% of patients were seen at this time point), 75% of both groups saw 20/20 or better without correction and 30% of the PRK eyes and 19% of the

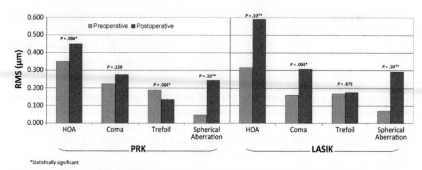

*Statistically significant

FIGURE 7.—Absolute preoperative to postoperative changes in HOA at 6 months (HOA = higher-order aberration; PRK = photorefractive keratectomy, n = 54; LASIK = laser in situ keratomileusis, n = 53). (Reprinted from Moshirfar M, Schliesser JA, Chang JC, et al. Visual outcomes after wavefront-guided photorefractive keratectomy and wavefront-guided laser in situ keratomileusis: prospective comparison. *J Cataract Refract Surg.* 2010;36:1336-1343, with permission ASCRS and ESCRS.)

LASIK eyes saw 20/15 or better without correction. While total higher-order aberrations were statistically significantly higher than preoperatively at 6 months in both groups, there was less-induced higher-order aberration after PRK than after LASIK ($P = .005$) (Fig 7). As similar laser treatments and ablation zones were used for both the PRK- and LASIK-treated eyes, the authors believe that the LASIK flap was the primary cause of the greater-induced higher-order aberrations after LASIK. This makes sense to me. Creation of a LASIK flap induces another variable into the equation. While LASIK has definite advantages over PRK, including less discomfort and faster visual recovery, more-induced higher-order aberrations may be a disadvantage.

C. J. Rapuano, MD

Meta-analysis: Clinical Outcomes of Laser-Assisted Subepithelial Keratectomy and Photorefractive Keratectomy in Myopia

Zhao L-Q, Wei R-L, Cheng J-W, et al (Xinhua Hosp Affiliated to Shanghai Jiao Tong Univ School of Medicine, China; Changzheng Hosp Affiliated to Second Military Med Univ, Shanghai, China)
Ophthalmology 117:1912-1922, 2010

Purpose.—To examine possible differences in clinical outcomes between laser-assisted subepithelial keratectomy (LASEK) and photorefractive keratectomy (PRK) for myopia.

Design.—Systematic review and meta-analysis.

Participants.—Patients from previously reported randomized controlled trials (RCTs) and comparative studies of LASEK and PRK with clinical outcomes.

Methods.—A comprehensive literature search was performed using the Cochrane Collaboration methodology to identify RCTs and comparative studies comparing LASEK and PRK for myopia.

Main Outcome Measures.—Primary outcome parameters included uncorrected visual acuity (UCVA) of 20/20 or better, manifest refractive spherical equivalent (SE) within ±0.50 diopters (D), final refractive SE, and final UCVA of 20/40 or worse. Secondary outcome parameters included healing time of corneal epithelium, postoperative pain, and corneal haze.

Results.—Twelve studies were identified and used for comparing PRK (499 eyes) with LASEK (512 eyes) for myopia. There were no significant differences in odds ratio (OR), weighted mean difference (WMD), and standardized mean difference (SMD) in the primary and secondary outcome measures. The final mean refractive SE (WMD, 0.00; 95% confidence interval [CI], −0.08 to 0.07; $P = 0.95$), manifest refractive SE within ±0.50 D of the target (OR, 0.90; 95% CI, 0.63−1.29; $P = 0.56$), patients achieving UCVA of 20/20 or better (OR, 0.86; 95% CI, 0.61−1.20; $P = 0.37$), final UCVA of 20/40 or worse (OR, 1.26; 95% CI, 0.63−2.51; $P = 0.52$), re-epithelialization time (WMD, 0.08; 95% CI, −0.44 to 0.59; $P = 0.77$), and postoperative pain (SMD, 0.26; 95% CI, −0.20 to 0.72; $P = 0.27$) were analyzed. However, LASEK-treated eyes showed less corneal haze at 1 month after surgery (WMD, 0.25; 95% CI, 0.10−0.39; $P = 0.0007$) and 3 months after surgery (WMD, 0.14; 95% CI, 0.01−0.26; $P = 0.03$) compared with PRK. No statistically significant difference was observed between the 2 groups at 6 months after surgery (WMD, 0.14; 95% CI, −0.02 to 0.30; $P = 0.08$).

Conclusions.—In this meta-analysis, LASEK-treated eyes had no significant benefits over PRK-treated ones with regard to clinical outcomes. Less corneal haze was observed in LASEK-treated eyes at 1 to 3 months after surgery.

▶ Meta-analyses are important tools that combine findings from multiple smaller studies to increase the power of the research. The problem is that most studies are not identical and direct comparisons are often difficult to make. These authors found 11 randomized controlled trials and 1 controlled trial comparing photorefractive keratectomy (all used mechanical epithelial scraping) and laser-assisted subepithelial keratectomy (LASEK) (all used alcohol to remove the epithelium). None of the studies used mitomycin C. One study was from the United States.

Taking all 12 studies into account, there were no differences between the 2 techniques in any clinical outcomes, including postoperative pain, epithelial healing time, uncorrected vision, and final refractive error. The only difference found was less corneal haze at 1 and 3 months in the LASEK group, but there was no difference in haze at 6 months. For me, the theoretical advantages of preserving the epithelium with LASEK or epilaser-assisted in situ keratomileusis just didn't pan out in reality, and I continue to discard it during my surface ablation procedures.

C. J. Rapuano, MD

Clinical outcomes of epi-LASIK: 1-year results of on- and off-flap procedures with and without mitomycin-C

Kim ST, Koh JW, Yoon GJ, et al (Chosun Univ College of Medicine, Dong-gu, Gwangju, Republic of Korea; Happy Eye Clinic, Gwangju, Republic of Korea)
Br J Ophthalmol 94:592-596, 2010

Aim.—To evaluate and compare the clinical outcomes of epi-laser in situ keratomileusis (LASIK) performed either on-flap or off-flap with or without 0.02% mitomycin-C (MMC) in terms of corneal haziness, pain scores and satisfaction scores.

Methods.—In this non-randomised comparative retrospective study, the charts of 198 patients (394 eyes) who had undergone an epi-LASIK procedure for myopia (-1.5 D to -8.0 D spherical equivalent) correction were reviewed. Patients were classified into four groups: Group I, on-flap without MMC, 181 eyes; Group II, on-flap with MMC, 52 eyes; Group III, off-flap without MMC, 93 eyes; Group IV, off-flap with MMC, 68 eyes. We compared the group outcomes on the first day, 1, 3 and 6 months and 1 year after the operation.

Results.—The mean uncorrected visual acuity was significantly better in the off-flap groups (III and IV) than in the on-flap groups (I and II) on day 1 (p=0.002). There was no significant difference in the spherical equivalent among all groups at 1 year (p=0.305). Some degree of haziness was present in 10 eyes (Grade II: 2; Grade I: 8), but the haziness level was not significantly different among groups at 1 year (p=0.533). Pain scores (0–10) were lower in the off-flap groups (III and IV) (p=0.010). Satisfaction scores (0–10) were higher in the off-flap groups (III and IV), but the difference was not statistically significant (p=0.248).

Conclusions.—Myopic correction by epi-LASIK surgery with all four methods showed stable visual results in terms of the 1-year postoperative clinical outcomes. Haziness levels revealed that treatment with 0.02% MMC was less effective than expected. Overall, the off-flap method offered faster visual recovery and less postoperative pain than the on-flap method (Fig 5).

▶ Pain and slow visual recovery are the bugaboos of surface ablation. Laser epithelial keratomileusis (LASEK) (laser surface ablation where alcohol is used to loosen the epithelium from the stroma; the epithelium is moved to the side, the excimer laser ablation is performed, and then the epithelium is replaced) was supposed to solve both of these problems. Since the epithelium was being replaced, there should be minimal to no pain and the vision should be good, just like in laser in situ keratomileusis (LASIK). However, that was not the case in practice. The alcohol damaged the epithelium too much, so it often wasn't viable, causing pain and slow recovery of vision. Epi-LASIK was developed to solve the alcohol problem. It uses a mechanical blunt blade microkeratome to separate the epithelium, theoretically preserving its viability. In its original iteration, the epithelium was replaced to decrease pain and speed visual

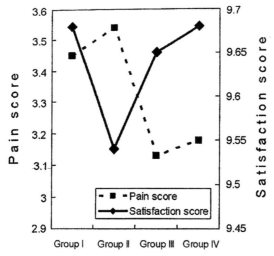

Group I   Group II   Group III   Group IV

FIGURE 5.—Comparison of overall subjective pain and satisfaction scores following epi-laser in situ keratomileusis surgery among the four groups. Postoperative pain, subjectively evaluated only on the second postoperative day using the Numeric Pain Intensity Scale (0, no pain to 10, worst possible pain), was significantly higher in the on-flap groups (Groups I and II) than in the off-flap groups (Groups III and IV) (p=0.010). The grades of postoperative patient satisfaction at 1 year after surgery, which were subjectively evaluated with a predetermined scale ranging from 0 (regret extremely for surgery) to 10 (satisfy perfectly for surgery), yielded similar results in Groups I, III and IV. The scores in Group II were lower than those of the other groups; however, no statistically significant differences were observed between any of the groups (p=0.248). (Reproduced from the British Journal of Ophthalmology, Kim ST, Koh JW, Yoon GJ, et al. Clinical outcomes of epi-LASIK: 1-year results of on- and off-flap procedures with and without mitomycin-C. *Br J Ophthalmol.* 2010;94:592-596, copyright 2010, with permission from BMJ Publishing Group Ltd.)

recovery. However, in practice, many surgeons believe removing the epithelium (off-flap) is better than replacing it (on-flap).

The authors of this article performed a retrospective study evaluating on-flap and off-flap epi-LASIK. They also looked at results with and without topical prophylactic mitomycin C (MMC). When used, the MMC was placed on the cornea for 2 minutes. They did not state why they used MMC in some eyes and not in other eyes.

The results in this large study (almost 400 eyes followed for 1 year) confirmed most surgeons impressions regarding replacing the epithelial flap. Leaving the flap off resulted in statistically significant less initial pain and faster visual recovery. Off-flap patients also tended to be more satisfied with their procedures (Fig 5). Not expected, at least by me, was that they found no difference in haze with or without MMC. Perhaps this was because they only used the MMC in high-risk eyes. Even so, they conclude, "MMC obviously reduces haze, although the optimal concentration and application time for MMC are debatable." This study supports my continued use of off-flap epi-LASIK as my preferred surface ablation technique. I use MMC 0.02% for 12 seconds in most eyes with greater than approximately −3.00 to −4.00 diopters of myopia or with moderate astigmatism.

C. J. Rapuano, MD

Keratocyte Density after Laser-Assisted Subepithelial Keratectomy with Mitomycin C

De Benito Llopis L, Drake P, Cañadas P, et al (Vissum Madrid, Spain)
Am J Ophthalmol 150:642-649, 2010

Purpose.—To study the effects of laser-assisted subepithelial keratectomy (LASEK) with mitomycin C (MMC) on the keratocyte population.

Design.—Prospective, nonrandomized, interventional, comparative case series.

Methods.—Fifty-six eyes treated at Vissum Santa Hortensia, Madrid, Spain, were included in the study. We compared 28 eyes treated with LASEK with intraoperative 0.02% MMC versus 28 non-treated eyes. Keratocyte density was measured 3 months after the surgery in the anterior, mid, and posterior stroma and was compared with the corresponding layers in the control eyes. The anterior layer in the LASEK group was compared with 2 layers in the control group: the most anterior stromal layer and the 80 μm-deep layer, because that was the mean ablation depth performed in eyes that underwent LASEK.

Results.—We found a statistically significantly lower keratocyte population in the most anterior stromal layer after LASEK with MMC compared with both the most anterior stromal layer and the 80 μm-deep layer in controls. On the contrary, the treated group showed a significantly higher keratocyte density in both the mid stroma and the deep stroma. The comparison between the average densities through the entire cornea showed a significantly higher keratocyte population in the LASEK with MMC group.

Conclusions.—LASEK with MMC seems to cause a decrease in the anterior stromal cells 3 months after the surgery compared with nonoperated corneas. There seems to be a compensating proliferation of keratocytes in the deeper corneal layers, suggesting that the ability of keratocytes to repopulate the cornea is maintained after the surgical procedure (Table 3).

▶ Mitomycin C (MMC) is an alkylating agent with cytotoxic and antiproliferative effects. It is used immediately after surface ablation to reduce the risk of postoperative haze by stopping corneal stromal keratocytes from activating, proliferating, and differentiating into myofibroblasts.

However, the effects of damaging keratocytes may have unintended consequences. This study used confocal microscopy to measure keratocyte density 3 months after surface ablation performed with MMC 0.02% for 30 seconds and compare it to normal unoperated corneas. While they found a decrease in keratocyte density in the anterior one-third of the cornea, there was an increase in keratocyte density in the posterior two-thirds of the cornea (Table 3). In fact, the mean keratocyte density of the entire cornea was higher in the surface ablation/MMC eyes than in the normal eyes ($P = .01$). It is nice to know that surface ablation with MMC doesn't prevent the keratocytes from repopulating

TABLE 3.—Comparison of Keratocyte Density in Normal Nonoperated Corneas (Control Group) and Uncomplicated Laser-Assisted Subepithelial Keratectomy Cases 3 Months after Surgery

	Control (n = 28)	LASEK (n = 28)	P Value
Anterior stroma (range), cells/mm^3	29 080.29 ± 5788.81 (19 934.64 to 41 830.06)	16 660.53 ± 7844.88 (6666.66 to 36 209.15)	.0001
Stromal bed (range), cells/mm^3	20 501.86 ± 2458.43 (16 470.58 to 25 228.75)	16 660.53 ± 7844.88 (6666.66 to 36 209.15)	.01
Mid stroma (range), cells/mm^3	18 144.25 ± 1955.88 (14 509.80 to 21 111.11)	30 179.73 ± 9117.64 (13 660.13 to 46 470.58)	.0001
Posterior stroma (range), cells/mm^3	18 076.56 ± 2097.73 (13 398.69 to 22 352.94)	29 675.24 ± 8158.77 (16 993.46 to 46 745.09)	.0001
Average (range), anterior-mid-posterior	21 767.04 ± 2676.74 (16 383.44 to 27 886.71)	25 505.17 ± 7052.47 (15 446.62 to 38 843.13)	.01

LASEK = laser-assisted subepithelial keratectomy.

the cornea without causing significant haze (not that we know exactly what happens if the keratocyte density remained low).

C. J. Rapuano, MD

Reduced Application Time for Prophylactic Mitomycin C in Photorefractive Keratectomy

Virasch VV, Majmudar PA, Epstein RJ, et al (Rush Univ Med Ctr, Chicago, IL)
Ophthalmology 117:885-889, 2010

Objective.—To determine whether the duration of mitomycin C (MMC) 0.02% application affects visual outcome or the incidence of subepithelial haze in patients undergoing photorefractive keratectomy (PRK) with prophylactic administration of MMC.

Design.—Retrospective, comparative case series.

Participants.—Two hundred sixty-nine eyes undergoing PRK.

Methods.—This was a retrospective comparative case series that included 269 eyes that underwent PRK with prophylactic MMC application for 120 seconds (group 1, n = 74), 60 seconds (group 2, n = 36), or 12 seconds (group 3, n = 159). The mean preoperative spherical equivalent was −6.49 diopters (D) in group 1, −6.77 D in group 2, and −7.10 D in group 3. Photorefractive keratectomy was performed using a modified nomogram. All eyes received a single intraoperative application of MMC (0.02%) after laser ablation for the above specified durations.

Main Outcome Measures.—Best-corrected visual acuity and corneal haze score.

Results.—Best-corrected visual acuity was 20/23 in group 1, 20/20 in group 2, and 20/21 in group 3. The mean haze score ± standard deviation (scale, 0.00—4.00) was 0.11 ± 0.31 in group 1, 0.14 ± 0.28 in group 2, and 0.07 ± 0.20 in group 3 throughout a mean follow-up of 31 months in group 1, 16 months in group 2, and 10 months in group 3. No eyes had a haze score of more than 1.00.

Conclusions.—There was no statistically significant difference in postoperative best-corrected visual acuity or haze scores among the 3 groups. Administration of prophylactic MMC 0.02% for 12 seconds after PRK seems to be equally efficacious for haze prophylaxis when compared with longer application times of 60 and 120 seconds.

▶ In 2000, the senior authors of this study published a groundbreaking article, also in *Ophthalmology*, regarding the successful use of topical mitomycin C (MMC) in the treatment of subepithelial fibrosis after corneal refractive surgery. Many corneal and refractive surgeons at that time were rather reluctant regarding using MMC, given the rare but devastating complications reported with its use after pterygium surgery. The current study, which was presented at the American Academy of Ophthalmology (AAO) meeting in 2007, was an important influence for many refractive surgeons. The authors described the results of 3 different application times of MMC 0.02% during photorefractive keratectomy (PRK) for moderate to high myopia. They included eyes that had a spherical equivalent over −6.0 diopter (D) and had a predicted depth of ablation of > 75 μm.

The study demonstrated the safety and efficacy of prophylactic MMC after PRK, even when applied for 2 minutes. But most importantly, it demonstrated equivalent efficacy when applied for only 12 seconds. The authors note that this study included 38 eyes with more than −9.0 D of attempted correction that received a 12-second application of MMC with a mean follow-up of 1 year. All but 2 of these eyes had no haze, and 2 had a haze grade of 0.5 out of 4.

While many refractive surgeons began to use topical MMC to treat under-lying haze after the 2000 article came out, many were still hesitant to use it prophylactically, especially for 1 to 2 minutes as often recommended at that time. After the 2007 presentation at the AAO meeting, many surgeons began using MMC prophylactically for approximately 12 seconds for their patients with higher myopia. As surgeons gained more and more experience with the use of MMC and additional studies demonstrated its safety and efficacy, many refractive surgeons have steadily lowered the amount of myopia at which time they begin to use MMC to approximately −3.0 to −4.0 D, and some surgeons use it in all cases of surface ablation. I generally use it for surface ablation when treating over approximately −3.0 to −4.0 D of myopia or if there is moderate to high astigmatism.

C. J. Rapuano, MD

Efficacy of Surface Ablation Retreatments Using Mitomycin C

De Benito-Llopis L, Teus MA (Vissum Madrid, Spain)
Am J Ophthalmol 150:376-380, 2010

Purpose.—To evaluate the visual and refractive results and the incidence of complications after laser subepithelial keratectomy (LASEK) enhancement using mitomycin C (MMC) after a previous LASEK procedure with MMC.

Design.—Retrospective, noncomparative, interventional case series.

Methods.—Setting was Vissum Santa Hortensia, Madrid, Spain. We performed a retrospective study of LASEK-treated eyes that received intra-operative MMC for 30 seconds and that needed an enhancement procedure. LASEK retreatment with MMC 0.02%, applied for 60 seconds, was performed 3 to 6 months after the initial surgery. We measured the visual and refractive results 3 months after the enhancement and the incidence of complications.

Results.—Eighty-two eyes were included in the study. The preoperative data were best spectacle-corrected visual acuity (BSCVA) 1.08 ± 0.19, sphere −4.68 ± 2.8 diopters (D), and cylinder −1.30 ± 1.20 D. Three to 6 months postoperatively, before enhancement, the uncorrected VA (UCVA) was 0.59 ± 0.2; the BSCVA, 0.976 ± 0.2; the residual sphere, +0.17 ± 0.7 D, and the cylinder, −0.39 ± 0.5 D. Three months after retreatment, the UCVA was 0.93 ± 0.1; the BSCVA, 0.977 ± 0.1; the residual sphere, 0.09 ± 0.3 D; and the residual cylinder, −0.2 ± 0.3 D.

The safety index after retreatment was 1.01 ± 0.1, and the efficacy index was 0.96 ± 0.1. No haze, no delay in epithelial healing, and no case of endothelial decompensation were detected.

Conclusion.—Surface ablation retreatment using MMC seems to be effective to correct residual refractive errors after an initial surgery with MMC.

▶ Adjunctive topical mitomycin C (MMC) has become the standard treatment to decrease the risk of haze after excimer laser surface ablation. While concentrations vary, most surgeons use 0.02% (0.2 mg/mL). Typical application times range from 12 seconds to 1-2 minutes. Single applications of MMC have been demonstrated to be safe and effective in multiple studies. However, there are little data on repeat applications of MMC.

This study reported on eyes that had undergone excimer laser surface ablation with MMC 0.02% for 30 seconds and then underwent an excimer laser surface ablation enhancement with MMC 0.02% for 60 seconds. The refractive results were very good. But perhaps more importantly, there were no epithelial healing problems, no stromal melts, and no cases of corneal edema. There was also no significant haze. Also of note, the authors contacted 80 of the 82 patients by telephone 1.5 to 3.5 years after the initial surgery, and no patient reported any corneal problems.

There is some evidence in the literature that using MMC along with alcohol removal of the epithelium increases keratocyte apoptosis and leads to lower keratocyte density 1 month after surgery compared with using MMC alone. It is nice to see that when alcohol and MMC were used twice, as in this series, the cornea seems to respond well clinically.

C. J. Rapuano, MD

Visually significant haze after retreatment with photorefractive keratectomy with mitomycin-C following laser in situ keratomileusis
Liu A, Manche EE (Stanford Univ School of Medicine, Palo Alto, CA)
J Cataract Refract Surg 36:1599-1601, 2010

Photorefractive keratectomy (PRK) with the adjunctive use of mitomycin-C (MMC) for the treatment of residual refractive error after laser in situ keratomileusis (LASIK) has been shown to be safe and effective, with no occurrences of visually significant postoperative haze reported. We report a case of visually significant haze after PRK with MMC for residual myopia following LASIK.

▶ Before the mitomycin C (MMC) era, surface ablation on a laser in situ keratomileusis (LASIK) flap had a high risk of developing significant corneal haze. After MMC was shown to significantly reduce the risk of haze after primary surface ablation, surgeons started using it for LASIK enhancements in which surface ablation was performed on the LASIK flap. Several studies reported minimal to no postoperative haze with the use of MMC for at least 30 seconds.

This case report describes severe (grade 3 out of 4) corneal haze after photo-refractive keratectomy over LASIK flap (which was performed approximately 6 years prior) for approximately −2.25 diopter of residual myopia. MMC 0.02% was used for 15 seconds.

The authors believe that 15 seconds of MMC application may not be long enough to prevent haze when performing surface ablation after LASIK. While I usually use MMC 0.02% for 12 seconds after primary surface ablation, I increase the application time to 30 seconds after LASIK.

C. J. Rapuano, MD

Refractive surgery in patients with accommodative and non-accommodative strabismus: 1-year prospective follow-up
Kirwan C, O'Keefe M, O'Mullane GM, et al (The Mater Private Hosp, Dublin, Ireland; The Children's Univ Hosp, Dublin, Ireland)
Br J Ophthalmol 94:898-902, 2010

Aim.—To determine the efficacy and safety of keratorefractive surgery in patients with accommodative and non-accommodative strabismus in a prospective study.

Methods.—Preoperative assessment included uncorrected (UCVA) and best-corrected visual acuity (BCVA), manifest and cycloplegic refraction and orthoptic examination. Laser in situ keratomileusis, laser epithelial keratomileusis and Artisan phakic intraocular lens implantation were performed. All treated eyes had a BCVA of at least 6/18 preoperatively. One year postoperatively, visual acuity, refractive error and ocular alignment were reassessed.

Results.—28 patients (nine male, 19 female) of mean age 33.0± 10.0 years (range 20−59) were included in the study. Esotropia was present in 16 patients; nine fully accommodative, three partially accommodative and four non-accommodative. Twelve patients had exodeviations; 10 exotropia and two exophoria and a history of strabismus surgery. Excellent visual and refractive outcomes were obtained postoperatively. There was no loss, and one eye gained a line of BCVA. Fully accommodative esotropes attained orthophoria or microtropia. Improved ocular alignment occurred in partially accommodative esotropes and myopic exotropes. No patient experienced decompensation of strabismus or diplopia.

Conclusions.—Refractive surgery may be performed successfully in patients with accommodative and non-accommodative strabismus. However, great care must be taken when determining patient suitability. This is of particular importance in young hyperopic patients to prevent decompensation of ocular alignment over time.

▶ There is nothing worse (almost) for the refractive surgeon than doing a perfect refractive surgery procedure and ending up with excellent refractive outcomes in both eyes but the patient being miserable from binocular diplopia. Fortunately, this is a rare occurrence. Higher risk patients include those with strabismus or a history of strabismus or strabismus surgery. The authors recommend "an orthoptic examination...in all potential refractive surgery patients with strabismus."

In this study, they describe 1-year outcomes of refractive surgery in 28 patients with both esodeviation and exodeviation. Overall, they report excellent results with no decompensation of strabismus or diplopia. Of note, fully accommodative esotropes attained excellent ocular alignment postoperatively, while ocular alignment improved in partially accommodative esotropes and most myopic exotropes. Some patients needed glasses to achieve optimal alignment postoperatively.

When refractive surgery and strabismus surgery are planned in the same patient, the authors feel that it is best to perform the refractive surgery first and then remeasure the ocular alignment, as it often changes before the strabismus surgery.

Whenever I have a question regarding ocular alignment in a potential refractive surgery candidate, I consult my strabismus surgery colleagues for their opinion. In addition, I perform a contact lens trial. If they do not develop symptoms and their alignment remains stable or improved with contact lens wear, they will likely do well with refractive surgery. Having said that, I counsel all these patients that there is no guarantee that their alignment won't breakdown sooner or later after refractive surgery.

C. J. Rapuano, MD

Refractive surgical practices in persons with human immunodeficiency virus positivity or acquired immune deficiency syndrome
Aref AA, Scott IU, Zerfoss EL, et al (Penn State Univ College of Medicine, Hershey, PA)
J Cataract Refract Surg 36:153-160, 2010

Purpose.—To evaluate current practices of refractive surgeons in terms of performing elective refractive surgery in persons with human immunodeficiency virus (HIV) positivity or acquired immune deficiency syndrome (AIDS).

Setting.—Penn State University College of Medicine, Hershey, Pennsylvania, USA.

Methods.—A link to an anonymous web-based survey was e-mailed to members of the International Society of Refractive Surgery. Surgeons were asked whether they considered persons with HIV or AIDS to be acceptable candidates for elective refractive surgery and specific precautions, if any, taken when operating on these individuals.

Results.—Of 1123 surgeons sent the link, 285 (25.4%) responded. Of respondents, 143 (50.2%) said they consider persons with HIV acceptable candidates for elective refractive surgery and 35 (12.5%) said they consider persons with AIDS acceptable candidates for elective refractive

TABLE 4.—Additional Precautions Taken During Elective Refractive Surgery in Persons With HIV Positivity or AIDS

Additional Precaution	Number (%)
Schedule patient for last on the surgery schedule	122 (51.3)
Wear a double layer of gloves	79 (33.2)
Prepare and drape the eyelids and the laser hand controls	71 (29.8)
Require OR staff to wear filter masks	66 (27.7)
No additional precautions taken	62 (26.1)
Evacuate the laser plume immediately after surgery	43 (18.1)
Perform unilateral surgery	35 (14.7)
Communicate patient status with OR staff	5 (2.1)
Increase sterilization time	3 (1.3)
Require extra postoperative visit	2 (0.8)

OR = operating room.

surgery. One hundred sixty-five (72.7%) respondents who perform elective refractive surgery in persons with HIV or AIDS said they take additional precautions when operating on these patients; precautions included performing unilateral surgery, scheduling the patient last on the surgery schedule for a given day, wearing a double layer of gloves, and evacuating the laser plume immediately after surgery.

Conclusions.—Approximately half of refractive surgeons said they consider HIV-positive persons acceptable candidates for elective refractive surgery; a much lower proportion considered patients with AIDS acceptable candidates. The majority of the surgeons recommended additional precautions when performing refractive surgery on patients with HIV or AIDS (Table 4).

▶ For me there are 2 important issues when thinking about performing refractive surgery in someone who is human immunodeficiency virus (HIV) positive or has AIDS: (1) patient safety and (2) surgeon and staff safety. As for patient safety, it is primarily an issue of increased risk of infection, given their immune status. For HIV-positive patients without AIDS, there is reason to believe their immune status is reasonable or they would have a history of opportunistic infections and therefore have AIDS. Once they have AIDS, their immune status is (or at least was at some point), by definition, compromised. While one can make a reasonable case for refractive surgery in either group (given appropriate informed consent), it is harder to justify in patients with AIDS than in those who are simply HIV positive. In fact, approximately 50% of surgeons polled in this study considered HIV-positive patients as acceptable candidates for refractive surgery, while only 12.5% said the same for AIDS patients.

As for surgeon and staff safety, the authors mention several experimental articles in which viruses the size of the HIV virus were subjected to excimer laser ablation and no live virus was detected in the plume, indicating a low risk to the surgeon and staff. The most interesting aspect of the article was the precautions taken by the surgeons surveyed (see Table 4). Over half scheduled the patients for the last procedure of the day, presumably to decrease the risk of viral transmission to other patients on the same day. Interestingly, only 15%

would perform unilateral surgery. If immune status is an issue and I am concerned about potential increased risk of infection (which I have already discussed with my patient), then unilateral surgery is going to be at the top of my list of precautions to take in these patients.

C. J. Rapuano, MD

IntraLase-Enabled Astigmatic Keratotomy for Post-Keratoplasty Astigmatism: On-Axis Vector Analysis
Kumar NL, Kaiserman I, Shehadeh-Mashor R, et al (Univ of Toronto, Ontario, Canada)
Ophthalmology 117:1228-1235, 2010

Purpose.—To determine the refractive predictability, stability, efficacy, and complication rate of femtosecond laser-enabled astigmatic keratotomy for post-keratoplasty astigmatism.

Design.—A retrospective case series (pilot study).

Participants.—Thirty-seven eyes of 34 patients.

Methods.—All eyes underwent IntraLase-enabled astigmatic keratotomy for high astigmatism (>5 diopters [D]) after penetrating keratoplasty.

Main Outcome Measures.—Uncorrected visual acuity (UCVA), best-corrected visual acuity (BCVA), manifest refraction, higher-order aberrations, and complications.

Results.—Mean follow-up was for 7.2 months. Uncorrected visual acuity improved from a mean of 1.08 ± 0.34 logarithm of the minimum angle of resolution preoperatively to a mean of 0.80 ± 0.42 postoperatively ($P=0.0016$). Best-corrected visual acuity improved from a mean of 0.45 ± 0.27 preoperatively to 0.37 ± 0.27 postoperatively ($P=0.018$). The defocus equivalent was significantly reduced by more than 1 D ($P=0.025$). The value of absolute astigmatism was reduced from 7.46 ± 2.70 D preoperatively to 4.77 ± 3.29 D postoperatively ($P=0.0001$). Higher-order aberrations were significantly increased. The efficacy index was 0.6 ± 0.6. There were no cases of perforation, wound dehiscence, or infectious keratitis. Three eyes (8%) experienced an episode of graft rejection. Overcorrection occurred in 9 eyes (24%).

Conclusions.—IntraLase-enabled astigmatic keratotomy is an effective treatment for high astigmatism after penetrating keratoplasty with an encouraging refractive predictability. Future studies may help refine the treatment parameters required to achieve reduction of cylinder with greater accuracy.

▶ Corneal surgeons have become pretty good at achieving a nice clear graft in the vast majority of patients with penetrating keratoplasty (PK). What we still are not very good at is achieving predictably low degrees of astigmatism. Telling a patient "Your graft looks great. I am sorry you can't see well" is analogous to the old medical school saying, "The surgery was a success but the patient died."

There are numerous ways to treat post-PK astigmatism ranging from glasses to contact lenses to manual astigmatic keratotomy to wedge resection to photo-refractive keratectomy/laser-assisted in situ keratomileusis, each with its own pros and cons. I personally favor manual astigmatic keratotomy in contact lens intolerant eyes with high astigmatism. However, even with advances in corneal imaging technology, I am frustrated by the unpredictable results. The femtosecond laser has brought us a highly reproducible accurate blade with great potential in corneal surgery.

The authors report results of IntraLase-enabled astigmatic keratotomy for high post-PK regular astigmatism in 37 eyes, with a minimum follow-up of 4 months and a mean follow-up of 7 months. Incisions were made 0.5 mm central to the graft-host junction to 90% corneal depth at the incision location. After several initial overcorrections (a few wounds had to be sutured), they used 40° to 60° arc length incisions for up to 6 diopters of astigmatism, 65° to 75° arc length incisions for 6 to 10 diopters of astigmatism, and 90° arc length incisions for astigmatism greater than 10 diopters.

After the nomogram adjustment (because of initial overcorrections), the results were fairly good overall, going from approximately 7.5 diopters to 4.75 diopters of absolute astigmatism. The initial decrease took approximately 6 weeks, with slight regression at 3 months after which it appeared stable. While encouraging, there was a statistically significant increase in higher order aberrations after the surgery ($P = .01$). The authors state that "Patients may experience greater glare and reduced contrast sensitivity" but don't offer a reason. I believe that this procedure has potential but still needs refinement.

C. J. Rapuano, MD

3 Glaucoma

An illuminated microcatheter for 360-degree trabeculectomy in congenital glaucoma: A retrospective case series

Sarkisian SR Jr (Univ of Oklahoma Health Sciences Ctr)
J AAPOS 14:412-416, 2010

Purpose.—To evaluate the efficacy of achieving a 360° ab externo trabeculectomy using an illuminated ophthalmic microcatheter for the treatment of primary congenital glaucoma.

Methods.—This retrospective, consecutive case series included 16 eyes of 10 patients ≤3 years of age at the time of surgery and diagnosed with primary congenital glaucoma. All patients underwent a trabeculectomy via microcatheter with the intent of catheterizing the full circumference of Schlemm's canal and rupturing the entire canal in a single procedure. The main outcome measure was the success rate of achieving a complete 360° as compared to a partial trabeculectomy. Secondary outcome measures included intraocular pressure (IOP), glaucoma medication usage, and adverse events. Clinical examination data are reported up to 12 months postoperatively.

Results.—Of 16 eyes included, 12 (75%) achieved a complete 360° trabeculectomy using the microcatheter; 4 of 16 eyes (25%) achieved a partial trabeculectomy. For all treated eyes the postoperative reduction in IOP from baseline was statistically significant at the 1-, 3-, and 6-month follow-up visits ($p < 0.001$). At 6 months, IOP was significantly lower in the complete as compared to the partial trabeculectomy cohort ($p = 0.03$).

Conclusions.—A complete or partial trabeculectomy was safely completed in eyes with primary congenital glaucoma using a microcatheter with an illuminated, atraumatic tip (Fig 1).

▶ This study shows that a lighted microcatheter may be used to aid the completion of trabeculotomy in congenital glaucoma. Compared with partial trabeculotomy, 360° trabeculotomy was associated with greater success in intraocular pressure reduction.

Although the article uses the term trabeculectomy, this term is usually used for guarded filtration surgeries. This procedure as described is similar to the suture trabeculotomy or Harms probe—assisted trabeculotomy: A tear is made from Schlemm canal through the trabecular meshwork into the anterior chamber. Trabeculotomy is the accepted terminology.

It is unclear that the results reported here are any better than those of suture trabeculotomy as described by Beck and Lynch.[1] However, it is very possible that

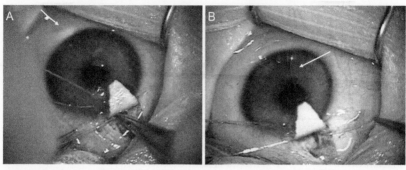

FIGURE 1.—A, Intraoperative photograph of the 1-flap surgical dissection and radial incision to access Schlemm's canal. The arrow indicates the beacon tip of the microcatheter in Schlemm's canal, which can be observed at the limbus transsclerally. B, After achieving a 360° catheterization, the microcatheter was used to gently rupture the entire canal inward. The arrow indicates the microcatheter passing through the trabecular meshwork into the anterior chamber. (Reprinted from Sarkisian SR Jr. An illuminated microcatheter for 360-degree trabeculectomy in congenital glaucoma: a retrospective case series. *J AAPOS.* 2010;14:412-416, Copyright 2010, with permission from the American Association for Pediatric Ophthalmology and Strabismus.)

the microcatheter may aid in the passage through Schlemm, as the visible tip helps to confirm that the tip has not moved into the suprachoroidal space and the ability to inject viscoelastic may help dilate and complete the pass through Schlemm.

Partial trabeculotomy was less effective than complete trabeculotomy. This is not a surprise. Opening less of the abnormal angle in congenital glaucoma would be expected to be less effective. Additionally, more diseased eyes would be expected to be associated with greater difficulty in catheter passage because of more anatomic abnormality. This could also be associated with worse outcomes.

It is very good to see surgical innovation. However, as suggested by the author, prospective studies are needed to analyze whether the cost and complexity of newer technology is justified by improved results, in novice or experienced hands.

J. S. Myers, MD

Reference

1. Beck AD, Lynch MG. 360 degrees trabeculectomy for primary congenital glaucoma. *Arch Ophthalmol.* 1995;113:1200-1202.

Association between Genetic Polymorphisms of Adrenergic Receptor and Diurnal Intraocular Pressure in Japanese Normal-Tension Glaucoma

Gao Y, Sakurai M, Takeda H, et al (Kanazawa Univ Graduate School of Med Science, Japan; et al)
Ophthalmology 117:2359-2364, 2010

Purpose.—To evaluate the relationship between genetic polymorphisms of the adrenergic receptor (ADR) and diurnal intraocular pressure (IOP) in Japanese normal-tension glaucoma (NTG) patients.

Design.—Prospective, comparative case series.

Participants.—Ninety-two untreated NTG patients.

Methods.—The IOP of both eyes was measured at 3-hour intervals from 0600 to 2400 hours over 2 consecutive days. We used IOP data from the eye with the greater visual field defect for statistical analysis. The mean IOP over 2 days was used for each time point. Genetic polymorphisms in α1A-, α2A-, α2B-, α2C-, β1-, β2-, and β3-ADR were determined mainly by direct DNA sequencing. The relationship between IOP and genetic polymorphisms was analyzed.

Main Outcome Measures.—The IOP and genotypes of genetic polymorphisms.

Results.—Diurnal mean IOP of the subjects was 14.8 ± 2.1 mmHg (mean value ± standard deviation). For Del 301-303 in α2B-ADR, insertion/insertion (I/I) had a significantly higher diurnal mean IOP ($P = 0.017$), peak IOP ($P = 0.038$), and trough IOP ($P = 0.046$) than deletion (D) carriers. For Del 322-325 in α2C-ADR, I/I had a significantly lower diurnal mean IOP ($P = 0.037$) and peak IOP ($P = 0.029$) than D carriers. For S49 G (A/G) in β1-ADR, A/A had a significantly higher diurnal mean IOP ($P = 0.023$), peak IOP ($P = 0.019$), and trough IOP ($P = 0.014$) than G carriers. For these 3 polymorphisms, repeated measures analysis of variance showed that the major homozygotes and minor carriers had parallel diurnal IOP curves, but significantly different diurnal IOP levels.

Conclusions.—Polymorphisms of the ADR gene may alter the untreated IOP level of patients with NTG (Table 2).

▶ Connections between the sympathetic nervous system and intraocular pressure (IOP) have been reported. Specifically, stimulation of ocular sympathetic nerves in rabbits by darkness may lead to increased IOP. Corresponding to the increase in IOP, aqueous humor levels of norepinephrine, the adrenergic neurotransmitter, and cyclic adenosine monophosphate (a messenger for β-adrenergic signal transduction) have been shown to increase. Furthermore, cervical ganglionectomy in rabbits suppressed nighttime elevation of IOP. Although the mechanism of increased IOP has not been conclusively determined, one theory is that stimulation of particular adrenergic receptors may lead to autoregulatory functions that limit release of neurotransmitters. Recently, genetic polymorphisms in adrenergic receptors were reported to affect response to antiglaucoma eye drops and correlate with risk of glaucoma. Therefore, the objective of this study was to find a possible correlation between genetic polymorphisms of adrenergic receptor subtypes and diurnal IOP in patients with glaucoma.

All subjects in this study were Japanese patients with normal tension glaucoma. No glaucoma therapy was used for at least 1 month prior to IOP measurement in the study. All patients had perimetric glaucoma with optic disc damage. History of ocular surgery was an exclusion criterion. IOP measurement was taken by Goldmann applanation tonometry in the sitting position. Seventeen total polymorphisms of the α- and β-adrenergic receptors were included in the study. Comparisons were made between subjects with inclusions and those with deletions of certain polymorphisms.

TABLE 2.—The Relationship between Diurnal Mean Intraocular Pressure (IOP), Peak IOP, Trough IOP, IOP Range and Genetic Polymorphisms

	Polymorphism	Genotype	Number n = 92(8)	Mean IOP[†]	P Value[†]	Peak IOP[†]	P Value[†]	Trough IOP	P Value[†]	IOP Range[‡]	P Value[‡]
α1A	R347C (C/T)	C/C	75 (6)	14.8±2.1	0.856	16.7±2.4	0.873	12.8±2.1	0.903	3.9±1.4	0.411
		T carriers	17 (2)	14.7±2.4		16.6±2.3		12.9±2.6		3.7±1.9	
α2A	G−1297C (G/C)	G/G	49 (5)	15.1±2.2	0.165	17.0±2.4	0.166	13.0±2.4	0.379	4.0±1.8	0.825
		C carriers	43 (3)	14.5±2.0		16.3±2.2		12.6±1.8		3.7±1.1	
	R365R (C/A)	C/C	40 (2)	14.8±2.2	0.990	16.8±2.3	0.760	12.7±2.4	0.588	4.1±1.7	0.321
		A carriers	52 (6)	14.8±2.1		16.6±2.4		13.0±2.0		3.7±1.4	
α2B	Del 301–303 (I/D) (G391G)	I/I	33 (5)	15.5±2.4	0.017*	17.4±2.6	0.038*	13.5±2.5	0.046*	3.9±1.7	0.928
		D carriers	59 (3)	14.4±1.9		16.3±2.1		12.5±1.9		3.8±1.4	
α2C	Del 322–325 (I/D)	I/I	78 (6)	14.6±2.1	0.037*	18.0±2.2	0.029*	12.7±2.1	0.093	3.8±1.3	0.943
		D carriers	14 (2)	15.9±2.2		16.6±2.3		13.8±2.5		4.2±2.4	
	A332A (G/A)	G/G	68 (4)	14.8±2.0	0.859	16.6±2.3	0.713	12.8±2.0	0.662	3.9±1.7	0.490
		A carriers	24 (4)	14.9±2.5		16.9±2.5		13.0±2.6		3.8±1.0	
β1	S49G (A/G)	A/A	65 (6)	15.1±2.2	0.023*	17.1±2.4	0.019*	13.2±2.3	0.014*	3.9±1.6	0.726
		G carriers	27 (2)	14.0±1.8		15.8±2.2		12.1±1.5		3.7±1.4	
	R389G (C/G)	C/C	54 (3)	14.7±2.0	0.395	16.5±2.3	0.332	12.6±1.9	0.142	3.9±1.7	0.952
		G carriers	38 (5)	15.0±2.3		17.0±2.5		13.3±2.5		3.7±1.3	
β2	T−47C (T/C) (T−20C)	T/T	72 (6)	14.9±2.0	0.611	16.7±2.3	0.871	13.0±2.1	0.381	3.8±1.5	0.198
		C carriers	20 (2)	14.6±2.5		16.6±2.5		12.5±2.5		4.2±1.5	
	R16G (A/G)	A/A	23 (2)	14.9±1.8	0.908	16.6±2.2	0.751	12.8±2.0	0.815	3.8±1.6	0.627
		G carriers	69 (6)	14.8±2.2		16.7±2.4		12.9±2.2		3.9±1.5	
	Q27E (C/G)	C/C	77 (6)	14.8±2.1	0.591	16.6±2.4	0.440	12.9±2.1	0.979	3.8±1.5	0.207
		G carriers	15 (2)	15.1±2.4		17.1±2.4		12.9±2.5		4.3±1.6	
	L84L (G/A)	G/G	36 (3)	14.7±2.1	0.658	16.5±2.3	0.486	12.6±2.3	0.317	3.9±1.6	0.866
		A carriers	56 (5)	14.9±2.1		16.8±2.4		13.0±2.1		3.8±1.5	
	R175R (C/A)	C/C	36 (3)	14.7±2.1	0.658	16.5±2.3	0.486	12.6±2.3	0.317	3.9±1.6	0.866
		A carriers	56 (5)	14.9±2.1		16.8±2.4		13.0±2.1		3.8±1.5	
β3	W64R (T/C)	T/T	63 (6)	14.7±2.2	0.402	16.7±2.5	0.765	12.7±2.3	0.341	3.9±1.6	0.576
		C carrier	29 (2)	15.1±2.0		16.8±2.1		13.2±2.0		3.6±1.3	

Data of IOP are expressed as mean ± standard deviation. Number of patients with IOP> 21 mmHg in at least one time point is shown in parentheses.
*P<0.05.
[†]Student t-test.
[‡]Mann-Whitney U test.

Three polymorphisms yielded statistically significant differences in mean, peak, and/or trough IOP between subjects with insertion versus deletion of the polymorphism (see Table 2). For 2 of the polymorphisms, insertion was correlated with higher mean and peak IOP. Of the 2 polymorphisms associated with higher IOP, 1 included statistically significantly higher trough IOP as well and 1 did not achieve statistical significance for trough IOP. For one of the polymorphisms, insertion was correlated with lower mean, peak, and trough IOP.

This article reports a correlation between genetic polymorphisms and diurnal IOP in patients with glaucoma. Given the well-established link between family history and risk of glaucoma, it is reasonable to expect the rapidly expanding field of medical genetics to elucidate the link between our DNA and glaucoma. However, as more detail becomes available, it may be difficult to place in a broad perspective. Statistically significant correlations are a crucial step toward understanding the role genetics plays in glaucoma. Hopefully, evidence regarding correlations will ultimately help to establish a causal link, if one exists, between the genetic code and glaucoma.

S. J. Fudemberg, MD

Bilateral Explantation of Visian Implantable Collamer Lenses Secondary to Bilateral Acute Angle Closure Resulting From a Non-pupillary Block Mechanism

Khalifa YM, Goldsmith J, Moshirfar M (Univ of Rochester, NY; Univ of Utah, Salt Lake City)
J Refract Surg 26:991-994, 2010

Purpose.—To report a case of bilateral non-pupillary block angle closure glaucoma after Visian Implantable Collamer Lens (ICL, STAAR Surgical) surgery.

Methods.—A 35-year-old woman with high myopia, white-to-white measurements of 11.8 mm in the right eye and 11.9 mm in the left eye, and anterior chamber depths >3 mm in both eyes underwent simultaneous bilateral ICL implantation with 13.2-mm lenses.

Results.—Persistent, bilateral acute angle closure developed despite multiple patent peripheral iridotomies and iridectomies. Visante anterior segment optical coherence tomography (AS-OCT, Carl Zeiss Meditec) revealed profound vaulting of the ICLs and angle closure. Both ICLs were explanted. After explantation, ultrasound biomicroscopy demonstrated a sulcus-to-sulcus diameter of 10.8 mm in the right eye and 11.2 mm in the left eye.

Conclusions.—The correlation between white-to-white and sulcus-to-sulcus measurements were poor in this patient, resulting in extreme vaulting of the ICL and angle closure from a non-pupillary block mechanism. Proper identification of the mechanism of angle closure is aided by AS-OCT. For non-pupillary block mechanisms, ICL extraction is necessary.

▶ The implantable collamer lens (ICL) is permanently implanted posterior to the iris and anterior to the native lens for correction of myopia. To avoid contact with the crystalline lens, the ICL vaults anterior. Given the high risk of pupillary block, prophylactic laser peripheral iridotomies are performed prior to implantation of the lens. Typically, 2 iridotomies are performed per eye in case one is imperforate or becomes blocked by ICL rotation. However, postoperative angle closure glaucoma may occur despite seemingly patent iridotomies.

This case report details a patient in whom postoperative angle closure glaucoma occurred despite seemingly patent laser peripheral iridotomies and in the presence of excessive anterior vaulting of an ICL. The authors theorize that the ICL was too large to be supported in a typical configuration as a result of mismatch between the estimated sulcus-to-sulcus diameter and the ICL size. Sulcus-to-sulcus diameter cannot be directly measured and must be extrapolated from external white-to-white horizontal diameter. Despite measurement of white-to-white diameter with calipers, IOLMaster, and Orbscan, use of the STAAR Surgical Calculator with standard downsizing protocol, and uneventful implantation, bilateral angle closure occurred on the first postoperative day. Placement of additional laser iridotomy, cycloplegia, and ultimately surgical iridectomy failed to break the attack. Further more, no evidence of ICL rotation was found. Anterior segment optical coherence tomography images indicated that vaulting of the ICL caused nonpupillary block acute angle closure glaucoma (Fig 1 in the original article). Explanation of the ICLs finally resolved the acute glaucoma.

White-to-white measurement of 11.8 mm in this patient indicates an estimated sulcus-to-sulcus diameter of 12.8 mm. Ultrasound biomicroscopy measurements of sulcus-to-sulcus diameter following explantation of the ICLs indicated that the actual diameter was closer to 10.8 OD and 11.2 OS. Measurements taken after implantation and explantation with intervening acute angle closure may not accurately reflect the preoperative value.

The incidence of nonpupillary block acute angle closure glaucoma is difficult to estimate because a paucity of literature exists. Nonetheless, this case supports consideration of unilateral ICL implantation since error in estimation of sulcus-to-sulcus diameter is likely to affect both eyes.

S. J. Fudemberg, MD

Bleb Morphology Characteristics and Effect on Positional Intraocular Pressure Variation
Weizer JS, Goyal A, Ple-Plakon P, et al (Univ of Michigan, Ann Arbor; et al)
Ophthalmic Surg Lasers Imaging 41:532-537, 2010

Background and Objective.—To study bleb morphology and positional intraocular pressure (IOP) change (IOP supine to IOP sitting).

Patients and Methods.—In this observational case series, blebs were graded for height, extent, vascularity, microcysts, and "ring of steel." Positional IOP change was analyzed using the paired *t* test. Associations between IOP change and bleb morphologies were evaluated by regression adjusting for inter-eye dependency.

Results.—Ninety-five eyes of 68 subjects were included. Decreased bleb height ($P = .05$), absence of microcysts ($P = .02$), and increased bleb vascularity ($P = .02$) were associated with larger positional IOP change. Twenty patients with a filter in one eye and a medically treated fellow eye had larger positional IOP change in the medically treated eye (6.1 vs 4.6 mm Hg, respectively; $P = .01$).

Conclusion.—Successful filtration surgery results in both lower IOP and less positional IOP change compared with medically treated eyes. Bleb features associated with smaller positional IOP change include higher elevation, microcysts, and less vascularity.

▶ A major weakness of glaucoma management may be the limited volume of intraocular pressure (IOP) measurement data used to guide management. Even with the use of diurnal curves, the total number of IOP measurements collected on an individual patient with glaucoma per year is relatively small. Compared with management of systemic hypertension, in which patients may monitor blood pressure at home, glaucoma care benefits only from information determined during an eye care provider visit. Fluctuations in IOP could play an important role in glaucoma progression. Also, the waxing and waning effect of antiglaucoma medicines may ineffectively temper IOP fluctuation. Understanding the impact of diurnal IOP variation and identifying means to stabilize IOP at an appropriate level could help reduce the risk of vision loss in patients with glaucoma.

The difference in IOP from supine to sitting is defined as positional change and has been shown to approximate diurnal IOP fluctuation. This article tests the hypothesis that in addition to lowering IOP, glaucoma filtration surgery stabilizes IOP by reducing fluctuation. All patients in this study had undergone glaucoma filtration surgery more than 4 months before enrollment and patients with glaucoma drainage devices or past cyclophotocoagulation were excluded. Of the 95 eyes included in the study, the majority underwent trabeculectomy with mitomycin C. However, 11.6% had trabeculectomy without antimetabolite, 9.5% had trabeculectomy with 5-fluorouracil, 6.3% had thermal sclerotomy, and 5.3% had trabeculectomy with mitomycin c and amniotic membrane. Mean number of glaucoma medicines was 1.0 ± 1.3. IOP measurements in the sitting position were performed by both pneumotonometry and Goldmann applanation tonometry. Supine measurements were performed by pneumotonometry alone. Bleb morphology was graded using the Indiana Bleb Grading Scale. Subjects with leaking blebs or completely scarred blebs were excluded.

A subset of 20 subjects in this study had unilateral filtering surgery with medical management of glaucoma in their fellow eye. The positional change in IOP among these patients was statistically significantly greater in medically treated eyes. Supine IOP measurements were greater than sitting IOP measurement. As well, indicators of poor bleb function, including decreased bleb height, absence of microcysts, and increased bleb vascularity, were statistically significantly associated with larger positional IOP change. However, bleb morphology is not necessarily a reliable measure of bleb function, and desired morphology depends on the goals and techniques of the surgeon.

The findings of this study support the concept that surgical glaucoma therapy yields a more stable IOP with less IOP fluctuation. Particularly as our understanding of hemodynamic factors at work in patients with glaucoma evolves, IOP fluctuation and its effect on ocular perfusion pressure may become even more important.

J. S. Myers, MD

Canaloplasty for primary open-angle glaucoma: long-term outcome
Grieshaber MC, Pienaar A, Olivier J, et al (Med Univ of Southern Africa, Pretoria, South Africa)
Br J Ophthalmol 94:1478-1482, 2010

Background/Aims.—To study the safety and effectiveness of 360° viscodilation and tensioning of Schlemm canal (canaloplasty) in black African patients with primary open-angle glaucoma (POAG).

Methods.—Sixty randomly selected eyes of 60 consecutive patients with POAG were included in this prospective study. Canaloplasty comprised 360° catheterisation of Schlemm's canal by means of a flexible microcatheter with distension of the canal by a tensioning 10-0 polypropylene suture.

Results.—The mean preoperative intraocular pressure (IOP) was 45.0 ± 12.1 mmHg. The mean follow-up time was 30.6 ± 8.4 months. The mean IOP at 12 months was 15.4 ± 5.2 mmHg (n=54), at 24 months

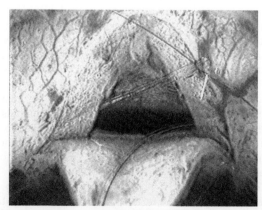

FIGURE 2.—After completing the cannulation of the entire canal length with the microcatheter, and with the distal tip exposed at the surgical cut down, a 10-0 polypropylene suture is tied to the distal tip and looped through the canal. (Reproduced from the British Journal of Ophthalmology, from Grieshaber MC, Pienaar A, Olivier J, et al. Canaloplasty for primary open-angle glaucoma: long-term outcome. *Br J Ophthalmol.* 2010;94:1478-1482, copyright 2010 with permission from BMJ Publishing Group Ltd.)

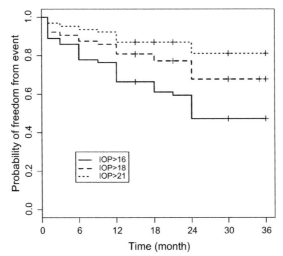

For IOP > 21 mmHg:

Time (months)	Number of eyes at risk	'Survival'	95% Confidence Interval
0	60	1.000	1.000 - 1.000
3	59	0.952	0.901 - 1.000
6	57	0.937	0.878 - 0.999
12	54	0.869	0.788 - 0.958
24	47	0.810	0.714 - 0.919
36	44	0.810	0.714 - 0.919

For IOP > 18 mmHg

Time	Number of eyes at risk	'Survival'	95% Confidence Interval
0	60	1.000	1.000 - 1.000
3	58	0.905	0.835 - 0.980
6	56	0.873	0.795 - 0.959
12	52	0.806	0.714 - 0.911
24	44	0.678	0.568 - 0.810
36	40	0.678	0.568 - 0.810

For IOP > 16 mmHg

Time	Number of eyes at risk	'Survival'	95% Confidence Interval
0	60	1.000	1.000 - 1.000
3	54	0.857	0.775 - 0.948
6	52	0.778	0.682 - 0.888
12	44	0.663	0.555 - 0.791
24	34	0.472	0.361 - 0.618
36	28	0.472	0.361 - 0.618

FIGURE 5.—Kaplan—Meier analysis for IOP. (Reproduced from the British Journal of Ophthalmology, from Grieshaber MC, Pienaar A, Olivier J, et al. Canaloplasty for primary open-angle glaucoma: long-term outcome. *Br J Ophthalmol.* 2010;94:1478-1482, copyright 2010 with permission from BMJ Publishing Group Ltd.)

16.3 ± 4.2 mmHg (n=51) and at 36 months 13.3 ± 1.7 mmHg (n=49). For IOP ≤21 mmHg, complete success rate was 77.5% and qualified success rate was 81.6% at 36 months. Cox regression analysis showed that preoperative IOP (HR=1.003, 95% CI=0.927 to 1.085; p=0.94), age (HR= 1.000, CI=0.938 to 1.067; p=0.98) and sex (HR=3.005, CI=0.329 to 27.448; p=0.33) were all not significant predictors of IOP reduction to ≤21 mmHg. Complication rate was low (Descemet's detachment n=2, elevated IOP n=1, false passage of the catheter n=2).

Conclusion.—Canaloplasty produced a sustained longterm reduction of IOP in black Africans with POAG independent of preoperative IOP. As a bleb-independent procedure, canaloplasty may be a true alternative to classic filtering surgery, in particular in patients with enhanced wound healing and scar formation (Figs 2 and 5).

▶ This article reports very good results for canaloplasty in a very challenging population of patients. Black Africans with high initial intraocular pressures (IOPs) were the subjects of this study, and they have a much greater risk of early failure because of excessive wound healing or other complications with trabeculectomy.

The results in this uncontrolled study show good pressure control at 3 years for most patients. However, the success rate by IOP goal (Fig 5) shows that there is loss of effect and success over time. Clearly, the average postoperative pressure is not as low as trabeculectomy. However, the safety profile and overall success were greater than would be expected for trabeculectomy.

This promising study should be read with caution. First, this phenotype of glaucoma, very high initial IOP in a black African population, is not what is seen in most of the world. Second, the authors themselves point out that they had reported before equally excellent results with viscocanalostomy in this same population and abandoned this procedure later because of disappointing long-term results. Canalostomy remains a promising alternative, but its exact role in the management of glaucoma will continue to evolve as studies demonstrate its strengths and weaknesses. Prospective controlled studies in particular will be of interest.

J. S. Myers, MD

Comparison of Comorbid Conditions between Open-Angle Glaucoma Patients and a Control Cohort: A Case-Control Study
Lin H-C, Chien C-W, Hu C-C, et al (Taipei Med Univ, Taiwan; Natl Yang-Ming Univ, Taipei, Taiwan; et al)
Ophthalmology 117:2088-2095, 2010

Objective.—To determine the prevalence of selected comorbidities in patients with open-angle glaucoma (OAG) and whether these comorbidities are more prevalent among individuals with OAG than those without OAG.

Design.—A retrospective, nationwide, case-control study using an administrative database.

Participants.—The study group comprised 76 673 OAG patients. The comparison group comprised 230 019 subjects matched to the study cohort.

Methods.—Data were collected retrospectively from the Taiwan National Health Insurance Research Database. The study cohort comprised all patients with a diagnosis of OAG (International Classification of Diseases, 9th Revision, Clinical Modification codes 365.1−365.11) in 2005 (n = 76 673). The comparison cohort comprised randomly

TABLE 3.—Crude and Adjusted Odds Ratios and 95% Confidence Intervals for Each of the 31 Medical Comorbidities between Open-Angle Glaucoma Patients and the Comparison Group (n = 306 692)

	Odds Ratio (95% Confidence Interval)	
Variable	Crude	Adjusted
Cardiovascular		
Hypertension	1.52* (1.48−1.56)	1.62* (1.58−1.67)
Ischemic heart disease	1.26* (1.16−1.37)	1.25* (1.15−1.36)
Hyperlipidemia	1.83* (1.78−1.88)	1.85* (1.80−1.91)
Congestive heart failure	1.30* (1.24−1.37)	1.31* (1.24−1.38)
Cardiac arrhythmias	1.34* (1.28−1.41)	1.35* (1.28−1.41)
Peripheral vascular disorders	1.46* (1.37−1.56)	1.46* (1.37−1.56)
Stroke	1.35* (1.30−1.41)	1.37* (1.32−1.43)
Neurologic		
Paralysis	0.89 (0.77−1.02)	0.89 (0.77−1.02)
Other neurologic disorders	1.34* (1.25−1.43)	1.33* (1.24−1.43)
Headaches	1.15* (1.12−1.19)	1.16* (1.12−1.19)
Migraines	1.21* (1.11−1.32)	1.21* (1.11−1.32)
Epilepsy	1.41* (1.22−1.63)	1.40* (1.21−1.62)
Dementia	1.19* (1.10−1.29)	1.19* (1.09−1.29)
Rheumatologic		
Rheumatoid arthritis	1.48* (1.40−1.57)	1.49* (1.40−1.57)
Systemic lupus erythematosus	2.04* (1.55−2.67)	2.05* (1.56−2.69)
Pulmonary		
Chronic obstructive pulmonary disease	1.30* (1.17−1.44)	1.29* (1.16−1.44)
Asthma	1.30* (1.24−1.37)	1.30* (1.24−1.37)
Pulmonary circulation disorders	0.98 (0.68−1.40)	0.97 (0.67−1.40)
Endocrine		
Diabetes	1.78* (1.74−1.84)	1.82* (1.77−1.88)
Hypothyroidism	1.69* (1.60−1.79)	1.70* (1.61−1.80)
Renal		
Renal failure	1.37* (1.28−1.47)	1.37* (1.28−1.47)
Fluid and electrolyte disorders	1.55* (1.41−1.71)	1.55* (1.41−1.71)
Gastrointestinal		
Liver diseases	1.44* (1.39−1.50)	1.45* (1.40−1.50)
Peptic ulcers	1.42* (1.37−1.46)	1.42* (1.38−1.47)
Viral/infectious		
Hepatitis B	1.32* (1.24−1.41)	1.32* (1.24−1.41)
Tuberculosis	1.20[†] (1.08−1.34)	1.19[†] (1.07−1.33)
Hematologic		
Deficiency anemias	1.29* (1.21−1.37)	1.29* (1.21−1.37)
Mental illness		
Depression	1.67* (1.57−1.76)	1.67* (1.58−1.76)
Psychosis	1.60* (1.49−1.71)	1.60* (1.49−1.72)
Oncologic		
Metastatic cancer excluding lymphomas	1.16 (0.92−1.47)	1.15 (0.91−1.46)
Solid tumor without metastasis	1.21* (1.14−1.28)	1.21* (1.14−1.28)

The odds ratios for patients with and without glaucoma were calculated by separate conditional regression analyses conditioned on patient age, gender, monthly income, and level of urbanization of the community in which the patient resided.
*$P<0.001$.
[†]$P<0.01$.

selected patients (3 for every 1 OAG patient; n = 230 019) matched with the study group in terms of age, gender, urbanization level, and monthly income. In total, 31 medical comorbidities were selected based mainly on the Elixhauser Comorbidity Index. Separate conditional logistic regression analyses were used to estimate the adjusted odds ratio for each of the medical comorbidities between patients with and without OAG.

Main Outcome Measures.—The prevalences of selected comorbidities.

Results.—More than half (50.5%) of the OAG patients had hypertension, and more than 30% had hyperlipidemia or diabetes (30.5% and 30.2%, respectively). The prevalences of 28 of 31 comorbidities were significantly higher for OAG patients than subjects without glaucoma after adjusting for age, gender, urbanization level, and monthly income. The adjusted odds ratio was more than 1.50 for hypertension, hyperlipidemia, systemic lupus erythematosus, diabetes, hypothyroidism, fluid and electrolyte disorders, depression, and psychosis. Among the studied comorbidities, the prevalence difference of the OAG group minus the control group was 3% or higher for hypertension, hyperlipidemia, stroke, diabetes, liver disease, and peptic ulcer.

Conclusions.—Open-angle glaucoma patients are significantly more likely to have comorbidities, many of which can be life threatening or can affect the quality of life appreciably (Table 3).

▶ This study from Taiwan of predominantly Chinese patients is notable for several reasons. First, it is a very large study, involving tens of thousands of subjects with glaucoma. Studies this large in glaucoma research are truly infrequent and should be considered carefully. The study is well designed, with careful consideration to maximize the likelihood that its findings will be correct.

This study shows increased prevalence of virtually all investigated comorbidities in subjects with glaucoma versus age- and income-matched controls. Hypertension and diabetes are not a surprise, as these relations have been shown in multiple other studies of other ethnic groups. Many believe that vasculopathic factors increase the risk of glaucoma and glaucomatous progression.

However, this study found that subjects with glaucoma were more likely to have all but 2 of the 31 comorbidities studied. The reasons for this are unknown, but clinicians have noted for years that patients with glaucoma in general seem to be less healthy than their peers.

These findings underscore how much we have yet to learn regarding the complicated physiology of glaucoma and the entire human body. They also emphasize the need to encourage patients with glaucoma to be closely and carefully monitored for systemic conditions.

J. S. Myers, MD

Determinants of Agreement between the Confocal Scanning Laser Tomograph and Standardized Assessment of Glaucomatous Progression
Vizzeri G, Bowd C, Weinreb RN, et al (Univ of California San Diego, La Jolla)
Ophthalmology 117:1953-1959, 2010

Purpose.—To estimate the agreement of confocal scanning laser tomograph (CSLT), topographic change analysis (TCA) with assessment of stereophotographs, and standard automated perimetry (SAP) for detecting glaucomatous progression and to identify factors associated with agreement between methods.

Design.—Observational cohort study.

Participants.—We included 246 eyes of 167 glaucoma patients, glaucoma suspects, and ocular hypertensives.

Methods.—We included CSLT series (n $\geq$4 tests; mean follow-up, 4 years), stereophotographs, and SAP results in the analysis. The number of progressors by guided progression analysis (GPA, "likely progression"), progressors by masked stereophotographs assessment and progressors by TCA as determined for 3 parameters related to the number of progressed superpixels within the disc margin was determined. Agreement between progression by each TCA parameter, stereophotographs and GPA was assessed using the Kappa test. Analysis of variance with post hoc analysis was applied to identify baseline factors including image quality (standard deviation of the mean topography), disc size and disease severity (pattern standard deviation [PSD] and cup area) associated with agreement/nonagreement between methods.

Main Outcome Measures.—Agreement in assessing glaucomatous progression between the methods including factors associated with agreement/nonagreement between methods.

Results.—Agreement between progression by TCA and progression by stereophotographs and/or GPA was generally poor regardless of the TCA parameter and specificity cutoffs applied. For the parameters with the strongest agreement, cluster size in disc ($CSIZE^{disc}$) and cluster area in disc ($CAREA^{disc}$), kappa values were 0.16 (63.9%, agreement on 134 nonprogressing eyes and 23 progressing eyes) and 0.15 (64.1%, agreement on 135 nonprogressing eyes and 22 progressing eyes) at 99% cutoff. Most of the factors evaluated were not significantly associated with agreement/nonagreement between methods (all $P>0.07$). However, SAP PSD was greater in the progressors by stereophotography only group compared with the progressors by TCA only group (5.8 ± 4.7 and 2.6 ± 2.2, respectively [$P = 0.003$] for $CSIZE^{disc}$ at 95% specificity and 5.4 ± 4.6 and 2.5 ± 2.3, respectively [$P = 0.002$] for $CAREA^{disc}$ at 99% specificity).

Conclusions.—Agreement for detection of longitudinal changes between TCA, stereophotography, and SAP GPA is poor. Progressors by stereophotography only tended to have more advanced disease at baseline than progressors by TCA only (Fig 1).

▶ Vizzeri et al report on a carefully performed study comparing scanning laser tomography (Heidelberg retina tomograph [HRT] II), visual fields, and stereophotography for the analysis of glaucomatous progression. The agreement among these methods is poor. The reasons for this discrepancy are likely many, including the divergence of structure and function, localized variability in structural imaging masking change, and factors as yet unknown.

In general, the HRT found many more eyes to be progressing towards glaucoma than the other methods found—on the order of 4 to 6 times more. This

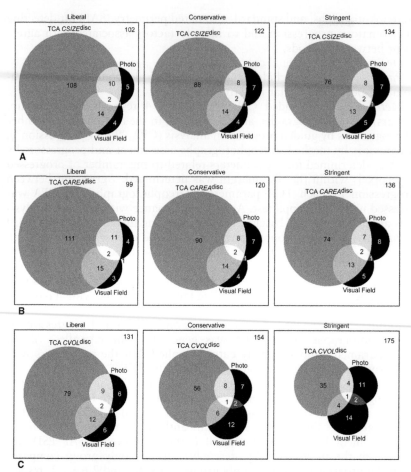

FIGURE 1.—Proportional Venn diagrams showing the agreement between progression TCA CSIZE^{disc} (**A**), TCA CAREA^{disc} (**B**), and TCA CVOL^{disc} (**C**) evaluated at 90% (liberal criteria), 95% (conservative criteria) and 99% (stringent criteria) specificity cutoffs and progression by stereophotography and visual field (SAP GPA). The number of eyes with all 3 tests stable is shown in the top right corner of each diagram. CAREA^{disc} = area of progressed superpixels in the largest cluster; CSIZE^{disc} = number of progressed superpixels in the largest cluster; CVOL^{disc} = volume of progressed superpixels in the largest cluster; GPA = guided progression analysis; SAP = standard automated perimetry; TCA = topographic change analysis. (Reprinted from Vizzeri G, Bowd C, Weinreb RN, et al. Determinants of agreement between the confocal scanning laser tomograph and standardized assessment of glaucomatous progression. *Ophthalmology.* 2010;117:1953-1959, copyright © 2010, with permission from the American Academy of Ophthalmology.)

may be because the HRT is truly much more sensitive to change, or these may be false-positive results. A previous report by Chauhan and coworkers had similar findings in this regard.[1] Only time and longitudinal studies will show whether these are true or false-positive results.

For now, there is no gold standard of glaucomatous progression, but clinicians must continue to seek the best concordance of evidence, relying on pressure, perimetry, structural evaluations, and patient symptoms to determine stability.

J. S. Myers, MD

Reference

1. Chauhan BC, McCormick TA, Nicolela MT, LeBlanc RP. Optic disc and visual field changes in a prospective longitudinal study of patients with glaucoma: comparison of scanning laser tomography with conventional perimetry and optic disc photography. *Arch Ophthalmol.* 2001;119:1492-1499.

Focusing on glaucoma progression and the clinical importance of progression rate measurement: a review
Rossetti L, Goni F, Denis P, et al (Lund Univ, Malmö, Sweden)
Eye 24:S1-S7, 2010

Purpose.—This review aims to provide guidance in managing glaucoma patients more effectively. It focuses on the importance of detecting progression and measuring its rate within the management of primary open-angle glaucoma today. Recent findings strongly indicate that continued monitoring of visual fields (VFs) and reassessment of target intraocular pressures (IOPs) depending on VF progression rates are mandatory in the management of glaucoma.

Methods.—Data on glaucoma progression from older as well as most recent literature findings are summarized in this article. In addition, the article elaborates on the scientific content from a series of lectures given by experts in the field during several international symposia on 'rate of progression' in 2008.

Results.—This review summarizes key findings on the natural history of glaucoma and known factors for disease progression. It highlights the visual function changes observed as glaucoma progresses and discusses disease impact on patients' quality of life. Findings support the need to obtain information on rate of progression and its importance for clinical management. Practical ways to measure rate of progression are given by new software options to help measure major parameters. Finally, on the basis of a patient's individual rate of progression therapeutic options are assessed, such as maximum medical therapy with fixed combinations.

Conclusions.—Estimating a patient's individual rate of VF progression by using newly developed analyses will be helpful to forecast the potential future development of the glaucoma. An individualized treatment approach then requires that in patients in whom the risk of becoming visually impaired or blind during their lifetime is higher, a more intensive medical IOP-lowering therapy such as fixed combinations can be considered as treatment option.

▶ This article discusses rate of change in glaucoma and its implications for care and outcomes. One of the key challenges in the clinical management of glaucoma is the assessment for progressive visual field loss or disc damage. Traditional methods of visual field assessment for progression have been based on evaluating the new field against a baseline and looking for sufficient change to be considered significant. Such criteria have included, for example, a cluster of 3 contiguous points depressed by 5 dB or more compared with the baseline field. This type of criterion is referred to as event-based change criteria. The Hodapp-Parrish-Anderson criteria for progression are of this type, as are the cutoff criteria for progression used in all of the major prospective trials, such as Ocular Hypertension Treatment Study (OHTS), Early Manifest Glaucoma Trial, Collaborative Initial Glaucoma Treatment Study, Advanced Glaucoma Intervention Study, and Collaborative Normal Tension Glaucoma Study.

As seen in OHTS, event-based criteria for visual field progression can yield unwanted results because of the inherent variability of visual field testing results. In OHTS, 85% of abnormal fields were judged normal on repeat. Of those who were abnormal on 2 consecutive tests, 65% were normal on the third test.

Trend-based visual field progression criteria assess a series of fields for the trend, overall, at each point, or in clusters of points. These techniques usually use linear regression analysis to look at the rate of change or slope. If the slope is negative and is statistically significantly different than a zero slope, progression is occurring. A key feature is the ability of linear regression analysis to assess for statistical significance of change based on the subjects' own intertest variability. This allows much greater confidence in the results for each patient. Also, the magnitude of the slope is clinically useful. For example, an eye with early glaucoma progressing at 2 dB of mean deviation per year in a young patient may go blind in 10 years if left unchecked. On the other hand, a 95-year old showing a 0.5 dB change per year is probably not in great danger.

Originally, these techniques were only used for research. However, the Progressor program was released a decade ago to allow progression criteria— based posttest analysis of visual fields by pointwise linear regression. Haag Streit/Octopus released software to allow global- and cluster-based analysis of change over time by linear regression years ago. More recently, Humphrey/Zeiss added a global linear regression—based analysis, the visual field index (VFI). The VFI is similar to mean deviation but emphasizes central points and starts at 100% and may go to 0% as vision is lost.

Research increasingly favors these linear regression techniques as robust tools to assess and compare glaucoma progression. These tools are now being used clinically and are especially useful with more frequent (twice yearly) visual field testing. Comparison of trend- and event-based change algorithms suggests a similar minimum number of fields in a series to be confident of change, given the inherent variability of fields.

J. S. Myers, MD

Glaucoma surgery: trainee outcomes and implications for future training: southeast Scotland
Welch J, Vani A, Cackett P, et al (Queen Margaret Hosp, Dunfermline, Fife, UK)
Eye (Lond) 24:1700-1707, 2010

Aim.—Postoperative outcome of trainee glaucoma surgery compared with glaucoma specialist consultant surgery. Survey of Scottish consultant ophthalmologists' views on trainee surgery.

Method.—Retrospective analysis of 128 trainee and 176 consultant trabeculectomies, with minimum postoperative follow-up of 2 years. Prospective postal survey of 80 Scottish consultant ophthalmologists.

Results.—Trainees operated mainly on cases of chronic open angle glaucoma, while consultants operated on significantly more complicated glaucomas $(P = 0.0004)$. Trainee cases had more bleb leaks $(P = 0.01)$, hypotony $(P = 0.05)$, early $(P = 0.01)$ and late $(P = 0.03)$ return to theatre, and bleb interventions $(P = 0.01)$. Trainee mitomycin trabeculectomies were associated with higher rates of return to theatre $(P = 0.002)$, and cataract extraction within the first postoperative year $(P = 0.002)$. Trainee cases of pseudoexfoliation had more early complications $(P = 0.024)$, and trainee cases of low tension required more bleb interventions $(P = 0.05)$. There was no significant difference $(P > 0.05)$ between average intraocular pressure control (IOP) at postoperative visit year 1 between consultant (14.3 mmHg) and trainee (13.9 mmHg) cases. More than 50% of the 80 Scottish ophthalmology consultants surveyed, indicated that glaucoma surgery training requirements should be retained.

Conclusions.—Trainee trabeculectomy cases showed significantly higher rates of early complications, return to theatres, and bleb interventions compared with consultant cases. Satisfactory IOP control was achieved in both groups at postoperative year 1. Trainee cases require careful preoperative selection, avoiding complicated glaucomas including pseudoexfoliation and low tension, and those that require mitomycin. The majority of Scottish consultants wish to retain glaucoma surgery within the remit of generic training (Tables 2 and 3).

▶ This study investigates outcomes of trabeculectomy performed by trainees and glaucoma specialists. Although the 1-year results are similar, the rate of complications, including reoperation, and cataract were much higher in the trainee group, even though the cases were lower risk.

The obligation to provide excellent care to patients while training the next generation of ophthalmologists is not always easy. Clear cornea phacoemulsification has reduced the experience of trainees in suturing and tissue manipulation compared to the extracapsular cataract extraction era. This further makes glaucoma surgical training a greater challenge. Simulators of phacoemulsification allow practice outside a living eye. Such simulations for glaucoma surgery are limited, as eyes recovered from organ donors do not allow practice on conjunctival suturing.

TABLE 2.—Early Trabeculectomy Complications

Complication	Consultant	%	95% CI	Trainee	%	95%CI	P-Value
Hyphaema	45	25.6	19.7–32.5	21	16.4	10.9–23.9	0.05
Leak	21	11.9	7.9–17.6	29	22.7	16.2–30.7	0.01
Choroidal effusions	17	9.7	6.0–15.0	21	16.4	10.9–23.9	0.08
Hypotony	25	14.2	9.8–20.2	29	22.7	16.2–30.7	0.05
Shallow AC	38	21.6	16.1–28.3	33	25.8	19.0–34.0	0.39
Iridocorneal touch	0	0.0	0.0–2.6	1	0.8	0.0–4.7	0.24
None	85	48.3	41.0–55.6	55	43.0	34.7–51.6	0.36

Abbreviation: CI, confidence interval.

TABLE 3.—Number of Postoperative Bleb Intervention Procedures and Patient Numbers

Interventions	Consultant	%	95% CI	Trainee	%	95% CI	P-Value
Suturelysis	15	8.5	5.1–13.7	14	10.9	6.5–17.6	0.48
5-FU injection	26	14.8	10.2–20.8	21	16.4	10.9–23.9	0.70
Bleb needling	14	8.0	4.7–13.0	12	9.4	5.3–15.8	0.66
Other	8	4.5	2.2–8.9	17	13.3	8.4–20.3	<0.01
Patients with interventions	40	22.7	17.1–29.5	50	39.1	31.0–47.7	<0.01
Patients without interventions	136	77.3	70.5–82.9	78	60.9	52.3–69.0	<0.01

Abbreviations: CI, confidence interval; 5-FU, 5-fluorouracil.

In many parts of the world, declining numbers of trabeculectomies coupled with increasing ranks of glaucoma specialists have led to greater proportions of trabeculectomies being performed by glaucoma specialists. Trabeculectomy remains challenging even in the most experienced hands. It is possible that newer simpler surgeries will replace trabeculectomy. However, until this occurs, the burden to patients of trainee surgery must be considered in light of the gain for society. If glaucoma specialists perform most trabeculectomies in the future, then the increased complications associated with training all residents in trabeculectomy will not be justified.

J. S. Myers, MD

Hypothyroidism and the Risk of Developing Open-Angle Glaucoma: A Five-Year Population-Based Follow-up Study

Lin H-C, Kang J-H, Jiang Y-D, et al (Taipei Med Univ, Taiwan; et al)
Ophthalmology 117:1960-1966, 2010

Objective.—To investigate the risk of open-angle glaucoma (OAG) after a diagnosis of hypothyroidism.

Design.—A retrospective, population-based follow-up study using an administrative database.

Participants.—The study group comprised 257 hypothyroidism patients. The comparison group included 2056 subjects.

Methods.—Data were retrospectively collected from the Taiwan Longitudinal Health Insurance Database. The study cohort comprised patients aged ≥60 who received a first diagnosis of hypothyroidism (International Classification of Diseases, Ninth Revision, Clinical Modification code 244.9) from 1997 to 2001 (n = 257). The comparison cohort consisted of randomly selected patients without hypothyroidism who were aged ≥60 and had no diagnosis of glaucoma before 2001 (8 for every OAG patient; n = 2056). Each sampled patient was tracked for 5 years from their index visit. Cox proportional hazard regressions were used to compute the 5-year OAG-free survival rate, after adjusting for possible confounding factors.

Main Outcome Measures.—The risk of developing OAG during the 5-year follow-up period.

Results.—Open-angle glaucoma developed in 7.4% of patients with hypothyroidism and 3.8% of patients in the comparison cohort during the follow-up period. Hypothyroid patients had a significantly lower 5-year OAG-free survival rate than patients in the comparison cohort. After adjusting for patients' age, gender, monthly income, urbanization level, and comorbid medical disorders, hypothyroidism patients were found to have a 1.78-fold (95% confidence interval [CI], 1.04—3.06) greater risk of developing OAG than the comparison cohort. This association remained significant in untreated hypothyroidism patients (adjusted hazard ratio [HR], 2.37; 95% CI, 1.10—5.09) and became statistically nonsignificant in patients treated with levothyroxine (adjusted HR, 1.73; 95% CI, 0.89—3.38).

Conclusions.—Hypothyroid patients had a significantly increased risk of OAG development during the 5-year follow-up period. Levothyroxine seemed to be protective (Fig 1).

▶ This is another study based on the Taiwan Longitudinal Health Insurance Database. It is one of the more systematic approaches to investigating a link between hypothyroidism and glaucoma. This study again confirms a possible link, with an increased risk of glaucoma in patients with hypothyroidism. Furthermore, the study shows an increased risk with untreated but not treated hypothyroidism. In a 5-year analysis, over 7% of patients with hypothyroidism developed glaucoma.

The authors refer to work that suggests hypothyroidism may be associated with reduced clearance of material from the trabecular meshwork, such as mucopolysaccharides, and other studies showing improved pressure control with treatment of hypothyroidism.

This association between hypothyroidism and glaucoma has been discussed for some time, but it is only more recently that thorough studies such as this have more conclusively demonstrated the link. The understanding of this

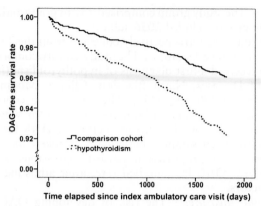

Time elapsed since index ambulatory care visit (days)

FIGURE 1.—Open-angle glaucoma-free survival rates for patients with hypothyroidism and patients in the comparison cohort, 1997–2001. OAG = open-angle glaucoma. (Reprinted from Lin H-C, Kang J-H, Jiang Y-D, et al. Hypothyroidism and the risk of developing open-angle glaucoma: a five-year population-based follow-up study. *Ophthalmology*. 2010;117:1960-1966, copyright © 2010, with permission from the American Academy of Ophthalmology.)

connection and the influence treatment for hypothyroidism may have on the development of glaucoma may be useful for clinicians in selected patients.

J. S. Myers, MD

Importance of Visual Acuity and Contrast Sensitivity in Patients With Glaucoma

Richman J, Lorenzana LL, Lankaranian D, et al (Wills Eye Inst of Jefferson Med College, Philadelphia, PA)
Arch Ophthalmol 128:1576-1582, 2010

Objective.—To determine which aspects of vision most influence the ability of patients with glaucoma to function.

Methods.—A total of 192 patients with a full range of glaucomatous visual loss were selected from the Glaucoma Service of Wills Eye Institute. Patients were evaluated clinically with standard visual assessments: visual acuity, contrast sensitivity, visual field, stereopsis, the Disc Damage Likelihood Scale, and intraocular pressure. Patients were evaluated objectively using a comprehensive performance-based measure of visual function, the Assessment of Disability Related to Vision (ADREV), and subjectively with the 25-item National Eye Institute Visual Function Questionnaire. Statistical analyses, including Spearman correlation coefficients and regression analysis, were performed on the data.

Results.—Performance on the ADREV was most strongly associated with binocular visual acuity ($r=-0.79$; $P<.001$) and binocular contrast sensitivity ($r=0.80$; $P<.001$). Monocular and binocular visual field test results correlated well with the ability to perform the ADREV tasks, but there was a significantly weaker association ($P<.05$) compared with visual acuity and contrast sensitivity.

Conclusion.—The aspects of visual function that best predict the ability of a patient with glaucoma to perform activities of daily living are binocular visual acuity and contrast sensitivity.

▶ Research has shown that quality-of-life questionnaires in visual diseases are affected by a host of issues in addition to a patient's vision. As a result, although strong statistical correlations exist between visual function and quality of life, any 2 patients may have widely different results on questionnaires with similar levels of visual function. This limits the clinical utility of these questionnaires.

Researchers at Wills Eye Institute have been developing instruments to measure functional vision in activities of daily living. These instruments in some ways bridge the gaps between clinical functional measures such as the visual field and patients' perception of function as assessed by questionnaires.

Not surprisingly, visual acuity was found in this study to be strongly correlated to performance on the tasks, as was contrast sensitivity. This relation appears to be true even at levels of visual impairment short of disability (better than 20/200). Clinically, it is not routine to measure contrast sensitivity, although among these glaucoma patients contrast sensitivity appears to have a significant impact. Prior research has shown that glaucoma patients lose contrast sensitivity with advancing disease.

This battery of functional tests is unlikely to be adopted clinically, but the results are improving the understanding of which clinical measures may be most helpful in assessing the impact of glaucoma. As yet, there are no concrete recommendations, but as this field evolves, we may see other tests gaining weight in the clinical management of glaucoma.

J. S. Myers, MD

Longitudinal and Cross-sectional Analyses of Visual Field Progression in Participants of the Ocular Hypertension Treatment Study

Artes PH, for the Ocular Hypertension Treatment Study Group (Dalhousie Univ, Halifax, Nova Scotia, Canada; et al)

Arch Ophthalmol 128:1528-1532, 2010

Objective.—To assess agreement between longitudinal and cross-sectional analyses for determining visual field progression in data from the Ocular Hypertension Treatment Study.

Methods.—Visual field data from 3088 eyes of 1570 participants (median follow-up, 7 years) were analyzed. Longitudinal analyses were performed using change probability with total and pattern deviation, and cross-sectional analyses were performed using the glaucoma hemifield test, corrected pattern standard deviation, and mean deviation. The rates of mean deviation and general height change were compared to estimate the degree of diffuse loss in emerging glaucoma.

Results.—Agreement on progression in longitudinal and cross-sectional analyses ranged from 50% to 61% and remained nearly constant across a wide range of criteria. In contrast, agreement on absence of progression ranged from 97.0% to 99.7%, being highest for the stricter criteria. Analyses of pattern deviation were more conservative than analyses of total deviation, with a 3 to 5 times lesser incidence of progression. Most participants developing field loss had both diffuse and focal changes.

Conclusions.—Despite considerable overall agreement, 40% to 50% of eyes identified as having progressed with either longitudinal or cross-sectional analyses were identified with only one of the analyses. Because diffuse change is part of early glaucomatous damage, pattern deviation analyses may underestimate progression in patients with ocular hypertension.

▶ This article reports the findings based on various analyses of a subset of the many visual fields taken as part of the Ocular Hypertension Treatment Study (OHTS). In the entire OHTS, 85% of abnormal fields were normal on repeat testing. Of those that were abnormal twice, 65% were normal on the third test. To overcome this variability, researchers in this report required the findings to be evident on 3 consecutive fields to establish change.

The analysis focuses on set criteria of abnormality (eg, an abnormal glaucoma hemifield test or a pattern deviation depressed at the $P < 1\%$ level) versus a pointwise evaluation of change compared with baseline field. This second approach, referred to as longitudinal analysis in this study, was of 2 types, one similar to the Humphrey Guided Progression Analysis (GPA) and the other to the Glaucoma Change Probability (GCP). The newer GPA is based on pattern deviation plots; the older GCP on total deviation plots.

Key findings include a reduced sensitivity in detecting change with the GCP and GCA when compared with the fixed criteria for abnormality (the so-called cross-sectional analysis). It is unclear from the data available if this reduced sensitivity is because of greater specificity (weeding out false-positives) or is just the result of missed true-positives. However, evidence suggested that the older total deviation–based GCP performed better than the newer GPA that is pattern deviation plot based. Perhaps related, the researchers saw evidence that many eyes showed diffuse loss related to glaucoma before focal loss, also emphasizing the importance of looking at total deviation plots and not just pattern deviation plots.

Please see also the commentary in this chapter on the article, "Focusing on glaucoma progression and the clinical importance of progression rate measurement: A review."

J. S. Myers, MD

Patterned Laser Trabeculoplasty

Turati M, Gil-Carrasco F, Morales A, et al (Association to Prevent Blindness in Mexico (APEC); et al)

Ophthalmic Surg Lasers Imaging 41:538-545, 2010

Background and Objective.—A novel computer-guided laser treatment for open-angle glaucoma, called patterned laser trabeculoplasty, and its preliminary clinical evaluation is described.

Patients and Methods.—Forty-seven eyes of 25 patients with open-angle glaucoma received 532-nm laser treatment with 100-µm spots. Power was titrated for trabecular meshwork blanching at 10 ms and subvisible treatment was applied with 5-ms pulses. The arc patterns of 66 spots rotated automatically after each laser application so that the new pattern was applied at an untreated position.

Results.—Approximately 1,100 laser spots were placed per eye in 16 steps, covering 360° of trabecular meshwork. The intraocular pressure decreased from the pretreatment level of 21.9 ± 4.1 to 16.0 ± 2.3 mm Hg at 1 month (n = 41) and remained stable around 15.5 ± 2.7 mm Hg during 6 months of follow-up (n = 30).

Conclusion.—Patterned laser trabeculoplasty provides rapid, precise, and minimally traumatic (sub-visible) computer-guided treatment with exact abutment of the patterns, exhibiting a 24% reduction in intraocular pressure during 6 months of follow-up (P < .01).

▶ The authors present the results of a trial of patterned laser trabeculoplasty. This technique uses the same wavelength as argon laser trabeculoplasty but smaller shorter applications delivered in a grid pattern over a 22.5° arc (16 grids per 360°).

The results in this limited cohort suggest that perhaps 65% or so of eyes achieve a 20% reduction of intraocular pressure at 6 months. This falls within the reported range of success of argon, diode, and selective laser trabeculoplasty.

To date, selective laser trabeculoplasty has been shown to have similar results to argon treatments, and perhaps the success rate of diode is not quite as good. Adequate studies are lacking on the newer micropulsed laser trabeculoplasty, but there are no data yet to suggest that it will be superior. This patterned laser trabeculoplasty approach is novel and interesting, but it remains to be seen if this innovation will result in improved outcomes for our patients.

J. S. Myers, MD

Randomised controlled trial of screening and prophylactic treatment to prevent primary angle closure glaucoma

Yip JLY, Foster PJ, Uranchimeg D, et al (London School of Hygiene and Tropical Medicine, UK; Health Sciences Univ, Ulaanbaatar, Mongolia; et al)
Br J Ophthalmol 94:1472-1477, 2010

Aims.—To determine if screening with an ultrasound A-scan and prophylactic treatment of primary angle closure (PAC) with laser peripheral iridotomy (LPI) can reduce the incidence of primary angle closure glaucoma (PACG) in Mongolia.

Methods.—A single-masked randomised controlled trial was initiated in 1999. 4725 volunteer Mongolian participants ≥50 years old from the capital Ulaanbaatar or the rural province of Bayankhongor were recruited, of which 128 were excluded with glaucoma. 4597 were randomly allocated to the control, no-screening arm or screening with ultrasound central anterior chamber depth (cACD), with the cut-off set at <2.53 mm. 685 screen-positive participants were examined and angle closure was identified by gonioscopy in 160, of which 156 were treated with prophylactic LPI. Primary outcome of incident PACG was determined using both structural and functional evidence from objective grading of paired disc photographs from baseline and follow-up, objective grading of follow-up visual fields and clinical examination.

Results.—Six years later, 801 (17.42%) participants were known to have died, and a further 2047 (53.92%) were traced and underwent full ophthalmic examination. In an intention to treat analysis using available data, PACG was diagnosed in 33 participants (1.61%, 95% CI 1.11% to 2.25%), of which 19 were in the screened group and 14 in the non-screened group (OR 1.29, 95% CI 0.65 to 2.60, p=0.47), indicating no difference between groups.

Conclusions.—We were not able to identify a reduction in the 6 year incidence of PACG after screening with cACD <2.53 mm and prophylactic treatment of PAC.

▶ This study used central anterior chamber depth (cACD) measurement for screening occludable angles. Over 4000 subjects were randomized to screening or no intervention. Eyes with cACD <2.53 mm in the screening group were treated with laser peripheral iridotomy.

After 6 years, this study shows evidence that laser iridotomy helps prevent acute angle closure glaucoma. However, the screened group had a similar (in fact greater, but not statistically so) number of conversions to primary angle closure glaucoma (PACG, this would have been called chronic angle closure glaucoma in the older terminology: elevated pressure with anterior synechiae or a narrow angle and disc damage).

In this Mongolian population, a single screening cACD depth as guidance for laser iridotomy was insufficient to prevent PACG. Reasons for this could include the inadequacy of this technique to assess who is at risk, the inadequacy of a single measurement to predict future angle closure glaucoma, the nature of PACG in Mongolian eyes, and bias introduced by the many subjects lost to follow-up.

Further studies are underway in Asia to look into these various issues. It is at least somewhat reassuring that laser iridotomy was seen to be safe in this trial and appeared effective in preventing acute angle closure glaucoma. However, clearly regular screening for glaucoma in people at risk is warranted.

J. S. Myers, MD

Reversal of Retinal Ganglion Cell Dysfunction after Surgical Reduction of Intraocular Pressure

Sehi M, Grewal DS, Goodkin ML, et al (Univ of Miami Miller School of Medicine, FL)
Ophthalmology 117:2329-2336, 2010

Purpose.—The pattern electroretinogram optimized for glaucoma screening (PERGLA) is a noninvasive method of objectively measuring retinal ganglion cell (RGC) function. This study was undertaken to quantify the RGC response to intraocular pressure (IOP) reduction after glaucoma surgery.

Design.—Prospective cohort study.

Participants.—Forty-seven eyes of 47 patients with uncontrolled IOP or progressive glaucomatous optic neuropathy receiving maximal medical therapy requiring trabeculectomy or aqueous drainage device implantation who met eligibility criteria.

Methods.—Eyes with visual acuity less than 20/30, corneal or retinal pathologic features, or unreliable standard automated perimetry (SAP) results were excluded. All patients underwent complete ocular examination, arterial blood pressure, SAP, and PERGLA at 2 sessions before surgery and at 3 months after surgery. Mean ocular perfusion pressure (MOPP) was calculated. Each measure of PERGLA amplitude and phase was an average of 600 artifact-free signal registrations.

Main Outcome Measures.—Intraocular pressure and PERGLA amplitude and phase.

Results.—Forty-seven eyes of 47 patients (mean age ± standard deviation [SD], 69.9 ± 11.3 years) were enrolled. Thirty-four eyes (72%) underwent trabeculectomy with antifibrosis therapy; 13 eyes (28%) underwent glaucoma drainage implant surgery. Mean ± SD postoperative IOP (10.4 ± 4.6 mmHg) was significantly ($P<0.001$) reduced compared with that before surgery (19.7 ± 8.6 mmHg). Mean ± SD postoperative PERGLA amplitude (0.46 ± 0.22 μV) was significantly ($P = 0.001$) increased compared with preoperative PERGLA amplitude (0.37 ± 0.18 μV). Mean ± SD postoperative PERGLA phase (1.72 ± 0.20 π-radian) was significantly ($P = 0.01$) reduced compared with preoperative PERGLA phase (1.81 ± 0.22 π-radian). Mean ± SD postoperative MOPP (53.1 ± 6.4 mmHg) was significantly ($P<0.001$) increased compared with mean ± SD preoperative MOPP (45.8 ±

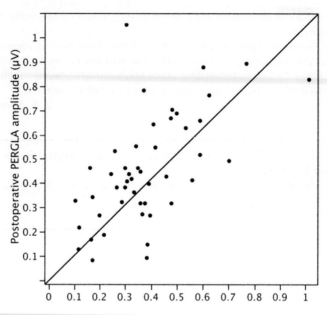

Preoperative PERGLA amplitude (μV)

FIGURE 3.—Scatterplot demonstrating the distribution of preoperative and postoperative amplitude values (μV) of pattern electroretinogram optimized for glaucoma screening (PERGLA). (Reprinted from Sehi M, Grewal DS, Goodkin ML, et al. Reversal of retinal ganglion cell dysfunction after surgical reduction of intraocular pressure. *Ophthalmology.* 2010;117:2329-2336, copyright © 2010, with permission from the American Academy of Ophthalmology.)

10.1 mmHg). No correlation (*P*>0.05) was identified between change in PERGLA amplitude and change in IOP or MOPP.

Conclusions.—Reversal of RGC dysfunction occurs after surgical reduction of IOP and may be quantified using PERGLA (Figs 3 and 6).

▶ The pattern electroretinogram optimized for glaucoma screening (PERGLA) is a mass response of the retina to flashes of light. The pattern is an alternating grid of on versus off squares, such that the total luminance is constant. This approach is thought to select for the signal from the retinal ganglion cell. PERGLA amplitudes have been shown to be reduced in glaucoma.

In this study, PERGLA parameters were improved 3 months after the surgical reduction of intraocular pressure. More patients showed improvement than reduction in PERGLA amplitude, and the overall change was statistically significant. Although the variability of PERGLA measures makes it possible that this could be a chance finding, that looks very unlikely.

Other studies have shown improved visual fields and other measures after intraocular pressure reduction, so it is conceivable that these findings could be real. Reduced pressure, through improved axoplasmic flow, blood flow, or other mechanisms, could be aiding the function of viable but distressed retinal ganglion cells.

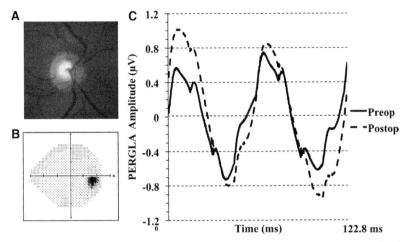

FIGURE 6.—The case of the right eye of a patient with ocular hypertension who underwent trabeculectomy for uncontrolled intraocular pressure. This patient had a central retinal vein occlusion in association with elevated intraocular pressure (IOP) in the fellow eye. A, Fundus photograph showing a normal optic disc. B, Standard automated perimetry results. In this patient, the mean IOP was reduced from 26 to 11 mmHg after surgery, the number of medications was reduced from 4 to 0, and (C) the average amplitude of pattern electroretinogram optimized for glaucoma screening (PERGLA) increased from 0.6 to 0.9 μV. Preop = before surgery; postop = after surgery. (Reprinted from Sehi M, Grewal DS, Goodkin ML, et al. Reversal of retinal ganglion cell dysfunction after surgical reduction of intraocular pressure. *Ophthalmology*. 2010;117:2329-2336, copyright © 2010, with permission from the American Academy of Ophthalmology.)

As research in glaucoma, like other neurodegenerative diseases, continues to seek neuroprotective modalities, the demonstration that there are reversibly affected ganglion cells, and the means to assess their function, is critical to the design of future studies on therapeutics.

J. S. Myers, MD

Structure—Function Relationships Using Spectral-Domain Optical Coherence Tomography: Comparison With Scanning Laser Polarimetry

Aptel F, Sayous R, Fortoul V, et al (Lyon 1 Univ, France)
Am J Ophthalmol 150:825-833, 2010

Purpose.—To evaluate and compare the regional relationships between visual field sensitivity and retinal nerve fiber layer (RNFL) thickness as measured by spectral-domain optical coherence tomography (OCT) and scanning laser polarimetry.

Design.—Prospective cross-sectional study.

Methods.—One hundred and twenty eyes of 120 patients (40 with healthy eyes, 40 with suspected glaucoma, and 40 with glaucoma) were tested on Cirrus-OCT, GDx VCC, and standard automated perimetry. Raw data on RNFL thickness were extracted for 256 peripapillary sectors of 1.40625 degrees each for the OCT measurement ellipse and 64 peripapillary sectors of 5.625 degrees each for the GDx VCC measurement ellipse. Correlations between peripapillary RNFL thickness in 6 sectors and visual field sensitivity in the 6 corresponding areas were evaluated using linear and logarithmic regression analysis. Receiver operating curve areas were calculated for each instrument.

Results.—With spectral-domain OCT, the correlations (r^2) between RNFL thickness and visual field sensitivity ranged from 0.082 (nasal RNFL and corresponding visual field area, linear regression) to 0.726 (supratemporal RNFL and corresponding visual field area, logarithmic regression). By comparison, with GDx-VCC, the correlations ranged from 0.062 (temporal RNFL and corresponding visual field area, linear regression) to 0.362 (supratemporal RNFL and corresponding visual field area, logarithmic regression). In pairwise comparisons, these structure—function correlations were generally stronger with spectral-domain OCT than with GDx VCC and with logarithmic regression than with linear regression. The largest areas under the receiver operating curve were seen for OCT superior thickness (0.963 ± 0.022; $P < .001$) in eyes with glaucoma and for OCT average thickness (0.888 ± 0.072; $P < .001$) in eyes with suspected glaucoma.

Conclusions.—The structure—function relationship was significantly stronger with spectral-domain OCT than with scanning laser polarimetry, and was better expressed logarithmically than linearly. Measurements with these 2 instruments should not be considered to be interchangeable (Figs 2 and 3).

▶ The structure-function relationship in glaucoma has long been appreciated. As every resident is taught, if the pattern of field loss does not correspond to changes on the optic nerve head, then a diagnosis other than glaucoma must be considered.

However, this relationship is far from simple. There is a huge variability in optic nerve head appearance and structure, and visual field loss is a complex phenomenon graded on a logarithmic scale. For this and other reasons, many nerves show advanced glaucomatous cupping before significant field loss, and other nerves, especially small nerves, may show relatively little glaucomatous change and have associated field loss.

There had been hope that nerve fiber layer thickness would prove to be more directly correlated with visual field loss, as it is less influenced by optic nerve head structure. However, research over the last decade has shown that there is significant variability in these measures as well at any given level of field damage. The newer spectral domain optical coherence tomography (OCT) had brought hope of better correlations with their greater data density and detail.

This report is notable for several reasons. First, it shows that nerve fiber layer thickness as measured by spectral domain OCT is not directly comparable to that measured by scanning laser polarimetry (GDx). This is not a surprise, as they are different technologies, and other reports have shown that different spectral domain OCTs do not fully match on nerve fiber layer measurements.

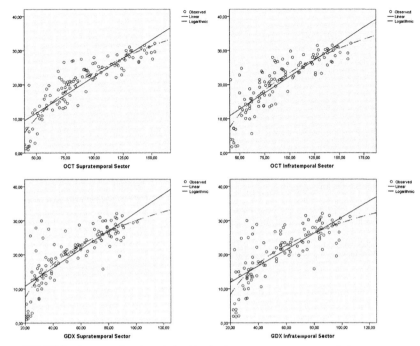

FIGURE 2.—Structure–function relationships in glaucomatous eyes, suspected glaucomatous eyes, and healthy eyes, as assessed using spectral-domain optical coherence tomography and scanning laser polarimetry. Scatter plots showing the relationships between visual field sensitivity (dB) and retinal nerve fiber layer thickness, as assessed by (Top left and Top right) Cirrus optical coherence tomography or (Bottom left and Bottom right) scanning laser polarimetry (GDx VCC). Measurements were made in the supratemporal and infratemporal peripapillary sectors, with linear and logarithmic fits. (Reprinted from Aptel F, Sayous R, Fortoul V, et al. Structure-function relationships using spectral-domain optical coherence tomography: comparison with scanning laser polarimetry. *Am J Ophthalmol.* 2010;150: 825-833, copyright 2010, with permission from Elsevier.)

In this report, the correlation of spectral domain OCT to field loss was slightly better than that for GDx, so some progress has been made. However, the correlation was generally limited, although statistically robust. From a clinical perspective, these machines will clearly suffer many of the same limitations for the discrimination of glaucoma from normal eyes that the last generation of machines suffered.

It is worth noting that the limitations of visual field testing also are likely part of the difficulty. The 24-2 perimetry pattern is not based on anatomic relationships: central test points represent much greater numbers of nerve fiber layer cells, and the scale is logarithmic (note that the best fit in this study was also logarithmic). Even without the issues surrounding subjective versus objective tests, there are plenty of factors that limit direct correlations between structure and this imperfect functional test. Other test patterns, with greater central versus peripheral test locations, are now favored by perimetry researchers but are infrequently used clinically.

There is continued hope that improved algorithms will be developed to analyze the very dense data that spectral domain OCTs collect and that this

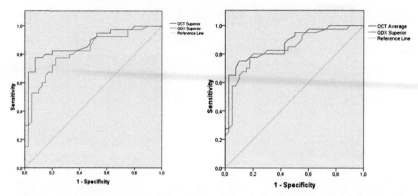

FIGURE 3.—Receiver operating curves illustrating the abilities of Cirrus optical coherence tomography and scanning laser polarimetry to distinguish (Left) glaucomatous or (Right) suspected glaucomatous eyes from healthy eyes. Receiver operating curves for the best parameters from each instrument are shown. (Reprinted from Aptel F, Sayous R, Fortoul V, et al. Structure-function relationships using spectral-domain optical coherence tomography: comparison with scanning laser polarimetry. *Am J Ophthalmol.* 2010;150:825-833, copyright 2010, with permission from Elsevier.)

will lead to progress in clinical use. It appears that this will be a gradual process, and spectral domain OCT has not yet provided a quantum leap in clinical management of glaucoma.

J. S. Myers, MD

The Relationship between Intraocular Pressure Reduction and Rates of Progressive Visual Field Loss in Eyes with Optic Disc Hemorrhage

Medeiros FA, Alencar LM, Sample PA, et al (Univ of California, San Diego; et al)
Ophthalmology 117:2061-2066, 2010

Purpose.—To evaluate rates of visual field progression in eyes with optic disc hemorrhages and the effect of intraocular pressure (IOP) reduction on these rates.

Design.—Observational cohort study.

Participants.—The study included 510 eyes of 348 patients with glaucoma who were recruited from the Diagnostic Innovations in Glaucoma Study (DIGS) and followed for an average of 8.2 years.

Methods.—Eyes were followed annually with clinical examination, standard automated perimetry visual fields, and optic disc stereophotographs. The presence of optic disc hemorrhages was determined on the basis of masked evaluation of optic disc stereophotographs. Evaluation of rates of visual field change during follow-up was performed using the visual field index (VFI).

Main Outcome Measures.—The evaluation of the effect of optic disc hemorrhages on rates of visual field progression was performed using

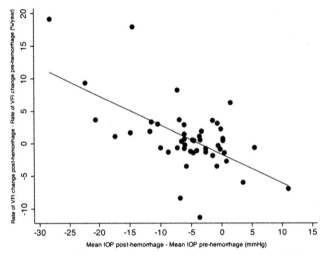

FIGURE 3.—Scatterplot of the relationship between change in the rate of visual field loss progression as measured by the VFI before and after hemorrhage and change in mean IOP levels. IOP = intraocular pressure; VFI = visual field index. (Reprinted from Medeiros FA, Alencar LM, Sample PA, et al. The relationship between intraocular pressure reduction and rates of progressive visual field loss in eyes with optic disc hemorrhage. *Ophthalmology.* 2010;117:2061-2066, copyright © 2010, with permission from the American Academy of Ophthalmology.)

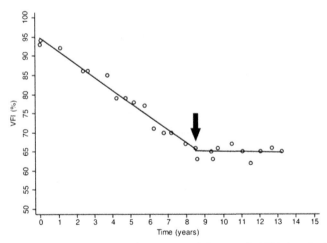

FIGURE 4.—Example of an eye that had a steep rate of change in the VFI before disc hemorrhage (−3.41%/year) with a mean IOP level of 18.6 mmHg. The mean IOP level was substantially decreased to 11.7 mmHg (37% reduction) after the episode of disc hemorrhage. Accordingly, the rate of visual field loss decreased to −0.07%/year after the episode of disc hemorrhage (*arrow*). VFI = visual field index. (Reprinted from Medeiros FA, Alencar LM, Sample PA, et al. The relationship between intraocular pressure reduction and rates of progressive visual field loss in eyes with optic disc hemorrhage. *Ophthalmology.* 2010;117:2061-2066, copyright © 2010, with permission from the American Academy of Ophthalmology.)

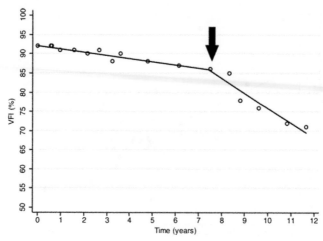

FIGURE 5.—Example of an eye that was progressing at a rate of VFI of −0.86%/year before disc hemorrhage. This rate increased to −4.13%/year after the episode of hemorrhage (*arrow*). The eye had no substantial change in mean IOP levels after the episode of hemorrhage compared with before hemorrhage (15.6 mmHg vs. 15.8 mmHg). VFI = visual field index. (Reprinted from Medeiros FA, Alencar LM, Sample PA, et al. The relationship between intraocular pressure reduction and rates of progressive visual field loss in eyes with optic disc hemorrhage. *Ophthalmology*. 2010;117:2061-2066, copyright © 2010, with permission from the American Academy of Ophthalmology.)

random coefficient models. Estimates of rates of change for individual eyes were obtained by best linear unbiased prediction (BLUP).

Results.—During follow-up, 97 (19%) of the eyes had at least 1 episode of disc hemorrhage. The overall rate of VFI change in eyes with hemorrhages was significantly faster than in eyes without hemorrhages (−0.88%/year vs. −0.38%/year, respectively, P<0.001). The difference in rates of visual field loss pre- and post-hemorrhage was significantly related to the reduction of IOP in the post-hemorrhage period compared with the pre-hemorrhage period (r = −0.61; P<0.001). Each 1 mmHg of IOP reduction was associated with a difference of 0.31%/year in the rate of VFI change.

Conclusions.—There was a beneficial effect of treatment in slowing rates of progressive visual field loss in eyes with optic disc hemorrhage. Further research should elucidate the reasons why some patients with hemorrhages respond well to IOP reduction and others seem to continue to progress despite a significant reduction in IOP levels. (Figs 3-5)

▶ The Ocular Hypertension Treatment Study, the Collaborative Normal Tension Glaucoma Study, the Canadian Glaucoma Study, and the Early Manifest Glaucoma Trial all reported increased progression of damage in eyes with disc hemorrhages. This large study also found that disc hemorrhages are associated with a greater rate of progression. In addition, further intraocular pressure (IOP) reduction following disc hemorrhage was associated with a reduced rate of progression.

In the Early Manifest Glaucoma Treatment Study, for every 1% of visits in which a disc hemorrhage was seen, the relative risk of progression went up 2%. This translates into a patient with 2 hemorrhages over 5 years at 3-month follow-up intervals going from a 20% risk of progression, for example, to a 24% risk. This is not a substantial increase.

In this study, however, using the Visual Field Index (VFI), the results were more striking. The VFI is a Humphrey visual field—based measure of visual function, similar to the mean deviation but placing more emphasis on central points, that ranges from 100% (normal) to 0% (vision completely lost on field testing). The rate of loss was more than twice as high in the disc hemorrhage group. Also, in subjects with further IOP reduction after hemorrhage, there were reduced rates of change.

This is a retrospective, nonrandomized study. It is possible that some of these results could be artifacts. However, the essential finding, that disc hemorrhages are associated with increased risk and may warrant increased intervention, is increasingly supported by experimental evidence.

J. S. Myers, MD

The Utility of the Monocular Trial: Data from the Ocular Hypertension Treatment Study

Bhorade AM, for the Ocular Hypertension Treatment Study Group (Washington Univ School of Medicine, St Louis, MO; et al)
Ophthalmology 117:2047-2054, 2010

Objective.—To determine whether adjusting the intraocular pressure (IOP) change of the trial eye for the IOP change of the fellow eye (i.e., monocular trial) is a better assessment of medication response than testing each eye independently.

Design.—Analysis of data from a prospective, randomized, clinical trial.

Participants.—Two hundred six participants with ocular hypertension randomized to the observation group and later started on a topical prostaglandin analog (PGA).

Methods.—Participants were started on a topical PGA in 1 eye and returned in approximately 1 month to determine medication response. The IOP response of the trial eye was determined by the IOP change between baseline and 1 month in the trial eye alone (unadjusted method) and by adjusting for the IOP change in the fellow eye between the same visits (adjusted method). Our "gold standard" for medication response was the IOP change in the trial eye between up to 3 pre- and 3 posttreatment visits on the same medication. Pearson correlation was used to compare the gold standard with the unadjusted and adjusted methods. In addition, symmetry of IOP response between trial and fellow eyes to the same medication was determined by correlating the trial eye IOP change between up to 3 pre- and 3 posttreatment visits to the fellow eye IOP change between the same visits.

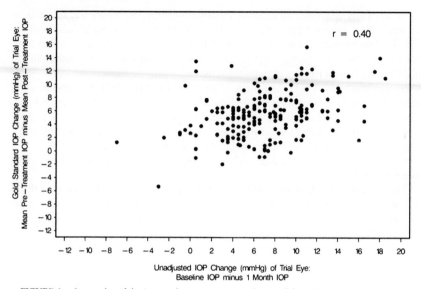

FIGURE 2.—Scatterplot of the intraocular pressure (IOP) change of the trial eye using the gold standard versus the unadjusted method. (Reprinted from Bhorade AM, for the Ocular Hypertension Treatment Study Group. The utility of the monocular trial: data from the ocular hypertension treatment study. *Ophthalmology.* 2010;117:2047-2054, copyright © 2010, with permission from the American Academy of Ophthalmology.)

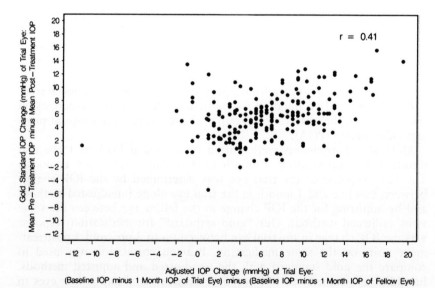

FIGURE 3.—Scatterplot of the intraocular pressure (IOP) change of the trial eye using the gold standard versus the adjusted method. (Reprinted from Bhorade AM, for the Ocular Hypertension Treatment Study Group. The utility of the monocular trial: data from the ocular hypertension treatment study. *Ophthalmology.* 2010;117:2047-2054, copyright © 2010, with permission from the American Academy of Ophthalmology.)

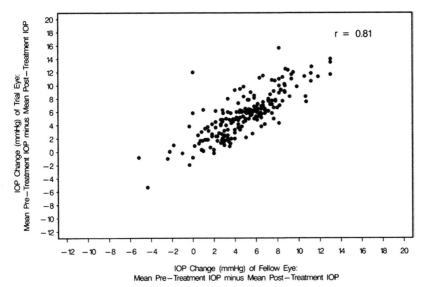

FIGURE 4.—Scatterplot of the intraocular pressure (IOP) change of trial and fellow eyes between up to 3 pre- and 3 posttreatment visits on the same topical prostaglandin analog medication. (Reprinted from Bhorade AM, for the Ocular Hypertension Treatment Study Group. The utility of the monocular trial: data from the ocular hypertension treatment study. *Ophthalmology.* 2010;117:2047-2054, copyright © 2010, with permission from the American Academy of Ophthalmology.)

Main Outcome Measures.—Correlations of IOP change of the trial eye using the gold standard to the IOP change of the trial eye using the unadjusted and adjusted methods.

Results.—The correlations of IOP change using the gold standard to the IOP change using the unadjusted and adjusted methods were $r = 0.40$ and $r = 0.41$, respectively. The correlation of IOP change of both eyes between the same pre- and posttreatment visits was $r = 0.81$.

Conclusions.—The monocular trial (i.e., adjusted method) appears equivalent to testing each eye independently (i.e., unadjusted method); however, neither method is adequate to determine medication response to topical PGAs. Both eyes have a similar IOP response to the same PGA. Further studies to understand IOP fluctuation are necessary to improve current methods of assessing medication response (Figs 2-4).

▶ The Ocular Hypertension Treatment Study has yielded a lot of useful science for treating physicians. This study examines carefully the monocular trial that used the contralateral eye to adjust for intervisit intraocular pressure fluctuations

This study finds that whether or not one adjusts for the fellow eye (monocular trial), there is little correlation between the prostaglandin pressure reduction as judged across 2 visits (immediately pretreatment and posttreatment) and the pressure reduction comparing 3 visits before and after the initiation of a prostaglandin. Both eyes had very similar responses to a single prostaglandin.

Although inconvenient for patients and clinicians, prolonged observation of intraocular pressure off and on new therapies appears to give a more accurate picture. Depending on the clinical situation, for example, if the current pressure is close to versus far from the target pressure, it may or may not be worthwhile to observe the pressure at additional visits before changing therapy.

J. S. Myers, MD

Trainee Glaucoma Surgery: Experience With Trabeculectomy and Glaucoma Drainage Devices
Connor MA, Knape RM, Oltmanns MH, et al (Univ of Florida College of Medicine, Gainesville)
Ophthalmic Surg Lasers Imaging 41:523-531, 2010

Background and Objective.—To examine outcomes of trabeculectomy with mitomycin C and glaucoma drainage device placement for uncontrolled glaucoma when performed by resident surgeons.

Patients and Methods.—This study included any patient who underwent a trabeculectomy with mitomycin C (n = 93) or a glaucoma drainage device (n = 60) by a resident surgeon between 2001 and 2006. Outcome measures at 3, 6, and 12 months included failure of treatment, number of follow-up appointments, complications, number of medications, and need for further surgery.

Results.—One year postoperatively, intraocular pressure averaged 12.1 ± 5.1 mm Hg in the trabeculectomy group and 13.0 ± 5.1 mm Hg in the glaucoma drainage device group (*P* = .31). Complications occurred in 30% of eyes with trabeculectomy and 10% of eyes with a glaucoma drainage device.

Conclusion.—During the first postoperative year, glaucoma drainage device surgery may have fewer complications and less morbidity than a trabeculectomy with mitomycin C when these surgeries are performed by resident surgeons. Final intraocular pressures were similar between the two groups.

▶ This retrospective study looks at tubes versus trabeculectomies performed by ophthalmology residents. The results are similar to those of the Tube versus Trab Study: similar intraocular pressure (IOP) at a year but fewer complications in the tube group.[1] Additionally, the tube group had fewer postoperative visits. It is important to note that the authors do not provide detailed information on prior surgical treatments in either group, so these results are not directly comparable to those of the Tube versus Trab Study.

Looking carefully at the baseline characteristics of the subjects enrolled, the trabeculectomy group had more favorable risk factors: more open-angle glaucoma, more whites, less diabetes. On the other hand, the baseline IOP was lower in the trabeculectomy group, which may have made the 20% IOP reduction success criterion more difficult to achieve in this group. Nonetheless, in resident hands, the trabeculectomy group had significant complications and greater failure for lack of IOP control or hypotony.

The role of tubes versus trabeculectomies in the management of glaucoma continues to evolve. However, experience affects surgical outcomes, and tubes may be simpler for the inexperienced surgeon. Additionally, as discussed in another section of this chapter, it is imperative that we train the next generation of surgeons in a manner that minimizes the burden to our patients.

J. S. Myers, MD

Reference

1. Gedde SJ, Schiffman JC, Feuer WJ, Herndon LW, Brandt JD, Budenz DL. Treatment outcomes in the tube versus trabeculectomy study after one year of follow-up. *Am J Ophthalmol.* 2007;143:9-22.

Videotaped Evaluation of Eyedrop Instillation in Glaucoma Patients with Visual Impairment or Moderate to Severe Visual Field Loss

Hennessy AL, Katz J, Covert D, et al (Glaucoma Specialists, Baltimore, MD; The Johns Hopkins Bloomberg School of Public Health, Baltimore, MD; Alcon Laboratories, Fort Worth, TX)
Ophthalmology 117:2345-2352, 2010

Purpose.—Objectively evaluate the ability of visually disabled glaucoma patients to successfully administer a single drop onto their eye.

Design.—Prospective, observational study.

Participants.—Experienced glaucoma patients with Early Treatment of Diabetic Retinopathy Study visual acuity (VA) of ≤6/18 (≤20/60) ≥1 eye, or moderate or severe visual field damage in ≥1 eye.

Methods.—Subjects were "low vision" (20/60 ≤VA <20/200) or "blind" (light perception <VA ≤20/200). They completed a survey about eyedrop use, and were video-recorded instilling 1 drop into their worst-seeing eye in their usual fashion, using a 5-ml bottle.

Main Outcome Measures.—Successful instillation of a single drop.

Results.—Of 204 glaucoma subjects (55% female; 74% Caucasian; 89% primary open-angle glaucoma; mean age, 68.8 ± 13.1 years), 192/204 (94%) used drops >6 months. Subjects used a mean of 1.9 ± 1.1 bottles of intraocular pressure-lowering medications to treat their glaucoma. Seventy-six percent (155/204) of subjects had severe visual field damage, with a mean deviation of −14.5 ± 8.0. Twenty-six percent (54/204) had acuity of ≤20/200 in ≥1 eye, and subjects had a mean logarithm of minimal angle of resolution acuity of 0.8 ± 0.9. Seventy-one percent of subjects were able to get a drop onto the eye; only 39% instilled 1 drop onto the eye without touching the ocular surface, instilling a mean 1.4 ± 1.0 drops, using 1.2 ± 0.6 attempts. Of the 142 subjects who denied touching the bottle to the ocular surface, 24% did touch the bottle to the eye. Multiple factors were tested for ability to predict successful application of an eyedrop; however, only age (<70 vs <70 years) was found to be a significant predictor for less successful instillation.

Conclusions.—In this video analysis of visually impaired glaucoma patients, we evaluated the difficulty this population has instilling eyedrops, most important, the use of multiple drops per instillation, potential contamination of a chronically used bottle, and poor patient understanding of the situation. Ability to self-administer eyedrops and cost considerations of wasted drops must be thought out before institution of glaucoma therapy. Efforts to determine better methods of eyedrop administration need to be undertaken.

▶ Adherence is the doses actually taken by a patient in a specific time period reported as a proportion of the doses prescribed during that period. Persistence refers to the accumulation of time from initiation to discontinuation of a therapy. These terms are common metrics for evaluating patient compliance with medical therapy. Numerous barriers exist to medication compliance, and shockingly, high rates of improper and inadequate medication use have been reported. Inability to effectively administer an eye drop may significantly affect adherence.

Glaucoma is often an asymptomatic disease. Therefore, motivation for medication compliance is dependent upon concern about the prospect of future vision loss. Intuitively, increased vision loss in patients with glaucoma should increase motivation and improve adherence as well as persistence. However, visual disability may also make drop administration more challenging. Interestingly, a recent study by Robin et al found serious problems with eye drop administration in a patient population with glaucoma with good visual status. In this study, Robin et al examine eye drop administration in patients with significant visual limitations.

Two hundred four patients were enrolled in this study. Subjects were all experienced in self-administration of eye drops and, on average, used multiple bottles of glaucoma eye drops daily. All subjects had visual acuity worse than 20/60 in 1 eye and/or met Hodapp-Parrish-Anderson criteria for moderate or severe visual field damage in 1 eye. While being video recorded, patients administered 1 artificial teardrop into their worse seeing eye. Subjects had access to a mirror and reclining chair and were allowed to perform the task in a manner consistent with their usual technique. A single investigator graded their performance by viewing the video.

The results of this study are impressive. Despite significant experience using eye drops, nearly one-third of subjects were unable to get a drop on the ocular surface, even with multiple attempts. Only half of subjects were able to hit the ocular surface on the first try. Only about one-third of subjects were able to hit the ocular surface without touching the bottle to the ocular surface. Furthermore, study subjects were either unaware or unwilling to admit that drop delivery is a problem. Eighty percent of subjects reported no difficulty instilling drops. Of the 36% of patients who report never missing a drop, 35% of them actually missed in the study. Twenty-four percent of people who denied touching ocular surface actually did touch it.

Decreased central vision and increased peripheral vision loss were not statistically significantly associated with successful drop administration. However, in light of the earlier study done by Robin et al on patients with relatively good vision, results from this study indicate that patients with visual impairment are less successful at drop administration.

Use of multiple attempts to hit the ocular surface in this group highlights a common complaint among patients with glaucoma. Pharmacy benefits often limit that amount of medication refills covered during a particular time interval. Patients who require multiple drops to hit the ocular surface may exhaust their supply of medicine before a new refill will be covered by their insurance. This problem adds to the financial burden of chronic glaucoma management.

It is possible the artificial circumstances in which subjects took their medicine during the study provoked performance anxiety or otherwise negatively affected their success with drop administration. However, this study population was highly experienced with self-administration of drops, and it's also possible that in the real world, there are many patients with less experience and even worse success administering drops.

This study demonstrates that poor adherence and persistence with glaucoma medications should not be underestimated.

J. S. Myers, MD

4 Cornea

Acupuncture for treating dry eye: a randomized placebo-controlled trial
Shin M-S, Kim J-I, Lee MS, et al (Korea Inst of Oriental Medicine, Daejeon; Kyung Hee Univ, Seoul, Korea; et al)
Acta Ophthalmol 88:e328-e333, 2010

Purpose.—To evaluate the efficacy and safety of acupuncture for ocular symptoms, tear film stability and tear secretion in dry eye patients.

Methods.—This is a randomized, patient-assessor blinded, sham acupuncture controlled trial. Forty-two participants with defined moderate to severe dry eye underwent acupuncture treatment three times a week for 3 weeks. Seventeen standard points (GV23; bilateral BL2, GB14, TE23, Ex1, ST1 and GB20; and unilateral SP3, LU9, LU10 and HT8 on the left for men and right for women) with '*de qi*' manipulation for the verum acupuncture group and seventeen sham points of shallow penetration without other manipulation for the sham group were applied during the acupuncture treatment. Differences were measured using the ocular surface disease index (OSDI), the visual analogue scale (VAS) of ocular discomfort, the tear film break-up time (BUT) and the Schimer I test with anaesthesia. In addition, adverse events were recorded.

Results.—There were no statistically significant differences between results on the OSDI, VAS, BUT or Schimer I tests from baseline between the verum and sham acupuncture groups. However, results from the within-group analysis showed that the OSDI and VAS in both groups and the BUT in the verum acupuncture group were significantly improved after 3 weeks of treatment. No adverse events were reported during this trial.

Conclusion.—Both types of acupuncture improved signs and symptoms in dry-eye patients after a 4-week treatment. However, verum acupuncture did not result in better outcomes than sham acupuncture.

▶ When I read the title of this article, I was immediately excited. Something new and different for dry eyes, which uses acupuncture, an increasingly accepted and sought-after Eastern therapy. Unfortunately, the findings were less hopeful than the title. In a randomized fairly controlled study of 42 participants with moderate to severe dry eye, there were no statistically significant differences in the ocular surface disease index, visual analogue scale, break-up time, or Schirmer tests from baseline between the acupuncture group and the sham group. Interestingly, there was a significant placebo effect of both treatments with improved signs and symptoms in both groups. This underscores what those of us who care for these patients observe: the real desire to be better. It also reinforces the need for any therapy to have a good control. There were a couple similar posters at this year's Association for Research in Vision and Ophthalmology meeting, demonstrating a lack of effectiveness of acupuncture on the tear film. We continue to search for the best way, through all philosophies, to treat these patients.

K. M. Hammersmith, MD
P. K. Nagra, MD

Comparison of Natamycin and Voriconazole for the Treatment of Fungal Keratitis

Prajna NV, Mascarenhas J, Krishnan T, et al (Aravind Eye Care System, Madurai, India; Aravind Eye Care System, Pondicherry, India; et al)
Arch Ophthalmol 128:672-678, 2010

Objective.—To conduct a therapeutic exploratory clinical trial comparing clinical outcomes of treatment with topical natamycin vs topical voriconazole for fungal keratitis.

Methods —The multicenter, double-masked, clinical trial included 120 patients with fungal keratitis at Aravind Eye Hospital in India who were randomized to receive either topical natamycin or topical voriconazole and either had repeated scraping of the epithelium or not.

Main Outcome Measures.—The primary outcome was best spectacle-corrected visual acuity (BSCVA) at 3 months. Other outcomes included scar size, perforations, and a subanalysis of BSCVA at 3 months in patients with an enrollment visual acuity of 20/40 to 20/400.

Results.—Compared with those who received natamycin, voriconazole-treated patients had an approximately 1-line improvement in BSCVA at 3 months after adjusting for scraping in a multivariate regression model but the difference was not statistically significant ($P=.29$). Scar size at 3 months was slightly greater with voriconazole after adjusting for scraping ($P=.48$). Corneal perforations in the voriconazole group (10 of 60 patients) were not significantly different than in the natamycin-treated group (9 of 60 patients) ($P>.99$). Scraping was associated with worse BSCVA at 3 months after adjusting for drug ($P=.06$). Patients with baseline BSCVA of 20/40 to 20/400 showed a trend toward a 2-line improvement in visual acuity with voriconazole ($P=.07$).

Conclusions.—Overall, there were no significant differences in visual acuity, scar size, and perforations between voriconazole- and natamycin-treated patients. There was a trend toward scraping being associated with worse outcomes.

Application to Clinical Practice.—The benefit seen with voriconazole in the subgroup of patients with baseline visual acuity of 20/40 to 20/400 needs to be validated in a confirmatory clinical trial.

Trial Registration.—clinicaltrials.gov Identifier: NCT00557362.

▶ Our experience with topical natamycin and voriconazole for the treatment of fungal keratitis has been very positive. The excellent oral bioavailability and broad spectrum of coverage make oral voriconazole a very attractive option in these difficult cases. However, the cost and availability remain major issues. This article, a combined effort from the Proctor Foundation and Aravind Eye Hospital, attempts to compare topical voriconazole and commercially available natamycin. Somewhat surprisingly, the overall findings had no significant differences in visual acuity, scar size, and perforations between these therapies. However, it is interesting to note that the subgroup of patients with baseline visual acuity of 20/40 to 20/400 appears to fare better with topical voriconazole. This certainly may be the group in which a significant difference can be detected. Those with better visual acuity likely have very small infections, which may be amenable to any topical antifungals. Those with worse baseline vision than 20/400 may be out of the range that topical medications can result in a cure and more likely to need a surgical intervention.

One fungal infection that may be resistant to voriconazole is Fusarium solani. This was reported at last year's Cornea Congress. In these cases, topical amphotericin, traditionally used for yeast organisms, may be a better alternative.

K. M. Hammersmith, MD

P. K. Nagra, MD

Corneal Regrafting After Endothelial Keratoplasty

Li JY, Wilhelmus KR (Devers Eye Inst, Portland, OR; Lions Eye Bank of Texas at Baylor College of Medicine, Houston)
Cornea 30:556-560, 2011

Purpose.—To determine the incidence of corneal regrafting after endothelial keratoplasty (EK) and to explore the possible reasons for repeat EK and subsequent penetrating keratoplasty (PK).

Methods.—This retrospective cohort study examined the occurrence of corneal regrafts among 803 eyes of 751 patients who underwent initial EK from January 2004 through February 2009 using donor corneas distributed by a single eye bank. Regression models and life tables evaluated the effects of donor corneal characteristics on the probability of a regraft.

Results.—Corneal regrafting after EK occurred in 119 eyes (15%), including 68 with repeat EK and 51 with subsequent PK. Ninety-five regrafts (80%) occurred within 1 year of EK, with 39 (33%) during the first postoperative month. Three years after EK, the cumulative probability of repeat EK was 11% and was 9% for subsequent PK. The secular trend in regrafting indicated an average 4% decline per year from 2005 to 2008. The odds of regrafting occurred less often ($P = 0.004$) with 202 eye bank-processed corneas than with 601 surgeon-prepared tissues. The cumulative probability of repeat EK was increased if donor corneas were maintained in preservation medium for more than 7 days ($P = 0.02$). Older donor age, death-to-preservation interval, or lower endothelial density was not significantly associated with repeat keratoplasty.

Conclusions.—Regrafting after EK is becoming less common, possibly because of surgical experience and technical innovations such as eye bank processing of precut tissues. Timely screening and distribution of donor corneas may foster graft survival.

▶ While endothelial keratoplasty (EK) has revolutionized corneal transplantation, the risk of early dislocation remains a troubling issue. The article, focusing on eye bank data, evaluates donor characteristics in patients who require regrafting following EK. Not surprisingly, the risk of regrafting decreased over the 5-year course of the study. Overall, 14.8% of eyes required regrafting, with 23% of EK requiring regrafts in 2004, dropping to 11% in 2008, the last full year of the study. Donor corneas with a preservation-to-surgery time of 1 to 7 days had lower rates of regrafting compared with 8 to 14 days, as did donor corneas removed from cadavers without refrigeration compared with refrigerated donors. Other factors, including death-to-preservation time, endothelial cell density, and donor age did not affect regraft rates. Interestingly, the authors found that eye bank—processed corneas were less likely to be associated with regrafts than surgeon-cut tissue. However, the center began using precut corneas in 2007, so these data are confounded by the fact that fewer regrafts overall were noted after 2007 compared with 2004 to 2007. Overall, this is an interesting study, highlighting high-risk characteristics for regraft, such as longer surgery-to-preservation time and refrigerated donors, but illustrating a lower regraft rate over time, as proficiency with this relatively new procedure increases.

K. M. Hammersmith, MD

P. K. Nagra, MD

Indications and Outcomes of Deep Anterior Lamellar Keratoplasty in Children

Harding SA, Nischal KK, Upponi-Patil A, et al (Great Ormond St Hosp for Children, London, UK)
Ophthalmology 117:2191-2195, 2010

Purpose.—To report our experience of deep anterior lamellar keratoplasty (DALK) in children.

Design.—Retrospective case note review.

Participants.—Nine patients (13 eyes) aged from 13 weeks to 14 years, 11 months at the Clinical and Academic Department of Ophthalmology, Great Ormond Street Hospital for Children National Health Service (NHS) Trust, London, United Kingdom.

Methods.—A study of all pediatric patients undergoing DALK from February 2002 to October 2008 was undertaken. Deep anterior lamellar keratoplasty was attempted in 9 children (13 eyes); the procedure was successful in

11 eyes, and 2 eyes progressed to penetrating keratoplasty (PKP). One eye underwent repeat DALK. Preoperative examination included electrophysiology, ultrasound biomicroscopy (UBM), and slit-lamp biomicroscopy.

Main Outcome Measures.—Complications and visual acuity at last follow-up.

Results.—Five patients had mucopolysaccharidoses (MPS), 3 patients had scarring presumed to be infectious, and 1 patient had keratoconus. Because of the failure of follow-up and loose sutures, 1 child with MPS had an epithelial rejection and the operation was repeated successfully. All grafts showed good graft clarity 10 to 80 months after grafting with visual acuities ranging from 0.28 to 1.0 logarithm of the minimum angle of resolution. Two children with nonspecific causes of scarring showed good visual acuities 24 to 51 months post-DALK. Two children who had conversion to PKP were lost to follow-up because they had moved abroad. In 4 of the 5 children with MPS, established techniques of DALK could not be performed because of excessive glycosaminoglycans (GAGs) in the stroma. Ultrasound biomicroscopy was used to guide trephination depth in the first instance. In 1 child with MPS, viscodissection was successfully used. All clinically diagnosed scars were histologically confirmed, and electron microscopy of corneal buttons confirmed the diagnosis in patients with MPS.

Conclusions.—Deep anterior lamellar keratoplasty should be considered in children with MPS and partial-thickness scars. In MPS, viscodissection and the "big bubble" technique may not be useful if there are excessive GAGs in the stroma.

▶ Improved deep anterior lamellar keratoplasty (DALK) techniques, such as big bubble technique, have led to a resurgence in anterior lamellar procedures over the past few years. In part, this may be because of the well-recognized benefits of DALK over penetrating keratoplasty, including decreased risk of rejection and no open-sky time, making it a safer surgery, although technically more demanding. This procedure is especially compelling in children, specifically because of the lifelong risks of rejection, recurrence of pathology and need for repeat surgery, compliance with medications, and risk of trauma and possible dehiscence. This retrospective analysis begins to give us insight into the use of DALK in this patient population. Although the study was small, with 11 eyes undergoing successful surgery, the authors found encouraging results, although limited vision most likely related to amblyopia. They found the standard big bubble technique was not applicable in most cases of mucopolysaccharidoses given the corneal opacification, but viscodissection was successful. Interestingly, the authors also found that patients were still at risk for stromal and epithelial rejection and stressed the importance of prophylactic use of steroids for prevention of rejection in DALK. While the study did not have any cases of trauma and dehiscence, we have had patients with DALK sustain trauma and have significant dehiscences involving rupture of their previously intact Descemet's membrane. While theoretically, having an intact Descemet's may provide some structural integrity to the eye, our experience suggests that this is not the case. Overall, however, based on the results of this article, DALK appears to be well tolerated in the pediatric population with good results.

K. M. Hammersmith, MD
P. K. Nagra, MD

Infectious Crystalline Keratopathy Treated With Intrastromal Antibiotics
Khan IJ, Hamada S, Rauz S (Univ of Birmingham, UK)
Cornea 29:1186-1188, 2010

An 84-year-old white female with nonprogressive conjunctival scarring developed infectious crystalline keratopathy (ICK) recalcitrant to topical therapy. After determination of the causative organism's antibiotic sensitivities, superficial keratectomy was performed with intrastromal corneal infiltration of cefuroxime into the affected cornea. Postoperatively, the ICK resolved completely, leading to an improvement in visual acuity and a reduction in ocular irritation. This case highlights the importance of a surgical approach in ICK and also demonstrates the possible benefit of a novel use of intracorneal antibiotics as an adjunct.

▶ Infectious crystalline keratopathy is often very difficult to treat. While, fortunately, it tends to be indolent and slowly progressive, getting antibiotics to penetrate through often-uninvolved anterior stroma and biofilm is very challenging. As the authors point out, the mediocre success with medical treatment may lead to surgical management with penetrating keratoplasty. The authors present a novel way to administer antibiotics to the corneal stroma. Similar to hydrating a cataract wound, they hydrate the stroma in the area of the infection with antibiotics. They achieved an excellent response to their treatment, with resolution of the ulcer and excellent uncorrected vision.

Definitive conclusions based on individual case reports are limited at best. However, this novel approach to antibiotic administration in the setting of infectious crystalline keratitis does warrant additional review.

K. M. Hammersmith, MD
P. K. Nagra, MD

Keratoconus and Normal-Tension Glaucoma: A Study of the Possible Association With Abnormal Biomechanical Properties as Measured by Corneal Hysteresis
Cohen EJ, Myers JS (Thomas Jefferson Univ, Philadelphia, PA)
Cornea 29:955-970, 2010

Purpose.—To test the hypothesis that patients with keratoconus and pellucid who have glaucoma or are glaucoma suspects have lower corneal hysteresis (CH) and/or corneal resistance factor (CRF) measurements compared with controls.

Methods.—A prospective study at a tertiary eye center of patients with keratoconus and pellucid, with glaucoma or suspect glaucoma and age-matched keratoconus and pellucid controls, was performed. After informed consent was obtained, corneal topography, ocular response analyzer (ORA; Reicher, Buffalo, NY), pachymetry, intraocular pressure, A scan measurements, Humphrey visual fields (VFs), and disk photographs were done. Analyses compared cases with controls on primary (CH and CRF) and secondary variables. Disk photographs and VFs were rated in a masked fashion.

Results.—The mean CH [8.2 (SD = 1.6) and 8.3 (SD = 1.5)] and CRF [7.3 (SD = 2.0) and 6.9 (SD = 2.1)] were low and did not differ significantly between 20 study (29 eyes) and 40 control patients (61 eyes), respectively. CH had a negative significant correlation with maximum corneal curvature by topography ($P < 0.002$) and positive significant correlation with central corneal thickness ($P < 0.003$). The mean cup to disk ratio was larger (0.54, SD = 0.20) among cases than in controls (0.38, SD = 0.20), $P = 0.003$. VFs were suspicious for glaucoma more often among the study eyes (11 of 29, 33.9%) than controls (8 of 60, 13.3%), $P = 0.019$.

Conclusions.—CH was low in study and control patients and was correlated with severity of keratoconus/pellucid but not with glaucoma/glaucoma suspect or control status. Evidence of glaucoma was more common in study eyes than in controls but was present in both.

▶ The diagnosis of glaucoma can be challenging in the setting of corneal diseases, which may alter intraocular pressure measurements (related to scars, thin corneas, or corneal edema/thick corneas), view to the optic nerve, and performance on visual field testing because of decreased vision. This study focused on the diagnosis of glaucoma in the setting of keratoconus and pellucid marginal degeneration. The authors hypothesized that patients with these ectatic corneal conditions have abnormal scleral rigidity, which may be related to the development of normal-tension glaucoma. Because of the difficulty assessing for and evaluating glaucoma with conventional methods, such as tonometry, visual field testing, and optic nerve evaluation, they evaluated whether a noninvasive noncontact method, the ocular response analyzer, used to measure corneal hysteresis (CH) and corneal resistance factor, may be helpful in these patients. While the study results suggested that CH was associated with the severity of ectasia, there was no association between CH and glaucoma. However, this study highlights the association between keratoconus/pellucid and normal-tension glaucoma, suggesting clinicians keep a high index of suspicion for this condition when evaluating patients with cornea ectatic disorders. Further, in spite of the difficulty in evaluating glaucoma, the authors found visual fields to be reliable, confirming this as an important tool for these patients, one that we should have a low threshold for performing.

K. M. Hammersmith, MD

P. K. Nagra, MD

Long-term Results of Riboflavin Ultraviolet A Corneal Collagen Cross-linking for Keratoconus in Italy: The Siena Eye Cross Study
Caporossi A, Mazzotta C, Baiocchi S, et al (Siena Univ, Italy; et al)
Am J Ophthalmol 149:585-593, 2010

Purpose.—To report the long-term results of 44 keratoconic eyes treated by combined riboflavin ultraviolet A collagen cross-linking in the first Italian open, nonrandomized phase II clinical trial, the Siena Eye Cross Study.

Design.—Perspective, nonrandomized, open trial.

Methods.—After Siena University Institutional Review Board approval, from September 2004 through September 2008, 363 eyes with progressive keratoconus were treated with riboflavin ultraviolet A collagen cross-linking. Forty-four eyes with a minimum follow-up of 48 months (mean, 52.4 months; range, 48 to 60 months) were evaluated before and after surgery. Examinations comprised uncorrected visual acuity, best spectacle-corrected visual acuity, spherical spectacle-corrected visual acuity, endothelial cells count (I Konan, Non Con Robo; Konan Medical, Inc., Hyogo, Japan), optical (Visante OCT; Zeiss, Jena, Germany) and ultrasound (DGH; Pachette, Exton, Pennsylvania, USA) pachymetry, corneal topography and surface aberrometry (CSO EyeTop, Florence, Italy), tomography (Orbscan IIz; Bausch & Lomb Inc., Rochester, New York, USA), posterior segment optical coherence tomography (Stratus OCT; Zeiss, Jena, Germany), and in vivo confocal microscopy (HRT II; Heidelberg Engineering, Rostock, Germany).

Results.—Keratoconus stability was detected in 44 eyes after 48 months of minimum follow-up; fellow eyes showed a mean progression of 1.5 diopters in more than 65% after 24 months, then were treated. The mean K value was reduced by a mean of 2 diopters, and coma aberration reduction with corneal symmetry improvement was observed in more than 85%. The mean best spectacle-corrected visual acuity improved by 1.9 Snellen lines, and the uncorrected visual acuity improved by 2.7 Snellen lines.

Conclusions.—The results of the Siena Eye Cross Study showed a long-term stability of keratoconus after cross-linking without relevant side effects. The uncorrected visual acuity and best spectacle-corrected visual acuity improvements were supported by clinical, topographic, and wavefront modifications induced by the treatment.

▶ Collagen cross-linking is an exciting potential treatment for keratoconus. Unlike all other treatments for this condition, cross-linking works to strengthen the cornea to induce and maintain stability for this condition and potentially reverse corneal steepening/ectasia. Unfortunately, most of us in the United States have limited to no experience with this treatment, and we look to our colleagues elsewhere for insight.

The authors present a prospective study of 44 patients with progressive keratoconus who underwent ultraviolet A collagen cross-linking and were followed for at least 48 months.

They demonstrated improvements in uncorrected and best corrected visual acuity, reduction in sphere and spherical equivalents, as well as mean keratometry readings. Further, no adverse events or significant side effects were noted. The authors also present guidelines for whom they recommend this treatment, specifically patients younger than 26 years with evidence of keratoconus progression, patients older than 26 years with documented evidence of progression, and any patient with contact lens intolerance. The focus of treatment in the first 2 groups is to stabilize the cornea, similar to the patients in this study. The last group with stabilization may benefit from the procedure with improved visual acuity, but the authors feel less confident regarding definite success in this group and recommend preparing patients for unpredictable or unsuccessful outcomes.

As we continue to see patients inquiring about this procedure and hopefully start to gain more firsthand experience with this treatment, this study may prove helpful in counseling patients regarding possible outcomes and benefits.

K. M. Hammersmith, MD
P. K. Nagra, MD

Optical Coherence Tomography for Corneal Diseases
Maeda N (Osaka Univ Graduate School of Medicine, Japan)
Eye Contact Lens 36:254-259, 2010

Anterior segment optical coherence tomography (OCT) is currently used for investigating the distribution of the corneal thickness, shape of the stromal interface after lamellar corneal surgery, association between host and corneal graft in keratoplasty, dimension of the anterior chamber, and lesions of the corneal diseases. In addition, the advances of OCT technology has enabled three-dimensional imaging, tissue imaging, cell imaging, and topographic analysis. In this review, examples of tissue imaging with 840-nm spectral-domain OCT, cell imaging with full-field OCT, and corneal topographic analysis with 1,310-nm swept-source OCT were introduced.

▶ The introduction of optical coherence tomography (OCT) of the cornea and anterior segment presents exciting potential for various applications for corneal and glaucoma specialists, anterior segment surgeons, and comprehensive ophthalmologists, but requires evaluation and testing to determine how to best use this potential. As we gain familiarity with this technology and the information it can provide, we can improve our visualization and knowledge of the cornea and anterior segment and hopefully provide better patient care as a result. This review article compares different modalities of OCT (time domain, spectrum domain, swept source, and full field) and presents examples of 3-dimensional imaging, tissue and cell imaging, and topographic analysis. Most impressive is the full-field OCT, with very high image resolution (2.0-2.4 μm), providing topographic and pachymetric evaluation of a Scheimpflug-based topographer, as well as the visualization of the cornea similar to confocal microscopy and specular microscopy. The author clearly demonstrates the remarkable advances in imaging quality and how this single instrument certainly shows great promise for clinical applications now and in the future.

K. M. Hammersmith, MD

P. K. Nagra, MD

Permanent Keratoprosthesis Combined With Pars Plana Vitrectomy and Silicone Oil Injection for Visual Rehabilitation of Chronic Hypotony and Corneal Opacity

Utine CA, Gehlbach PL, Zimmer-Galler I, et al (The Johns Hopkins Univ School of Medicine, Baltimore, MD)

Cornea 29:1401-1405, 2010

Purpose.—To present outcomes of combined pars plana vitrectomy, silicone oil (SO) injection, and permanent keratoprosthesis (Kpro) procedure in prephthisical eyes.

Methods.—All 3 patients were monocular with chronic severe hypotony, aphakia, and total corneal opacity in their vital eye. Preoperative visual acuity ranged from light perception to counting fingers at 1 foot. Two patients had a history of failed corneal grafts because of SO, and one had funnel retinal detachment. Pars plana vitrectomy and long-term SO tamponade were performed, and a permanent Boston type 1 Kpro was used in lieu of a donor corneal transplantation.

Results.—No unexpected intraoperative complications were encountered. Patients were followed for a period of 11—13 months. All patients had anatomic success with an attached retina and a clear visual axis. The procedures resulted in increased visual function in all patients ranging from hand motions to 20/800. No case has progressed to phthisis bulbi during the follow-up period. At the last visit, biomicroscopic examination revealed clear Kpro with an attached retina.

Conclusions.—Boston type 1 Kpro implantation, as the primary corneal procedure with pars plana vitrectomy and intraocular SO, may be a viable option in selected patients with prephthisical eyes.

▶ This article gives a glimmer of hope to patients with chronic hypotony and failed corneas. Dealing with this group of patients is very depressing, as we have had nothing to offer. Dr Dohlman and colleagues have had poor experiences in the past with the Boston keratoprosthesis and silicone oil, based on the development of severe retroprosthetic membranes and inflammation. However, the group from Wilmer presents on a few patients who were able to recover ambulatory vision. Encouraged by this experience, I performed a similar surgery in a young woman last month. The surgery was quite difficult because the eye was so small, barely accommodating the pediatric-size back plate. The patient has been ecstatic with her visual recovery (20/400), but I remain guarded about the future, given the short follow-up and mixed literature. The latest iteration of the Boston keratoprosthesis may involve a titanium back plate, which has been shown to have fewer retroprosthetic membranes.[1] This may be especially beneficial in these "Hail Mary" cases.

K. M. Hammersmith, MD

P. K. Nagra, MD

Reference

1. Todani A, Ciolino JB, Ament JD, et al. Titanium back plate for a PMMA keratoprosthesis: clinical outcomes. *Graefes Arch Clin Exp Ophthalmol.* 2011 Apr 26 [Epub ahead of print].

Prevalence and Features of Keratitis with Quantitative Polymerase Chain Reaction Positive for Cytomegalovirus
Kandori M, Inoue T, Takamatsu F, et al (Osaka Univ Med School, Suita, Japan)
Ophthalmology 117:216-222, 2010

Purpose.—To assess corneal scrapings and aqueous humor samples analyzed by polymerase chain reaction (PCR) that were positive for cytomegalovirus (CMV) in patients with keratitis of unknown origin and to investigate their clinical manifestations.

Design.—Retrospective, interventional case series.

Participants.—Seventy-eight patients with epithelial (n = 37), stromal (n = 12), or endothelial keratitis (n = 29) of unknown origin examined at the Osaka University Medical Hospital.

Methods.—Clinical examination and tears, corneal scrapings, and aqueous humor specimens were evaluated by real-time PCR for CMV.

Main Outcome Measures.—Quantification of CMV DNA at the diagnosis of each type of keratitis with unknown origin and monitoring during the therapeutic course for CMV-positive cases.

Results.—No cases of epithelial or stromal keratitis had CMV DNA. Seven of 29 corneal endotheliitis cases (24.1%) were positive for CMV. Cytomegalovirus-positive cases of corneal endotheliitis characterized by localized corneal edema and keratic precipitates included 4 patients who had undergone penetrating keratoplasty and were refractory to the treatment for graft rejection and 3 patients with idiopathic endotheliitis. Cytomegalovirus DNA copy numbers were estimated and ranged from 6.3×10^4 to 3.6×10^6/ml. In all positive cases, the numbers of CMV DNA copies decreased within weeks during treatment with systemic and topical ganciclovir (GCV) combined with a topical steroid. Five eyes (62.5%) had clinical improvement. In cases of endothelial keratitis, diabetes mellitus was significantly higher in patients positive for CMV (71.4%) than in patients negative for CMV (18.2%, $P=0.016$, chi-square test).

Conclusions.—A total of 24.1% of cases with corneal edema of unknown origin were CMV positive and should be included in the differential diagnosis of idiopathic corneal endotheliitis or graft edema after penetrating keratoplasty, especially for bullous keratopathy. Real-time

PCR for CMV, based on the diagnosis and monitoring of the clinical course, may be useful. Cytomegalovirus corneal endotheliitis requires early appropriate treatment using GCV. Because clinical remission after GCV may depend on the area of normal endothelium, early diagnosis and therapy are important for CMV corneal endotheliitis.

▶ Cytomegalovirus (CMV) is well known to cause chorioretinitis in the immunocompromised patient. However, there is a growing body of evidence that CMV may be an important pathogen in causing anterior uveitis and endotheliitis in immunocompetent patients. This article looks at patients with keratitis of unknown cause (a frustrating group) and analyzes for the prevalence of CMV by polymerase chain reaction. This is a very nice study, comparing CMV rates in an unaffected group (none detected) and in different forms of keratitis. The authors find that none of the cases of epithelial or stromal keratitis had CMV. However, nearly a quarter of patients with endotheliitis demonstrated CMV. These patients were treated with ganciclovir (mostly oral, some topical and oral) and steroids. The CMV copy numbers declined with treatment and many corneas cleared. Perhaps the most interesting finding is that a large number of the patients with CMV had coexisting diabetes, which begs the question, "Are these patients truly immunocompetent?" Unfortunately, anterior chamber paracentesis is not available to all or convenient for most. But this article certainly makes a case that we should consider CMV in the differential of unknown endotheliitis, especially in individuals with diabetes.

K. M. Hammersmith, MD

P. K. Nagra, MD

Subconjunctival bevacizumab for corneal neovascularization
Zaki AA, Farid SF (Res Inst of Ophthalmology, Giza, Egypt; Cairo Univ, Egypt)
Acta Ophthalmol 88:868-871, 2010

Purpose.—This work aimed to study and evaluate the effect of subconjunctival bevacizumab injection in patients with corneal neovascularization (CNV) resulting from different ocular surface disorders.

Methods.—Ten eyes with CNV caused by different ocular surface disorders were studied. All eyes had both major and minor vessel CNV caused by factors such as healed corneal ulcers, long-standing chronic inflammatory diseases and corneal ischaemia (caused by contact lenses). All eyes received a single subconjunctival injection of 2.5 mg (0.1 ml) bevacizumab. Morphological changes in the major and minor vessels were evaluated using slit-lamp biomicroscopy and corneal photography.

Results.—Conspicuous recession of the minor vessels of CNV was observed in all eyes at 2 weeks post-injection. The extent of CNV of the major vessels was significantly decreased at 2 weeks post-injection. The level of CNV continued to decrease noticeably for 3 months and then stabilized for the remainder of the 6-month follow-up period. Parameters used for evaluation included the total area of CNV, which amounted to 14.0 ± 5.4% of the corneal surface pre-injection, compared with 9.4 ± 3.9% post-injection (p < 0.01), reflecting a mean decrease in CNV of 33 ± 8%, and the extent of neovascularization, which decreased from 4.3 ± 1.5 clock hours pre-injection to 2.4 ± 1.1 clock hours post-injection (p < 0.01). During the 6-month follow-up, none of the 10 eyes showed any complication that could be related to subconjunctival bevacizumab injection.

Conclusions.—Bevacizumab can be used safely and effectively for CNV resulting from different ocular surface disorders. It represents an effective treatment for minor vessel neovascularization caused by long-standing chronic inflammation (e.g. trachoma) or long-standing corneal ischaemia (e.g. contact lenses), as well as for major vessel neovascularization resulting from different causes. Bevacizumab was well tolerated over the 6-month follow-up period.

▶ The early success of bevacizumab for age-related macular degeneration suggests exciting potential for applications to the cornea and anterior segment neovascularization. The authors of this prospective study looked at the effects of a single subconjunctival injection of 2.5 mg of bevacizumab and found improvement in both major and minor vessels (although the definition of major and minor vessels was not clear). Interestingly, they found that the effect from the single dose was still noted 6 months later, and the medication was well tolerated in their patients without significant side effects. Unfortunately, we have experienced significant side effects from topical, not subconjunctival, bevacizumab at Wills Eye Institute in the past few years, with 2 cases of extreme corneal thinning. Overall, this article adds to our current knowledge base, but additional studies are certainly necessary to help elucidate the most effective dose, when to repeat the medication, whether topical bevacizumab is as effective as subconjunctival injection, and the most responsive indications.

K. M. Hammersmith, MD

P. K. Nagra, MD

The Associations of Floppy Eyelid Syndrome: A Case Control Study

Ezra DG, Beaconsfield M, Sira M, et al (Moorfields Eye Hosp NHS Foundation Trust, London, UK; Western Eye Hosp, London, UK)
Ophthalmology 117:831-838, 2010

Objective.—To describe the demographic features of a large series of patients with floppy eyelid syndrome (FES) and to investigate the associations of the condition with keratoconus, obstructive sleep apnea hypopnea syndrome (OSAHS), and a variety of upper and lower eyelid features.

Design.—Case control study.

Participants.—The test group comprised 102 patients with FES. A control group of 102 patients were recruited from a diabetic retinopathy clinic and matched on a 1:1 basis on age, gender, and body mass index (BMI).

Methods.—A full medical and ophthalmic history was taken. Patients also underwent a full ocular examination, including an assessment of upper and lower lid laxity and upper lid levator function. Keratoconus grading was made using the Oculus Instruments Pentacam imaging system (Oculus Optikgerate GmbH, Wetzlar, Germany). Patients were screened for OSAHS using the Epworth daytime somnolence score. Matched statistical analysis of dichotomous data was made using Mantel–Haenszel methods for odds ratios and McNemar's test. Analysis of continuous data was performed using a matched t test and tests for symmetry of larger tables were made using the McNemar–Bowker test.

Main Outcome Measures.—The significance of association of FES with keratoconus, OSAHS, smoking history, medial and lateral canthal laxity of the upper and lower lids, levator function, lash ptosis, and dermatochalasis.

Results.—Significant associations were found between FES and OSAHS ($P = 0.0008$), keratoconus ($P<0.0001$), lash ptosis ($P<0.0001$), dermatochalasis ($P = 0.02$), upper lid medial canthal laxity ($P = 0.02$), upper lid distraction ($P = 0.001$), palpebral aperture ($P = 0.004$), and levator function ($P = 0.005$).

Conclusions.—Floppy eyelid syndrome seems to be a condition strongly associated with OSAHS and keratoconus. As well as providing a platform for an etiologic hypothesis for the condition, these findings should also encourage clinicians to be aware of these associations and to direct further treatment.

▶ As physicians, it is important to recognize associations between different conditions, such as the potential association between floppy eyelid syndrome (FES), obstructive sleep apnea-hypoxia syndrome (OSAHS), and keratoconus. While several studies have suggested this association, most series were small, and the strength of the association is unclear. Further, some have suggested that obesity is the common variable, and there is not a direct association between FES and OSAHS, including a recent study by Fowler and Dutton.[1]

The authors of this study evaluated the associations with FES in a case-control manner, with 102 patients in the test group and patients from a diabetic retinopathy clinic serving as a matched control group. Clinical features found associated with patients with FES included lash ptosis, medial canthal laxity, upper lid distraction, blepharoptosis, and reduction in levator function. Further, a strong association with keratoconus and OSAHS were found. Of note, the patients were corrected for weight, suggesting that factors other than obesity may be involved. Such an association is particularly important for the ophthalmologist, who may be the initial clinician to evaluate the patient. This recognition may improve the quality of care we provide to our patient, as we can affect their overall health by referring patients with floppy eyelid syndrome for a sleep study and treatment of OSAHS, a condition with potentially significant cerebrovascular morbidity.

K. M. Hammersmith, MD

P. K. Nagra, MD

Reference

1. Fowler AM, Dutton JJ. Floppy eyelid syndrome as a subset of lax eyelid conditions: relationships and clinical relevance (as ASOPRS thesis). *Ophthal Plast Reconstr Surg.* 2010;26:195-204.

The outcome of deep anterior lamellar keratoplasty in herpes simplex virus-related corneal scarring, complications and graft survival

Awan MA, Roberts F, Hegarty B, et al (Gartnavel General Hosp, Glasgow, UK; Western Infirmary, Glasgow, UK)

Br J Ophthalmol 94:1300-1303, 2010

Aims.—To determine the visual outcome, graft survival and complications after deep anterior lamellar keratoplasty (DALK) in patients with herpes simplex virus (HSV)-related corneal scarring.

Methods.—A retrospective analysis of the patients who had DALK for HSV-related corneal scarring between January 2004 and February 2007 was performed. Mean follow-up was 30 months (range 16—48 months). The statistical significance of host corneal vascularisation was determined using Fisher's exact test.

Results.—There were 18 eyes from 18 patients and the mean age was 57 years. Preoperative visual acuity ranged from hand movements (HM) to 6/12. Fifty per cent of the eyes achieved visual acuity of 6/12 or better postoperatively. Six eyes (33%) had recurrence of HSV-related inflammation, eight eyes (including four eyes with recurrence of HSV-related inflammation) developed graft rejection and four eyes (including two eyes with recurrence of HSV-related inflammation) had bacterial keratitis. The graft survival rate was 83%. Three eyes developed glaucoma and one eye required trabeculectomy. Immunohistochemistry revealed that HSV was focally positive or equivocal in four recipient corneal buttons, and transmission electron microscopy showed intracellular HSV virions in two of them.

Conclusions.—This is the largest series of DALK for herpetic corneal scarring that shows a comparable visual outcome and better graft survival rate than penetrating keratoplasty. There is significant risk of recurrence of HSV-related inflammation and graft rejection that requires timely recognition and adequate management.

▶ Penetrating keratoplasty in patients with herpes simplex virus (HSV) may present challenges postoperatively with healing, rejection, and reactivation of the virus. The authors evaluated deep anterior lamellar keratoplasty (DALK) as an alternative to full-thickness corneal transplantation as a treatment option in these patients with good results. They assessed 18 patients, making this the largest case series to date of DALK performed in patients with HSV, and found improved graft survival with DALK. However, compared with reported rates of rejection following DALK (between 0% and 10%), they found significantly more rejection in these patients with a history of HSV (33%). Furthermore, they remain at risk for recurrence of HSV, although they found a recurrence rate of only 5% in the first year, during which time patients remained on acyclovir, with most reported recurrences occurring the second year after acyclovir was discontinued. Interestingly, they were able to detect HSV by immunohistochemistry in 4 patients and transmission electron microscopy in 2 patients. Of importance, this study makes a case for long-term treatment with acyclovir after penetrating keratoplasty or DALK. Other studies have also shown a benefit of long-term anti-viral prophylaxis, beyond the first year, in preventing reactivation of HSV.[1,2]

With penetrating keratoplasty, the postoperative course for patients with HSV can be rocky with delayed healing, rejection, and HSV recurrence. While DALK does not eliminate or even greatly minimize any of these risks, the results suggest that it is a good procedure for these patients.

K. M. Hammersmith, MD

P. K. Nagra, MD

References

1. Goodfellow JF, Nabili S, Jones MN, et al. Antiviral treatment following penetrating keratoplasty for herpetic keratitis. *Eye (Lond)*. 2011 Jan 28 [Epub ahead of print].
2. Jansen AF, Rijneveld WJ, Remeijer L, et al. Five-year follow-up on the effect of oral acyclovir after penetrating keratoplasty for herpetic keratitis. *Cornea*. 2009; 28:843-845.

Treatment of Ocular Graft-Versus-Host Disease With Topical Cyclosporine 0.05%

Malta JB, Soong HK, Shtein RM, et al (Univ of Michigan Med School, Ann Arbor)

Cornea 29:1392-1396, 2010

Purpose.—To evaluate the efficacy of topical cyclosporine-A 0.05% (CsA) in the treatment of dry eye syndrome in ocular graft-versus-host disease after bone marrow transplantation (BMT) of hematopoietic stem cells.

Methods.—One-hundred five patients were enrolled in a retrospective, comparative, interventional case series. Eighty-one patients received topical CsA starting 1 month before BMT (treatment group), and 24 patients did not receive CsA until at least 6 months after the transplantation (control group). Mean follow-up time was 17.5 ± 11.0 months (range: 6.0–49.0 months). Clinical history, ocular surface disease index questionnaire, slit-lamp examination, lissamine green and fluorescein staining of the ocular surface, tear breakup time, and Schirmer test with topical anesthesia were obtained to create a composite dry eye-grading score.

Results.—Dry eye symptoms were significantly more severe in the control group at 3 months, 1 year, and 2 years ($P < 0.05$). There was no correlation with type of stem cell transplant (related vs. unrelated donor), presenting indication for BMT, or concurrent systemic immunosuppressive medications.

Conclusions.—Pre-BMT initiation of topical CsA may reduce the inflammatory response in the lacrimal glands that may be responsible for the development of post-BMT keratitis sicca.

▶ Dry eye syndrome in ocular graft-versus-host disease (GVHD) can be among the most challenging conditions we treat. Because dry eye symptoms often develop 6 months following bone marrow transplantation (BMT), there can be a delay in presentation and institution of treatment by the ophthalmologist. The authors of this study presented a retrospective case series comparing dry eye signs and symptoms in patients who received Restasis 1 month prior to BMT with patients who started the medication at least 6 months after BMT and found a definite benefit in patients who started Restasis early. Patients who start Restasis at least 6 months after BMT had more severe dry eyes, assessed by the dry eye—grading score. While Schirmer scores were higher in the early treatment group at 1 year, there was no difference in visual acuity and staining.

The authors recognize the possible implications of these results in supporting earlier referral to ophthalmology by the patients' oncologist, internist, etc. By intervening early with Restasis, we may be helping prevent or minimize inflammatory damage to the ocular surface from this condition. The authors conclude that a prospective, randomized, placebo-controlled clinical trial is warranted to confirm these findings. We have growing experience with GVHD, as more patients are having hematopoietic stem cell transplant and survival rates are improving. It is a very frustrating disease, as patients are thankful to be alive but resentful of the chronic ocular sequelae. Any intervention that can ameliorate some of these dreaded consequences is important. We look forward to additional evidence from a larger controlled study.

K. M. Hammersmith, MD

P. K. Nagra, MD

Trends in Fungal Keratitis in the United States, 2001 to 2007

Gower EW, Keay LJ, Oechsler RA, et al (The Johns Hopkins Univ, Baltimore, MD; The George Inst, Sydney, Australia; Univ of Miami, FL; et al)
Ophthalmology 117:2263-2267, 2010

Objective.—Fungal keratitis is a serious ocular infection that is considered to be rare among contact lens wearers. The recent *Fusarium* keratitis outbreak raised questions regarding the background rate of *Fusarium*-related keratitis and other fungal keratitis in this population.

Design.—Retrospective, multicenter case series.

Participants.—Six hundred ninety-five cases of fungal keratitis cases who presented to 1 of 10 tertiary medical centers from 2001 to 2007.

Methods.—Ten tertiary care centers in the United States performed a retrospective review of culture-positive fungal keratitis cases at their centers between January 2001 and December 2007. Cases were identified using microbiology, pathology, and/or confocal microscopy records. Information was collected on contact lens status, method of diagnosis, and organism(s) identified. The quarterly number of cases by contact lens status was calculated and Poisson regression was used to evaluate presence of trends. The Johns Hopkins Medicine Institutional Review Board (IRB) and the IRBs at each participating center approved the research.

Main Outcome Measures.—Quarterly number of fungal keratitis cases and fungal species.

Results.—We identified 695 fungal keratitis cases; 283 involved the use of contact lenses. The quarterly number of *Fusarium* cases increased among contact lens wearers (CLWs) during the period that ReNu with MoistureLoc (Bausch & Lomb, Rochester, NY) was on the market, but returned to prior levels after withdrawal of the product from the market. The quarterly frequency of other filamentous fungi cases showed a statistically significant increase among CLWs comparing October 2004 through June 2006 with July 2006 through December 2007 with January 2001 through September 2004 (*P*<0.0001).

Conclusions.—The quarterly number of *Fusarium* fungal keratitis cases among CLWs returned to pre-Renu with Moistureloc levels after removal of the product from the market. However, the number of other filamentous fungal keratitis cases, although small, seems to have increased among refractive CLWs. Reasons for these apparent increases are unclear.

▶ This large retrospective review of fungal keratitis from 10 academic ophthalmic centers in the United States helps put the recent ReNu with MoistureLoc-related *Fusarium* outbreak into perspective. The authors identified a total of 695 cases of fungal keratitis, 283 of which were associated with contact lens wear. While a well-documented spike was noted in cases of *Fusarium* keratitis during the time ReNu with MoistureLoc was on the market, they found a decline back to baseline following withdrawal of this product. However, a more worrisome trend was noted in the increase of non-*Fusarium* fungal keratitis, in both contact lens wearers and non—contact lens wearers. We also found a similar increase in rates of fungal keratitis in a recent retrospective review of fungal keratitis spanning almost 10 years at Wills Eye Institute.[1] Further, we have noted an increase in unusual fungal species, specifically *Alternaria* and *Paecilomyces*, associated with fungal keratitis in contact lens wearers.[2] No reason for this apparent trend could be identified, but it certainly warrants additional investigation.

K. M. Hammersmith, MD

P. K. Nagra, MD

References

1. Yildiz EH, Abdalla YF, Elsahn AF, et al. Update on fungal keratitis from 1999 to 2008. *Cornea.* 2010;29:1406-1411.
2. Yildiz EH, Ailani H, Hammersmith KM, Eagle RC Jr, Rapuano CJ, Cohen EJ. Alternaria and paecilomyces keratitis associated with soft contact lens wear. *Cornea.* 2010;29:564-568.

5 Retina

A Prospective Randomized Trial of Intravitreal *Bevacizumab or Laser Therapy* in the Management of Diabetic Macular Edema (BOLT Study): 12-Month Data: Report 2

Michaelides M, Kaines A, Hamilton RD, et al (Moorfields Eye Hosp, London, UK; et al)
Ophthalmology 117:1078-1086, 2010

Purpose.—To report the findings at 1 year of a study comparing repeated intravitreal bevacizumab (ivB) and modified Early Treatment of Diabetic Retinopathy Study (ETDRS) macular laser therapy (MLT) in patients with persistent clinically significant diabetic macular edema (CSME).

Design.—Prospective, randomized, masked, single-center, 2-year, 2-arm clinical trial.

Participants.—A total of 80 eyes of 80 patients with center-involving CSME and at least 1 prior MLT.

Methods.—Subjects were randomized to either ivB (6 weekly; minimum of 3 injections and maximum of 9 injections in the first 12 months) or MLT (4 monthly; minimum of 1 treatment and maximum of 4 treatments in the first 12 months).

Main Outcome Measures.—The primary end point was the difference in ETDRS best-corrected visual acuity (BCVA) at 12 months between the bevacizumab and laser arms.

Results.—The baseline mean ETDRS BCVA was 55.7 ± 9.7 (range 34–69) in the bevacizumab group and 54.6 ± 8.6 (range 36–68) in the laser arm. The mean ETDRS BCVA at 12 months was 61.3 ± 10.4 (range 34–79) in the bevacizumab group and 50.0 ± 16.6 (range 8–76) in the laser arm ($P = 0.0006$). Furthermore, the bevacizumab group gained a median of 8 ETDRS letters, whereas the laser group lost a median of 0.5 ETDRS letters ($P = 0.0002$). The odds of gaining ≥ 10 ETDRS letters over 12 months were 5.1 times greater in the bevacizumab group than in the laser group (adjusted odds ratio, 5.1; 95% confidence interval, 1.3–19.7; $P = 0.019$). At 12 months, central macular thickness decreased from 507 ± 145 µm (range 281–900 µm) at baseline to 378 ± 134 µm (range 167–699 µm) ($P < 0.001$) in the ivB group, whereas it decreased to a lesser extent in the laser group, from 481 ± 121 µm (range 279–844 µm) to 413 ± 135 µm (range 170–708 µm) ($P = 0.02$). The median number of injections was 9 (interquartile range [IQR] 8–9) in the ivB group, and the median number of laser treatments was 3 (IQR 2–4) in the MLT group.

Conclusions.—The study provides evidence to support the use of bevacizumab in patients with center-involving CSME without advanced macular ischemia.

▶ Although there have been many reports on the effectiveness of intravitreal bevacizumab (IVB) for diabetic macular edema, very few have been prospective comparative trials. This is such a trial and is worth analyzing closely. The authors have concluded that repeated IVB is superior to focal laser in terms of reducing edema and improving vision. There are some critical considerations. First, all of these eyes had prior focal laser and had persistent/recurrent edema centrally with ≤20/40 vision. Thus, injections as primary treatment cannot be recommended based on this article. Second, over 75% of patients treated with injections had at least 8 injections (essentially at every 6-week visit) in 1 year and still had a mean central foveal thickness of 378 microns. In other words, it is likely that ongoing injections will be needed with no obvious end point. This leads to the third consideration, which is safety. If injections are to be continued indefinitely, then infrequent adverse events such as endophthalmitis become more likely. Other concerns such as elevation of intraocular pressure and systemic effects may also become apparent with more experience. While it is tempting to turn toward injections earlier and more often, we should be mindful of these matters before jumping in with both feet.

J. F. Vander, MD

A Randomized Controlled Trial of Alleviated Positioning after Small Macular Hole Surgery

Tadayoni R, Vicaut E, Devin F, et al (Université Paris Diderot, France; Centre Paradis-Monticelli, Marseille, France; et al)
Ophthalmology 118:150-155, 2011

Objective.—To establish whether the success rate of surgery for small idiopathic macular holes (diameter, ≤400 μm) is significantly reduced if facedown positioning is replaced by simply taking care to avoid the supine position.

Design.—Randomized, controlled, parallel-assignment, open-label, interventional, multicenter clinical trial.

Participants.—Sixty-nine patients from 6 specialized vitreoretinal units, randomized into 2 parallel groups and followed up after surgery for 3 months.

Methods.—All patients underwent pars plana vitrectomy, peeling of any epiretinal membrane, and 17% C_2F_6 gas filling. Patients then were advised randomly to observe either strict facedown positioning for 22 of 24 hours or simply to avoid the supine position for 10 days.

Main Outcome Measures.—The primary outcome measure was the rate of anatomic closure 3 months after surgery. Main secondary measurements included Early Treatment Diabetic Retinopathy Study (ETDRS) visual acuity, progression of cataract, and frequency of complications.

Results.—The mean size of macular holes was approximately 300 μm in both groups. Closure rates were more than 90% in both groups: 32 (91.4%) of 34 eyes in the alleviated positioning group versus 32 (94.1%) of 35 eyes in the facedown positioning group (lower margin of 95% confidence interval of difference, −14.88%). The ETDRS scores at 3 months increased in both groups by 10.23 ± 14.64 and 10.52 ± 14.54 letters, respectively. Progression of cataract and the rate of other complications were not significantly different in the 2 groups.

Conclusions.—The success rate of surgery for idiopathic macular holes of 400 μm or smaller is not significantly reduced if facedown positioning is replaced by simply taking care to avoid the supine position. These macular holes can be treated by streamlined surgery, that is, with no internal limiting membrane peeling and no facedown positioning (only avoidance of the supine position) with a closure rate of more than 90% and a mean gain in visual acuity of more than 2 ETDRS lines at 3 months.

▶ As macular hole techniques have evolved, the success rates have steadily improved. Part of this evolution has involved the need, or lack thereof, for facedown positioning postoperatively. Many patients with this diagnosis are so concerned about the positioning requirements that they decline attempted repair. This report adds more evidence to support the trend toward reducing the positioning requirements postoperatively. A large majority of patients, at least those with relatively small holes, will be successfully repaired with essentially no positioning requirements at all. If there is a difference in the success rates with and without positioning, it would appear to be fairly small. It is important to recall, however, that the best chance for visual improvement is with successful initial hole closure. Hole closure may be achieved with reoperation as in this study, but no visual results are offered. Previous studies have suggested that the results in such cases are not as favorable. There is also evidence that hole closure occurs within 3 to 4 days in almost all cases so that the 10 days recommended in this study may be unnecessarily prolonged. It is possible that a small improvement in success could be achieved (which could be missed by this study because of sample size) with just a few days of positioning. If such positioning is possible, then the added effort might be worth it for a few patients even if most patients didn't need it.

J. F. Vander, MD

A Treat and Extend Regimen Using Ranibizumab for Neovascular Age-Related Macular Degeneration: Clinical and Economic Impact
Gupta OP, Shienbaum G, Patel AH, et al (Thomas Jefferson Univ, Philadelphia, PA)
Ophthalmology 117:2134-2140, 2010

Purpose.—To evaluate the visual outcome, number of injections, and direct medical cost of a "treat and extend" regimen (TER) in managing neovascular age-related macular degeneration (nAMD) with intravitreal ranibizumab.

Design.—Retrospective, interventional, consecutive case series.

Participants.—Ninety-two eyes of 92 patients met the entry criteria from May 2006 to May 2008.

Methods.—All patients with treatment-nave nAMD were treated monthly until no intraretinal or subretinal fluid was observed on optical coherence tomography (OCT). The treatment intervals were then sequentially lengthened by 2 weeks until signs of exudation recurred. The interval was individualized for each patient in an attempt to maintain an exudation-free macula.

Main Outcome Measures.—Change from baseline visual acuity, proportion of eyes losing <3 lines and gaining ≥3 lines at 1 year of follow-up, annual mean number of injections, change from baseline OCT central retinal thickness (CRT), maximum period of extension, and adverse ocular and systemic events.

Results.—The mean follow-up was 1.52 years. Mean Snellen visual acuity improved from 20/135 at baseline to 20/77 at 1 year follow-up ($P<0.001$) and 20/83 at 2 years follow-up ($P = 0.002$). The proportion of eyes that lost <3 Snellen visual acuity lines at final follow-up was 96% and the proportion that gained ≥3 Snellen visual acuity lines was 32%. The mean OCT CRT decreased from 303 μm at baseline to 238 μm at 1 year follow-up ($P<0.001$). The mean number of injections over the first year and between years 1 and 2 was 8.36 and 7.45, respectively. The mean maximum period of extension was 79.9 days. No adverse ocular or systemic events were reported during the follow-up period. The direct annual medical cost per patient was $16 114.52 for the TER. The direct annual medical cost per patient ranged from $15 880.07 to $28 314.16 based on previous clinical trial protocols.

Conclusions.—Eyes with nAMD experienced significant visual improvement when managed with intravitreal ranibizumab using a TER. This treatment approach also was associated with significantly fewer patient visits, injections, and direct annual medical cost compared with monthly injections such as in the phase III clinical trials.

▶ The introduction of anti—vascular endothelial growth factor treatment for wet age-related macular degeneration (ARMD) transformed the practice of retina practically overnight. How to incorporate this treatment into practice and the specific strategy to be used for delivering this care were areas of great uncertainty for most physicians. It very quickly became apparent that the rigid exam, testing, and dosing schedules used in the clinical trials leading to the approval of ranibizumab, for example, were not necessarily the ideal approaches in terms of results, cost, and patient compliance. As the introduction in this article points out, nearly 90% of treating physicians use an individualized strategy when caring for patients with wet ARMD. The treat-and-extend strategy is probably the most widely used, yet there was virtually nothing in the peer-reviewed literature on the subject until this publication. It is probably not appropriate to consider this a breakthrough or landmark article, in that it is a fairly small retrospective summary of a technique already widely used. Nevertheless, it is important to critically review this technique, and the authors have done so. These results suggest that over a 2-year period, a thoughtful systematic approach to patients with wet ARMD may produce results nearly equal to the regimented approach in the initial trials with fewer visits and injections. This means a substantial cost reduction, theoretically reduced risk of injection complications (eg, endophthalmitis), and potentially enhancing a patient's quality of life as a result.

J. F. Vander, MD

Antagonism of Vascular Endothelial Growth Factor for Macular Edema Caused by Retinal Vein Occlusions: Two-Year Outcomes
Campochiaro PA, Hafiz G, Channa R, et al (The Johns Hopkins Univ School of Medicine, Baltimore, MD)
Ophthalmology 117:2387-2394, 2010

Purpose.—To determine the long-term effects of intraocular antagonism of vascular endothelial growth factor (VEGF) in patients with macular edema caused by retinal vein occlusions (RVOs).

Design.—Prospective randomized trial.

Participants.—Twenty patients with macular edema caused by branch RVOs (BRVOs) and 20 patients with central RVOs (CRVOs).

Methods.—After the month 3 primary end point, patients were seen every 2 months and received injections of an anti-VEGF agent as needed for recurrent edema.

Main Outcome Measures.—Mean change from baseline best-corrected visual acuity (BCVA) at month 24 with assessment of other parameters of visual function and center subfield thickness (foveal thickness [FTH]).

Results.—For 17 patients with BRVO who completed 2 years of follow-up, the mean improvement from baseline in BCVA at month 24 was 17.8 letters compared with 15.6 letters at month 3. Improvement by at least 6, 3, or 2 lines occurred in 18%, 59%, and 76% of patients, respectively. The Snellen equivalent BCVA at month 24 was 20/40 or better in 10 patients. With an average of 2 injections of ranibizumab during year 2, the mean FTH at month 24 was 245.8 μm compared with 217.1 μm at month 3 and 481.5 μm at baseline. For 14 patients with CRVO who completed 2 years of follow-up, the mean improvement in BCVA at month 24 was 8.5 letters compared with 12.0 letters at month 3. Improvement by at least 6, 3, or 2 lines occurred in 14%, 21%, and 43% of patients, respectively. The Snellen equivalent BCVA at month 24 was 20/40 or better in 4 patients. With an average of 3.5 injections of ranibizumab in year 2, mean FTH at month 24 was 338 μm compared with 278 μm at month 3 and 533 μm at baseline. Duration of RVO >1 year at study entry and nonperfusion of perifoveal capillaries for 360 degrees correlated with reduced visual outcomes.

Conclusions.—Antagonism of VEGF provides substantial long-term benefit to patients with macular edema caused by RVO, but frequent injections are required in some patients with BRVO and most patients with CRVO.

▶ The staggering changes in the management of retinal disorders over the past few years have occurred so rapidly that there is often a lag between the public dissemination of new information and the appearance of that information in a peer-reviewed publication. This report describes the results of a clinical trial initiated in 2006 with results published in 2010. Since initiation of the trial, much larger efforts, including the BRAVO and CRUISE trials, were undertaken, and ranibizumab is now approved for treatment of branch retinal vein occlusions (BRVOs) and central retinal vein occlusions (CRVOs). The rapid and widespread acceptance of intravitreal injection with this agent has taken place even though this report is the first to describe a substantial series with 2 years of follow-up. The results are encouraging for both entities. Most patients had improvement of at least 2 lines of acuity with BRVO, and a sizable minority did so with CRVO. These are better results than those achieved in the BRVO and CRVO laser studies completed many years ago. It is also encouraging that these results can be sustained over 2 years, although ongoing treatment is likely going to be necessary, especially for CRVO patients. It seems that the treatment burden for CRVO patients in year 2 is still substantial if maximizing vision is desired. We do not know what happens beyond 24 months, and it is possible that a considerable amount of ongoing treatment will be necessary. At least it appears that the benefits of this further treatment are meaningful.

J. F. Vander, MD

Antibiotic Resistance of Conjunctiva and Nasopharynx Evaluation Study: A Prospective Study of Patients Undergoing Intravitreal Injections
Kim SJ, Toma HS, Midha NK, et al (Vanderbilt Univ School of Medicine, Nashville, TN; et al)
Ophthalmology 117:2372-2378, 2010

Purpose.—To determine the baseline antibiotic susceptibility patterns of conjunctival and nasopharyngeal flora isolated from patients undergoing intravitreal (IVT) injections for choroidal neovascularization (CNV).

Design.—Prospective, observational study.

Participants.—Forty-eight eyes of 24 patients undergoing unilateral IVT injections for CNV.

Methods.—Bilateral conjunctival and unilateral nasopharyngeal cultures on the treatment side were taken before application of any topical medications.

Main Outcome Measures.—Bacterial isolates were identified and tested for antibiotic susceptibility to 16 different antibiotics using the Kirby-Bauer disc diffusion technique.

Results.—A total of 57 bacterial isolates were obtained from the conjunctiva of 48 eyes. Coagulase-negative staphylococci (CNS) accounted for 37 of the 57 isolates (65%). The most common CNS organisms were *Staphylococcus epidermidis* and *Staphylococcus lugdunensis* accounting for 73% and 11% of CNS isolates, respectively. More than half of *S. epidermidis* isolates demonstrated some level of resistance to ofloxacin and levofloxacin, and 33% and 37% of isolates showed some level of resistance against gatifloxacin and moxifloxacin, respectively. Some 60% and 30% of CNS isolates were resistant to ≥ 3 and ≥ 5 antibiotics, respectively. Among the 24 nasopharyngeal cultures, 8 (33%) grew *Staphylococcus aureus*, and 1 of the 8 isolates (13%) was resistant to all penicillin, cephalosporin, macrolide, and fluoroquinolone antibiotics tested.

Conclusions.—Our results demonstrate subtantial levels of resistance to third- and fourth-generation fluoroquinolones and multiresistance among ocular CNS isolated from patients undergoing IVT injections for CNV.

▶ The rate of bacterial endophthalmitis after intravitreal injection is very low, but because of the enormous number of injections being given, particularly for exudative macular degeneration, the absolute number of infected eyes is substantial. Prophylactic use of topical antibiotics is a common, though unproven, practice. Critical unanswered questions include whether prophylactic antibiotic use reduces the rate of infection and if so, which medications are best. This study cannot directly answer these questions, but it at least provides indirect evidence that one commonly employed class of medication may not be a wise choice. The patient's conjunctival flora is believed to be the source of most cases of endophthalmitis. *Staphylococcus* species, particularly coagulase negative, are the most common cause of infection and, as shown in this paper, the organisms most frequently found on the conjunctiva in this population. What is striking is the relatively poor activity demonstrated by the fluoroquinolones against *Staphylococcus* organisms. This class of antibiotics is probably used more than any other for this purpose and yet its coverage is among the worst of all antibiotic types. There are more effective drugs commercially available which are also likely to be considerably cheaper. We still can't say whether using drops prophylactically is useful but if they are prescribed we should at least be more thoughtful as to which drugs to recommend.

J. F. Vander, MD

Clinical Trial of Lutein in Patients With Retinitis Pigmentosa Receiving Vitamin A

Berson EL, Rosner B, Sandberg MA, et al (Harvard Med School, Boston, MA; et al)
Arch Ophthalmol 128:403-411, 2010

Objective.—To determine whether lutein supplementation will slow visual function decline in patients with retinitis pigmentosa receiving vitamin A.

Design.—Randomized, controlled, double-masked trial of 225 non-smoking patients, aged 18 to 60 years, evaluated over a 4-year interval. Patients received 12 mg of lutein or a control tablet daily. All were given 15 000 IU/d of vitamin A palmitate. Randomization took into account genetic type and baseline serum lutein level.

Main Outcome Measures.—The primary outcome was the total point score for the Humphrey Field Analyzer (HFA) 30-2 program; prespecified secondary outcomes were the total point scores for the 60-4 program and for the 30-2 and 60-4 programs combined, 30-Hz electroretinogram amplitude, and Early Treatment Diabetic Retinopathy Study acuity.

Results.—No significant difference in rate of decline was found between the lutein plus vitamin A and control plus vitamin A groups over a 4-year interval for the HFA 30-2 program. For the HFA60-4 program, a decrease in mean rate of sensitivity loss was observed in the lutein plus vitamin A group ($P = .05$). Mean decline with the 60-4 program was slower among those with the highest serum lutein level or with the highest increase in macular pigment optical density at follow-up ($P = .01$ and $P = .006$, respectively). Those with the highest increase in macular pigment optical density also had the slowest decline in HFA 30-2 and 60-4 combined field sensitivity ($P = .005$). No significant toxic effects of lutein supplementation were observed.

Conclusion.—Lutein supplementation of 12 mg/d slowed loss of mid-peripheral visual field on average among nonsmoking adults with retinitis pigmentosa taking vitamin A.

Application to Clinical Practice.—Data are presented that support use of 12 mg/d of lutein to slow visual field loss among nonsmoking adults with retinitis pigmentosa taking vitamin A.

Trial Registration.—ClinicalTrials.gov Identifier: NCT00346333.

▶ This trial describes the third major report in a series dating back to a controversial study published in 1994. The initial report described a benefit obtained 15 000 IU of vitamin A in patients with retinitis pigmentosa (RP). Many researches in the field disputed the validity of the claim that vitamin supplementation slowed progression of RP. Much of the controversy resulted from grouping of data and analysis of secondary end points. Seventeen years later, this study assessing the use of adding lutein to a regimen of vitamin A supplementation can be criticized for similar reasons. (In fact, the claims are disputed fairly strongly in an editorial that appears in the same issue.) No significant difference was found in the primary end point of slowing central visual field loss. Analysis of several secondary end points took place, and for one of them (changes in 60° field), a difference was found. Given that there is no known treatment for this devastating condition, it is tempting to create treatment guidelines based on a reasonable rationale and some encouraging data. It is useful to bear in mind, however, that this study does not provide compelling proof that there is a therapeutic effect achieved with lutein supplementation, and recommending such a strategy may not be warranted.

J. F. Vander, MD

Comparison of Persistent Submacular Fluid in Vitrectomy and Scleral Buckle Surgery for Macula-Involving Retinal Detachment

Kim Y-K, Woo SJ, Park KH, et al (Seoul Natl Univ College of Medicine, Korea)
Am J Ophthalmol 149:623-629, 2010

Purpose.—To compare the frequency of persistent submacular fluid (SMF) and sequential visual outcomes after pars plana vitrectomy (PPV) and scleral buckling (SB) in recent-onset macula-involving rhegmatogenous retinal detachment (RD), and thus to determine the role of persistent SMF on visual outcome with different surgical methods.

Design.—Observational case series.

Methods.—Sixty-one patients (61 eyes) who underwent successful PPV (16 patients) or SB (45 patients) underwent thorough ophthalmologic examinations including optical coherence tomography at 1 month after surgery, as well as every 3 months until SMF disappeared. The SB group was divided into 2 groups according to the presence (SB-SMF+) or absence (SB-SMF−) of persistent SMF at 1 month after surgery. Preoperative and postoperative best-corrected visual acuities were compared among the different surgical groups and also were analyzed depending on the RD duration (acute, symptom duration ≤ 7 days; subacute, symptom duration > 7 and ≤ 30 days).

Results.—Persistent SMF at 1 month after surgery was more frequent in the SB group (55.6%) than it was in the PPV group (6.25%; $P = .006$). The SB-SMF+ group showed worse postoperative best-corrected visual acuity than the PPV or SB-SMF− groups at 6 to 12 months after surgery, whereas there were no significant differences in the final visual acuity among the groups. This difference in visual recovery was not observed in patients with subacute RD.

Conclusions.—The similar visual recovery patterns seen in the PPV and SB-SMF− groups suggest that persistent SMF is a more important prognostic factor than surgical method is in the setting of acute onset and successful RD surgery.

▶ There has been an enormous shift in the preferred method for repair of primary retinal detachment (RD) over the past 10 to 15 years. Pars plana vitrectomy is now used in most cases, and in some training programs, the ratio of vitrectomy versus buckle for treatment of primary RDs is so high that newly trained retinal fellows often have limited experience in performance of primary scleral buckles. Before we declare the scleral buckle to be a procedure without an indication, we should carefully consider articles such as this one. Although the number of patients is not large and the data are retrospective, the critical conclusion of this article is that the final visual results for patients with macula-involving RDs were the same whether treated with buckle or vitrectomy. The resolution of submacular fluid may be slower in the buckle group, but ultimately, the recovery was comparable to the primary vitrectomy group. Furthermore, none of the patients with phakic buckle required cataract surgery, whereas nearly all of the vitrectomy group did. This is not a trivial matter when dealing with a young myope with a clear lens in the fellow eye, a common scenario for this diagnosis. It is noteworthy that the buckle patients were more likely to have an inferior RD than the vitrectomy group. The subretinal fluid in such cases is often much more viscous than with superior RDs, as symptoms frequently develop with acute extension of a more chronic detachment. Potentially further confounding this result is that the author did not drain subretinal fluid when using a buckle. While this avoids the potential complications seen with drainage, it may at least partially explain the delayed resolution of subretinal fluid seen in this setting. In any case, it is reassuring to know that visual results were similar between the 2 groups despite the variability in optical coherence tomography findings. It appears that scleral buckling for repair of primary RD is still a procedure worth having in the surgeon's armamentarium.

J. F. Vander, MD

Cryotherapy vs Laser Photocoagulation in Scleral Buckle Surgery: A Randomized Clinical Trial

Lira RPC, Takasaka I, Arieta CEL, et al (State Univ of Campinas, Recife, Brazil)
Arch Ophthalmol 128:1519-1522, 2010

Objective.—To compare the reattachment rate and visual acuity results among patients with rhegmatogenous retinal detachment who underwent scleral buckle surgery with retinopexy by intraoperative cryotherapy (cryopexy) vs postoperative (1 month later) laser photocoagulation (laserpexy).

Methods.—Eighty-six patients with rhegmatogenous retinal detachment scheduled for scleral buckle surgery were randomly assigned to the cryopexy or laserpexy group.

Main Outcome Measures.—The primary outcome was the 1-week reattachment rate. Other outcome measures included later reattachment rate (1 month and 6 months), best-corrected visual acuity, rate of subsequent operations, and postoperative complications.

Results.—The 1-week, 1-month, and 6-month anatomical success rates were similar in the 2 groups: 93% (40 patients), 100%, and 100% in the cryopexy group and 95% (41 patients), 100%, and 100% in the laserpexy group, respectively. Three patients in the cryopexy group and 2 in the laserpexy group underwent 1 additional rhegmatogenous retinal detachment surgery (pars plan vitrectomy) after primary failure at 1-week follow-up. The types of post-operative complications were similar in both groups, except for eyelid edema. Visual recovery was slower in the cryotherapy group, but the difference in visual acuity after 6 months was not significant.

Conclusions.—In patients with uncomplicated retinal detachment, both techniques of retinopexy have shown satisfactory anatomical and functional success. Laserpexy offers faster visual acuity recuperation with fewer postoperative complications but requires a second intervention and costs more than cryotherapy.

Application to Clinical Practice.—Laserpexy is a successful alternative to cryopexy in creating chorioretinal adhesion for scleral buckle surgery.

Trial Registration.—clinicaltrials.gov Identifier: NCT01068379.

▶ This study was nicely designed and well executed. The authors sought to determine if there is a difference between using intraoperative cryotherapy versus postoperative laser for simple retinal detachments (RDs) treated with scleral buckle. The answer is that there is no significant difference in terms of retinal reattachment rates or final visual results. Postoperative lid edema was, not surprisingly, much less in the laser group. The trade-off is that the laser patients had to undergo a second procedure 1 month after initial repair. Perhaps of more interest is that the reattachment rates were equally high between the groups receiving retinopexy (cryo) and those not treated for 1 month (laser). This reaffirms the now classic theory behind scleral buckling that relief of vitreoretinal traction with mechanical support of a retinal break is the essential step in RD repair. Retinopexy MAY help to reduce the rate of late onset recurrence of RD, but it has nothing to do with the primary reattachment of the retina.

J. F. Vander, MD

Effects of Medical Therapies on Retinopathy Progression in Type 2 Diabetes

The ACCORD Study Group and ACCORD Eye Study Group (Natl Insts of Health [NIH], Bethesda, MD; Wake Forest Univ School of Medicine, Winston-Salem, NC; Univ of Wisconsin, Madison; et al)
N Engl J Med 363:233-244, 2010

Background.—We investigated whether intensive glycemic control, combination therapy for dyslipidemia, and intensive blood-pressure control would limit the progression of diabetic retinopathy in persons with type 2 diabetes. Previous data suggest that these systemic factors may be important in the development and progression of diabetic retinopathy.

Methods.—In a randomized trial, we enrolled 10,251 participants with type 2 diabetes who were at high risk for cardiovascular disease to receive either intensive or standard treatment for glycemia (target glycated hemoglobin level, <6.0% or 7.0 to 7.9%, respectively) and also for dyslipidemia (160 mg daily of fenofibrate plus simvastatin or placebo plus simvastatin) or for systolic blood-pressure control (target, <120 or <140 mm Hg). A subgroup of 2856 participants was evaluated for the effects of these interventions at 4 years on the progression of diabetic retinopathy by 3 or more steps on the Early Treatment Diabetic Retinopathy Study Severity Scale (as assessed from seven-field stereoscopic fundus photographs, with 17 possible steps and a higher number of steps indicating greater severity) or the development of diabetic retinopathy necessitating laser photocoagulation or vitrectomy.

Results.—At 4 years, the rates of progression of diabetic retinopathy were 7.3% with intensive glycemia treatment, versus 10.4% with standard therapy (adjusted odds ratio, 0.67; 95% confidence interval [CI], 0.51 to 0.87; P = 0.003); 6.5% with fenofibrate for intensive dyslipidemia therapy, versus 10.2% with placebo (adjusted odds ratio, 0.60; 95% CI, 0.42 to 0.87; P = 0.006); and 10.4% with intensive blood-pressure therapy, versus 8.8% with standard therapy (adjusted odds ratio, 1.23; 95% CI, 0.84 to 1.79; P = 0.29).

Conclusions.—Intensive glycemic control and intensive combination treatment of dyslipidemia, but not intensive blood-pressure control, reduced the rate of progression of diabetic retinopathy. (Funded by the National Heart, Lung, and Blood Institute and others; ClinicalTrials.gov numbers, NCT00000620 for the ACCORD study and NCT00542178 for the ACCORD Eye study.)

▶ We have known for several years that tight glycemic control is effective in reducing the rate of retinopathy progression among patients with type 1 diabetes. This large randomized trial demonstrates a significant effect for the much larger population of patients with type 2 diabetes, at least over a 4-year period. The measured difference is from around 10% to 7%. This represents a 30% reduction in risk. Because the overall incidence of progression in the standard group (ie, hemoglobin A1C between 7 and 8) is quite low, very aggressive treatment is needed for a very large number of patients to achieve an apparent benefit for a relatively small number of individuals. Given the practical implications of trying to achieve a hemoglobin A1C of < 6, including the risks of hypoglycemic episodes, which can be dangerous, such an ambitious treatment goal may not be right for every patient.

J. F. Vander, MD

Intravitreal infliximab for the treatment of sight-threatening chronic noninfectious uveitis
Farvardin M, Afarid M, Mehryar M, et al (Shiraz Univ of Med Sciences, Iran)
Retina 30:1530-1535, 2010

Purpose.—Tumor necrosis factor-alpha is known to play an important role in various immune-mediated ocular diseases. Infliximab, a chimeric monoclonal antibody against tumor necrosis factor-alpha, has been used for the treatment of various chronic systemic and ocular inflammatory diseases. The purpose of this study was to evaluate the effect of intravitreal injection of infliximab on the visual acuity and central macular thickness in patients with chronic noninfectious uveitis.

Methods.—Ten eyes of 7 patients with chronic persistent noninfectious uveitis who were nonresponsive to conventional previous medications during the previous 3 months were included in this study. The patients received intravitreal injection of 1.5 mg/0.15 mL infliximab. Mean best-corrected visual acuity and mean central macular thickness 1 day before and 4 weeks after the injection were evaluated and compared.

Results.—Mean logarithm of the minimum angle of resolution before and after injection was 1.37 ± 0.43 and 0.67 ± 0.56, respectively, with statistically significant improvement after injection ($P = 0.005$). The mean central macular thickness before and after injection was 673.20 ± 338.39 μm and 456.40 ± 317.46 μm, respectively, with a significant decrease in the central macular thickness after the injection ($P = 0.005$).

Conclusion.—Intravitreal injection of infliximab may improve the visual acuity and decrease the central macular thickness in patients with chronic noninfectious uveitis and significant visual loss and central macular edema.

▶ As retinal specialists are increasingly comfortable with the use of intravitreal injections for the management of a variety of retinal pathologies, it is inevitable that attention will turn toward exploration of alternative medications for use with this method of delivery. When managing posterior uveitis, corticosteroids remain the mainstay of treatment, but the safety profile, especially elevation of intraocular pressure, can sometimes make its use problematic. This pilot study represents the first human use of this agent via intravitreal administration for management of uveitis. The authors determined the dose based on experimental animal data. In this small series, the drug was well tolerated and showed a therapeutic effect for at least 1 month. A much larger series will be necessary to ensure safety, quantify efficacy, and determine ideal dosing in terms of amount of drug per injection and frequency of injections. Nevertheless, for patients with refractory uveitis, this could prove an exciting new option for the future.

J. F. Vander, MD

Long-term Temporal Changes of Macular Thickness and Visual Outcome after Vitrectomy for Idiopathic Epiretinal Membrane

Kim J, Rhee KM, Woo SJ, et al (Seoul Natl Univ College of Medicine, Korea; Univ of Adelaide Med School, Australia)
Am J Ophthalmol 150:701-709, 2010

Purpose.—To evaluate the long-term correlation of visual outcome and macular thickness after vitrectomy for idiopathic epiretinal membrane and to identify prognostic factors for good visual outcome.

Design.—Retrospective, observational case series.

Methods.—We reviewed the records of 52 patients with idiopathic epiretinal membrane who were treated with vitrectomy and could be followed up for more than 12 months. The main outcome measures were best-corrected visual acuity (BCVA) and central macular thickness at baseline; at 1, 3, 6, and 12 months after surgery; and at the final follow-up visit. The correlation between BCVA and central macular thickness was analyzed and the receiver operating characteristic curve analysis was performed to obtain cutoff values for visual prognosis.

Results.—Most of the changes in BCVA and central macular thickness took place during the first 3 months and reached a plateau at 12 months after surgery. Despite the lack of changes in BCVA after 12 months of follow-up, significant reduction in central macular thickness could still be observed over 12 months after surgery. The final BCVA was correlated significantly with preoperative BCVA and central macular thickness and early postoperative central macular thickness. Among them, the postoperative central macular thickness at 1 month showed the largest area under the receiver operating characteristic curve.

Conclusions.—Given the removal of the confounding effect of cataract, postoperative follow-up of 12 months may be sufficient to reach the final BCVA after surgery. However, more time is needed to achieve final central macular thickness. Because of the significant correlation between final BCVA and early postoperative central macular thickness, serial optical coherence tomography images in the early postoperative period were needed to predict visual outcome after epiretinal membrane removal.

▶ Most studies that attempt to study macular thickness and its relationship to visual acuity have found a strong correlation across several disease states. This study is somewhat unusual in that while the initial correlation between reduction in macular thickness and improvement in visual acuity in the first 3 months after peeling of epiretinal membrane is high, this correlation diminishes somewhat over time. Most of the visual improvement that occurs after surgery takes place in the first 3 months with a lesser degree of recovery after month 12. Virtually no visual improvement occurs beyond the first year. In contrast, while much of the reduction in edema takes place early, there is ongoing resolution of edema and restoration of macular anatomy based on optical coherence tomography (OCT) images beyond month 12. The authors hypothesize why this disconnect might occur in the late phases on recovery, but the answer remains unknown. While OCT findings are in general a reasonable surrogate for visual acuity data, this study reminds us that this is not inevitably the case.

J. F. Vander, MD

Macular Hole Surgery and Cataract Extraction: Combined vs Consecutive Surgery
Muselier A, Dugas B, Burelle X, et al (Dept of Ophthalmology Univ Hosp, Dijon, France; Dept of Ophthalmology Univ Hosp, Nancy, France)
Am J Ophthalmol 150:387-391, 2010

Purpose.—To compare the functional and the anatomic outcomes of a combined surgery and consecutive surgery for macular hole and cataract extraction.

Design.—Multicenter, retrospective, comparative case series.

Patients.—One hundred twenty patients (120 eyes) with an idiopathic macular hole and cataract were operated on in 1 or 2 sessions in 2 academic centers, Dijon University Hospital and Nancy University Hospital. Combined surgery (n = 64) and consecutive surgery (n = 56) were performed between 2006 and 2007. All patients underwent pars plana vitrectomy with internal limiting membrane peeling and gas tamponade. Cataract extraction was performed with phacoemulsification followed by a posterior chamber intraocular lens implantation. The main outcome measures were near and far visual acuity at 6 and 12 months, and the rate of closure of macular hole evaluated with optical coherence tomography.

Results.—After a 12-month follow-up, the postoperative best-corrected visual acuities significantly improved in both the combined and the consecutive surgery groups (near and far vision in both groups, $P < .0001$). However the improvement of far visual acuity was not significant in the consecutive surgery group at 6 months ($P = .06$) while such an improvement was observed in the combined surgery group ($P < .0001$). The rates of closure, 100% and 96% in the combined and the consecutive groups respectively, and the complications did not differ significantly between groups.

Conclusion.—Both combined and consecutive surgeries are safe and effective methods to treat macular hole and cataract with equivalent functional and anatomic results in both procedures. However, combined surgery shortened the delay for visual recovery.

▶ With recent advancements in vitreous surgery, macular hole repair has become a very common highly successful procedure. In particular, the widespread adoption of internal limiting membrane peeling has brought closure rates up close to 100%, even with much less onerous face down postoperative positioning than initially used. Most patients experience substantial visual recovery. This retrospective nonrandomized series assessed the timing of cataract extraction for these patients. Given that nearly all phakic patients will ultimately require cataract surgery, this is an important clinical question. The results suggest that in terms of final visual result, it doesn't really matter whether surgery is combined with the hole repair or delayed until later. Economic considerations make combining the surgery attractive. However, there are a few additional considerations. Placement of a vitreous gas bubble is essential for hole closure. This is generally not an issue if the intraocular lens (IOL) is placed in the capsular bag with a fairly small capsulorrhexis. If there is an issue with the capsule, however, it is not uncommon that intravitreal gas will cause iris capture or other IOL positioning problems postoperatively. This small series did not describe this problem, but in a larger series, it could prove to be an issue. The logistics of retinal surgeons either performing cataract surgery or bringing in an anterior segment surgeon to share the procedure was also not addressed. Surgeon and patient preference will likely determine the approach used given the similarity in results.

J. F. Vander, MD

Obstructive Sleep Apnea Among Patients With Retinal Vein Occlusion

Glacet-Bernard A, Leroux les Jardins G, Lasry S, et al (Intercommunal and Henri Mondor Hospitals/Assistance Publique des Hôpitaux de Paris, France; Paris XII University, France)

Arch Ophthalmol 128:1533-1538, 2010

Objective.—To evaluate the possible involvement of obstructive sleep apnea (OSA) in retinal vein occlusion (RVO).

Methods.—From the medical records of 63 consecutive patients with RVO, 30 patients with 2 of the 3 following risk factors for OSA were selected for further screening from February 1, 2008, through March 31, 2009: associated cardiovascular disease, snoring, or daytime sleepiness.

Results.—Of the 30 selected patients, 23 (77%) had OSA. If all 33 of the unscreened patients did not have OSA, the OSA prevalence would have been 37%. Among the patients with OSA, the mean apnea-hypopnea index (AHI) was 21; OSA was mild (AHI <15) in 13 patients, moderate in 5 patients (AHI 15-30), and severe (AHI >30) in 5 patients. The AHI was correlated with body mass index ($P = .02$).

Conclusions.—We found a higher than expected prevalence of OSA in a series of patients with RVO. Our findings suggest that OSA could be an additional risk factor that plays an important role in the pathogenesis of RVO or at least that it is a frequently associated condition that could be a triggering factor. This association may explain why most patients discover visual loss on awakening. It is too early to assess whether OSA treatment could improve visual outcome of RVO, but it seems vital to recognize OSA in RVO for the general health of the patient.

▶ Patients with retinal vein obstructions will often ask why, and frequently, the reply is one of uncertainty. As with other vascular diseases, ocular and otherwise, the correct answer is probably multifactiorial. This report highlights a potentially important contributing factor, and unlike some factors (eg, genetics and age), it is potentially treatable. While it may not be necessary to perform formal sleep studies in every patient with a retinal vein occlusion, at the very least, it would seem prudent to include the appropriate questions when taking a history from such patients. If a family member can confirm breathing issues while sleeping or if chronic fatigue is reported, then formal studies would seem warranted, if only to minimize risk for fellow eye or other systemic vascular problems.

J. F. Vander, MD

Polypoidal Choroidal Vasculopathy Masquerading as Neovascular Age-Related Macular Degeneration Refractory to Ranibizumab

Stangos AN, Gandhi JS, Nair-Sahni J, et al (Royal Liverpool Univ Hosp, UK; et al)
Am J Ophthalmol 150:666-673, 2010

Purpose.—To report a neovascular age-related macular degeneration pattern refractory to ranibizumab.

Design.—Retrospective, observational case series.

Methods.—Between March and May 2009, cases with neovascular age-related macular degeneration refractory to ranibizumab were investigated with indocyanine green angiography. We identified 12 eyes of 12 patients with polypoidal choroidal vasculopathy. Refractory to treatment were defined cases with persistent subretinal or intraretinal fluid, or both, after 3 or more consecutive monthly ranibizumab injections regardless of best-corrected visual acuity.

Results.—All patients identified were white, of whom 6 were male. Mean age ± standard deviation at presentation was 75 ± 5.6 years (range, 64 to 81 years); diagnosis, based on fluorescein angiography, comprised occult choroidal neovascularization (CNV) in 8 eyes, and 1 case each of classic-no-occult CNV, minimally classic CNV, predominantly classic CNV, and retinal angiomatous proliferation. Eight cases had switched from courses of other therapy (5 pegaptanib, 1 photodynamic therapy, 1 photodynamic therapy then pegaptanib, 1 bevacizumab). After a mean follow-up of 10.2 ± 4.8 months (range, 3 to 18 months) and 7.6 ± 3.9 ranibizumab injections (range, 3 to 14 injections), indocyanine green angiography revealed polypoidal choroidal vasculopathy lesions in all cases.

Conclusions.—Neovascular age-related macular degeneration refractory to a course of ranibizumab injections may harbor polypoidal choroidal vasculopathy. In such cases, indocyanine green angiography is a valuable tool for revealing polypoidal lesions (Fig 2).

▶ Intravitreal injections of anti—vascular endothelial growth factor medications have transformed the care of exudative age-related macular degeneration. Most patients will respond to an injection with rapid resolution of fluid regardless of the precise nature of the lesion causing the exudation. Whereas retinal specialists historically studied fluorescein angiograms carefully to determine the exact location and character of choroidal neovascularization in macular degeneration, there is now a sense among some ophthalmologists that this level of scrutiny is no longer warranted. While that strategy may work most of the time, this report reminds us that for some patients, this degree of attention can make a big difference. Polypoidal choroidal vasculopathy is an exudative maculopathy that can easily be mistaken for typical wet age-related macular degeneration. This condition can sometimes be diagnosed with fluorescein angiography but in some cases will require indocyanine green angiography to confirm the exact nature of the leakage (Fig 2). Furthermore, while ranibizumab injections may help

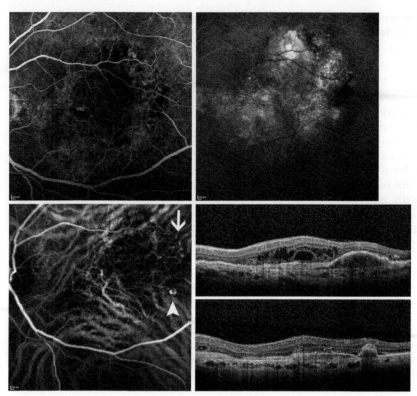

FIGURE 2.—Images of the left eye of Case 1 after 6 consecutive pegaptanib and 14 consecutive monthly ranibizumab intravitreal injections for neovascular age-related macular degeneration. (Top left) Early phase of the fluorescein angiogram showing minimally classic choroidal neovascularization, (Top right) with leakage at the late phase. (Bottom left) Indocyanine green angiography performed the same day revealing a single extrafoveal polypoidal choroidal vasculopathy (PCV) lesion (white arrow-head) as well as an extrafoveal cluster of 4 PCV lesions (white arrow). (Middle right) Spectral-domain optical coherence tomography scan of the clustered PCV lesion and (Bottom right) the single PCV lesion showing a relative hyperreflectivity under the retinal pigment epithelium detachment, suggestive of the polypoidal lesions, with concomitant intraretinal and subretinal fluid. (Reprinted from Stangos AN, Gandhi JS, Nair-Sahni J, et al. Polypoidal choroidal vasculopathy masquerading as neovascular age-related macular degeneration refractory to ranibizumab. *Am J Ophthalmol.* 2010;150:666-673, copyright 2010, with permission from Elsevier.)

reduce edema, treatment with photodynamic therapy, perhaps combined with ranibizumab, is usually far more effective. It is essential to recognize this entity in order to ensure that the ideal treatment strategy is used. Using an "if it's wet, inject" strategy for all exudative maculopathies does a disservice to this important segment of our patient population.

J. F. Vander, MD

Retinal Toxicity Associated With Hydroxychloroquine and Chloroquine: Risk Factors, Screening, and Progression Despite Cessation of Therapy
Michaelides M, Stover NB, Francis PJ, et al (Oregon Health & Science Univ, Portland)
Arch Ophthalmol 129:30-39, 2011

Objective.—To report the detailed clinical findings of patients with retinal toxicity that developed secondary to the use of hydroxychloroquine sulfate (n = 13), chloroquine phosphate (n = 2), or a combination of the agents (n = 1).

Methods.—Ophthalmologic examination, fundus photography, visual field testing, and detailed electrophysiologic assessment were undertaken in all 16 affected patients. Selected patients also had spectral domain optical coherence tomography (n = 6) and fundus autofluorescence imaging (n = 4).

Results.—Sixteen women (mean age, 67 years; range, 44-85) were monitored for 7 years. The mean duration of hydroxychloroquine therapy was 13 years (range, 2-20). In patients in whom the daily dosage of hydroxychloroquine could be estimated (12 of 13), when using actual body weight, 8 were taking 6.5 mg/kg or less and 4 were taking greater than this recommended dosage. However, if lean body weight was used, 3 patients were taking 6.5 mg/kg or less and 9 were taking greater than this daily dosage. The most common (n = 10) presenting symptom was difficulty with reading; 4 women were asymptomatic. Two patients had preexisting retinal disease, 2 were obese, and none had renal or liver dysfunction. Fundus findings ranged from mild retinal pigment epithelial changes to bull's-eye maculopathy; 3 patients had a normal-appearing macula. Two patients had full-field electroretinograms that showed no abnormalities and 6 showed evidence of generalized retinal dysfunction with reduced rod and cone responses. All 15 patients who underwent multifocal electroretinography testing had evidence of bilateral macular cone dysfunction. Four patterns of visual field abnormality were observed in the 15 patients with abnormal visual fields, the most common (n = 10) being isolated central loss. Repeat electrophysiologic and visual field assessment provided evidence of disease progression despite cessation of medication in 6 patients, with documented progression for 7 years in 1 woman.

Conclusions.—Sustained visual improvement following cessation of drug therapy was not observed in any patient in this series, and our identification of 6 patients with objective evidence of progression serves to remind physicians of the potentially devastating visual consequences of antimalarial-related retinal toxicity. It is also of note that profound abnormalities detected with visual field and multifocal electroretinography testing can be observed in the presence of a normal macular appearance, and our findings suggest that lean body weight should be used for all patients when calculating daily dosage.

▶ This report provides a nice update on the issue of hydroxychloroquine toxicity. There is not a great deal of new information per se, but because this is an uncommon condition, putting together a series of this size while considering the latest screening tools is helpful. It should be pointed out that in this retrospective case series, one cannot learn anything about the rate of toxicity in the relevant population. The authors assert that toxicity may be more common than previously thought, but they do not provide any information on the source population for this series of patients, thereby suggesting that this supposition is purely speculative. Nevertheless, the extremely high rate of abnormalities on multifocal electroretinography suggests that this may be the best way to pick up early toxicity. There is insufficient information regarding spectral domain optical coherence tomography to discern whether that has enough sensitivity to justify routine use. The relatively high rate of progressive injury even years after discontinuation of the drug along with the lack of recovery in any patient is concerning and serves to emphasize the importance of regular screening. Attention to the daily dose relative to lean body mass is also worth remembering, with a target dose of less than 6.5 mg/kg/d.

J. F. Vander, MD

Risk of Iatrogenic Peripheral Retinal Breaks in 20-G Pars Plana Vitrectomy
Ramkissoon YD, Aslam SA, Shah SP, et al (Moorfields Eye Hosp, London, UK)
Ophthalmology 117.1025 1830, 2010

Purpose.—To estimate the frequency and risk factors for entry site and other peripheral iatrogenic retinal breaks in eyes undergoing standard 20-G 3-port pars plana vitrectomy.

Design.—Single-center, retrospective, interventional case series.

Participants.—A total of 645 eyes undergoing pars plana vitrectomy at Moorfields Eye Hospital during the period June 1, 2005, to June 1, 2006, for indications excluding rhegmatogenous retinal detachment.

Methods.—Case note review. Exclusion criteria were preexisting retinal breaks or rhegmatogenous retinal detachment, previously vitrectomized eyes, and iatrogenic breaks posterior to the equator.

Main Outcome Measures.—Frequency, anatomic location, and risk factors associated with iatrogenic peripheral retinal breaks and rate of postoperative rhegmatogenous retinal detachment.

Results.—Iatrogenic peripheral retinal breaks occurred in 98 of 645 eyes (15.2%) intraoperatively. Eleven of 645 cases (1.7%) experienced postoperative rhegmatogenous retinal detachment caused by undetected or new peripheral retinal breaks. Breaks were most common during surgery for tractional retinal detachment (22.2%), macular hole (18.1%), dislocated intraocular lens implants (16.7%), and epiretinal membrane (13.9%). Overall, breaks were more common in the superior retina ($P<0.01$), with 41.5% occurring in the 10 and 2 o'clock positions. Eyes requiring surgical induction of a posterior vitreous detachment had 2.9 times greater odds of developing iatrogenic peripheral retinal breaks (95% confidence interval, 1.8—4.7, $P<0.001$) than eyes with preexisting posterior vitreous detachment. Similarly, phakic eyes had 2.4 times higher odds (95% confidence interval, 1.42–3.96, $P = 0.001$) of break formation.

Conclusions.—Iatrogenic peripheral retinal breaks caused by vitrectomy are more common than previously indicated. Approximately 4 in 10 breaks are related to traction at sclerotomy entry sites. Eyes undergoing surgery for tractional retinal detachment seemed to have the highest risk for break formation. Similarly, phakic eyes and eyes that require induction of a posterior vitreous detachment have more than double the risk for break formation.

▶ There have been numerous reports published over the years on the subject of iatrogenic peripheral retinal tears in eyes undergoing vitrectomy. The rate of over 15% published in this retrospective review is indeed higher than most other reports and it is not clear as to why that is. As the authors acknowledge in their discussion, nearly half of the breaks are tractional in nature and found at the sclerotomy entry sites. It is likely that attention to minimizing this traction would reduce the rate of tear formation. In fact, the higher rate found in this report suggests that variation in technique may be vital in the prevention of this complication. Experienced vitreoretinal surgeons know that avoiding sudden alteration of fluid flow through the sclerotomies, meticulous trimming of gel near the sclerotomies, and careful insertion of certain instruments prone to tear formation such as scissors are among the subtleties that help prevent this problem. Of particular interest is whether the recent shift to small incision vitrectomy with 23- or 25-gauge cannulas helps to avoid retinal tear formation. If so then this would indicate a meaningful advantage to this newer technique.

J. F. Vander, MD

6 Oculoplastic Surgery

Imiquimod 5% cream for the treatment of periocular Basal cell carcinoma
Carneiro RC, de Macedo EM, Matayoshi S (Univ of São Paulo School of Med, Brazil)
Ophthal Plast Reconstr Surg 26:100-102, 2010

Purpose.—The objective of this pilot study was to evaluate the efficacy and safety of 5% imiquimod cream in the treatment of periocular basal cell carcinoma (BCC) through the analysis of a case series.

Methods.—Eight subjects with primary nodular BCC of the eyelid were recruited. Treatment lasted 10 to 16 weeks. The average follow-up time was 11.7 months.

Results.—Of a total of 10 lesions, 80% resolved clinically and histologically and have remained asymptomatic since.

Conclusion.—Imiquimod cream 5% was shown to be an attractive alternative to surgical treatment of periocular BCC. Future studies with larger samples and longer follow-up periods are expected to provide more accurate information on the efficacy and safety of the drug.

▶ This article from Brazil treats 10 patients with a basal cell carcinoma of their eyelid with 5% imiquimod cream. The results were good with 8 of 10 lesions disappearing, and the 2 that did not go away were reduced in size and then underwent surgical excision.

Imiquimod cream has been used with success for the treatment of basal cell carcinoma on the skin. The use for eyelid lesions has been limited by the concern that imiquimod may have a toxic effect on the eye. Although this study only involved 10 patients, it did not find any significant ocular side effects or toxicity from 5% imiquimod cream when used on the eyelids. It should be noted that each time 5% imiquimod cream was used, the eye was protected with ointment prior to application of the imiquimod cream on the eyelid lesion. In addition, if the cream did get in the eye, the eye was washed out with eyewash. Artificial tears were used 4 times per day for all patients.

This article is a small study that suggests imiquimod may be safe to use around the eye. This should be used cautiously, and it must be remembered that 5% imiquimod cream causes skin irritation, so it certainly may irritate the eye. This is not the new standard of care but is an option that can be considered in patients with small basal cell carcinomas of the eyelid who are not surgical candidates.

R. B. Penne, MD

Targeted biological therapies for Graves' disease and thyroid-associated ophthalmopathy. Focus on B-cell depletion with Rituximab
Hegedüs L, Smith TJ, Douglas RS, et al (Odense Univ Hosp, Odense C, Denmark; Univ of Michigan, Ann Arbor; et al)
Clin Endocrinol 74:1-8, 2011

Based on experience from the treatment of other autoimmune diseases and because of the limitations imposed by existing therapeutic options for Graves' disease (GD) and thyroid-associated ophthalmopathy (TAO), rituximab (RTX) was recently proposed as a novel therapy option. Here, we summarize the rationale for using RTX; give an overview of the possible mechanisms of action; and give an account of its effects and side-effects when used in GD and TAO. Scant evidence, originating from only a few methodologically inhomogeneous studies, suggests that RTX may prolong remission for hyperthyroidism over that seen with antithyroid drugs, at least in mild GD. Furthermore, in patients with TAO, who are unresponsive to conventional immunosuppressive therapy, RTX seems efficacious. As we wait for larger-scale randomized studies, RTX, should be considered experimental and reserved for patients who do not respond favourably to conventional therapy. It is the first in what is likely to be a series of new and emerging treatments specifically targeting relevant components of the immune system. Further studies will hopefully

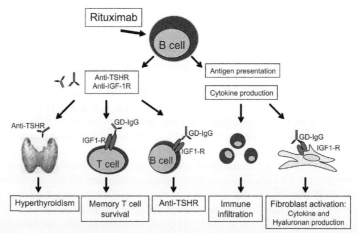

FIGURE 1.—The multifaceted role of B cells in Graves' disease (GD). Rituximab specifically eliminates peripheral CD20⁺ B cells. B cells produce autoantibodies to the TSHR and IGF-1R, which leads to hyperthyroidism and potentially fibroblast activation. B and T cells from Graves' patients display increased expression of the IGF-1R and activation of this receptor via GD-IgG enhances B-cell autoantibody production and T-cell survival. Furthermore, B cells are excellent antigen-presenting cells and produce cytokines which may be central to immune infiltration and the exuberant inflammatory response demonstrated in patients with GD. (Reprinted from Hegedüs L, Smith TJ, Douglas RS, et al. Targeted biological therapies for Graves' disease and thyroid-associated ophthalmopathy. Focus on B-cell depletion with Rituximab. *Clin Endocrinol.* 2011;74:1-8, with permission from Blackwell Publishing Ltd.)

lead to improved and better tailored, individualized therapy for GD and especially TAO (Fig 1).

▶ This article nicely summarizes our current knowledge on how rituximab works to treat thyroid-associated ophthalmopathy (TAO) and is worth reading. The depletion of B lymphocytes by rituximab seems to be the mechanism, as the presentation of antigens by the B lymphocyte is important in the immune reaction in TAO (Fig 1). It is important to remember that this therapy at this point is not a mainstream therapy. With further studies, its usefulness will become clear. I doubt that rituximab will be the final medication that is used for the treatment of TAO. There are many more potential medications on the horizon that target a specific area of the immune process.

R. B. Penne, MD

Rituximab for thyroid eye disease
Silkiss RZ, Reier A, Coleman M, et al (California Pacific Med Ctr, San Francisco)
Ophthal Plast Reconstr Surg 26:310-314, 2010

Purpose.—To assess the efficacy and safety of rituximab-mediated B-lymphocyte depletion as treatment for thyroid eye disease (TED).

Methods.—Prospective, open-label, interventional clinical trial evaluating 12 patients with TED and Clinical Activity Scores (CAS) (VISA [vision, inflammation, strabismus and appearance/exposure] classification) of 4 or greater followed for 1 year after rituximab (1000 mg) treatment, administered intravenously on days 1 and 15. CAS, peripheral B-lymphocyte levels, thyroid autoantibody levels, and thyroid function tests were recorded at baseline, 4 weeks, 8 weeks, 12 weeks, 24 weeks, 36 weeks, and 52 weeks after the second infusion. The primary endpoint was a change from baseline in CAS. Thyroid-stimulating immunoglobulin and thyroid-stimulating hormone levels were also monitored over the 12-month postinfusion observation period.

Results.—CAS scores demonstrated a statistically significant decrease from baseline at each of the follow-up visits. Thyroid-stimulating immunoglobulin and thyroid-stimulating hormone levels demonstrated no statistically significant change from baseline. B-cell depletion was observed within 1 month after rituximab treatment, and peripheral B-lymphocyte counts started to increase 36 weeks after the infusion. B-cell depletion was well tolerated, and there were no adverse effects of the rituximab infusions.

Conclusions.—CAS scores were significantly reduced over time in this group of 12 patients and appeared to be associated with rituximab infusion. The variable natural history of TED makes it difficult to definitively assign efficacy. The results support the continued investigation of rituximab for TED in a larger placebo-controlled trial.

▶ This is a small but exciting study showing efficacy of rituximab for the treatment of active thyroid eye disease (TED). This is a small number of patients (12), but they all had a positive response to rituximab without any significant side effects.

The move to try and target the immune mechanism of TED for treatment is exciting, and this seems to be a step toward preventing the scarring rather than treating the scarring after it has occurred. It needs to be emphasized that this is a small number of patients, and a larger study needs to be done before this should be considered for all patients. There still are issues in getting insurance companies to cover this treatment. The exact way that rituximab works is outlined in another article reviewed.[1] However, this appears to be an alternative to radiation, steroids, and surgery that have promise for the treatment of TED. Targeted immune therapy for TED is a hope for treatment that may offer prevention and intervention before there is significant deformity and dysfunction of the ocular tissues.

R. B. Penne, MD

Reference

1. Hegedüs L, Smith TJ, Douglas RS, Nielsen CH. Targeted biological therapies for Graves' disease and thyroid-associated ophthalmopathy. Focus on B-cell depletion with Rituximab. *Clin Endocrinol.* 2011;74:1-8.

Wooden intraorbital foreign body injuries: clinical characteristics and outcomes of 23 patients
Shelsta HN, Bilyk JR, Rubin PA, et al (Jefferson Univ Hosp, Philadelphia, PA)
Ophthal Plast Reconstr Surg 26:238-244, 2010

Purpose.—To describe the clinical characteristics, interventions, and visual outcomes of orbital injuries associated with wooden foreign bodies.

Methods.—A retrospective case review of orbital injuries managed at Wills Eye Institute and Massachusetts Eye and Ear Infirmary was conducted between 1992 and 2006.

Results.—The clinical course and management for a total of 23 intraorbital wooden foreign body injuries were reviewed. The distribution of wood included pencil (39%), tree branch/plant matter (35%), and other treated wood (26%). About half of the subjects (52%) presented with preoperative vision between 20/20 and 20/40. Almost all [corrected] of the subjects with preoperative vision between 20/20 to 20/40 retained vision in that range postoperatively (92%). [corrected] Time from injury to presentation was highly variable, ranging from 24 hours to 17 months (mean, 62 days; median, 3 days). Forty-three percent of subjects presented within 24 hours of injury. The site of foreign body found within the orbit was superior (26%; n = 6), medial 30% (n = 7), inferior (26%, n = 6), posterior (9%; n = 2), and lateral (4%; n = 1). Preliminary radiographic interpretation for foreign body was definite in 61% (n = 14), possible in 22% (n = 5), and absent in 13% (n = 3).

Conclusions.—Young men are at particularly high risk for wood intra-orbital foreign body. There was a relatively equal distribution of wood type. The time from injury to presentation was variable, ranging from <1 day to over a year. Almost half of the subjects presented within 24 hours of injury. In patients with a known site of penetration, almost half occurred in the conjunctiva, notably without presence of eyelid laceration, emphasizing the need to check the conjunctiva and fornices closely. Preliminary radiographic readings often miss or are inconclusive in detecting the foreign body. The shape, location, serial examinations, and particularly the use of quantitative CT are extremely helpful in distinguishing retained wood foreign body from other low-density signals of air or fat.

▶ This article reviews 23 cases of wooden intraorbital foreign bodies and makes recommendations for diagnosis and treatment. These cases are not common, which is seen from the fact that only 23 cases were found over 14 years in 3 busy oculoplastic practices.

The real point to be taken from these cases is you must always suspect a foreign body. If the presentation is such that a wooden foreign body is possible, then careful CT imaging must be done. An entrance wound may not be obvious, especially on the conjunctival surface. If the index of suspicion is high and the CT is not helpful, MRI may be helpful (do not do an MRI unless a CT has ruled out a metallic foreign body first). Finally, surgical exploration may be required to ultimately rule out a wooden foreign body.

Much of this urgency to diagnose and remove a wooden foreign body is because of the risk of infection. Organic material like wood can cause infection quickly or on a delayed basis. Removal lessens this risk, but empiric antibiotics when a foreign body is suspected should be used and be continued even after removal. Finally, wood is often splintered, so the patient and family need to be counseled pre- and postoperatively that there can be splinters left behind that can later cause an infection or require additional surgery for removal.

R. B. Penne, MD

Secondary intention healing in lower eyelid reconstruction – a valuable treatment option

Morton J (Whiston Hosp, Prescot, Merseyside, UK)
J Plast Reconstr Aesthet Surg 63:1921-1925, 2010

Secondary intention healing – or laissez-faire technique – is the first rung on the reconstructive ladder but may often be overlooked in favour of more elegant reconstructive options. Whilst the nose and medial canthus of eye have long been considered suitable sites for secondary intention healing, most plastic surgeons would hesitate to employ this technique with full-thickness lower eyelid wounds. There are currently no reports in the plastic surgery literature advocating its use, but the technique is gaining credence in the field of oculoplastics as a genuinely useful alternative to formal reconstruction.

Four cases are presented where tumours excised from the lower eyelid were allowed to heal by secondary intention. The largest involved 75% of the lid margin. All were elderly patients in whom formal reconstruction was either declined by the patient or considered unwise by the surgeon.

The cosmetic and functional results were quite remarkable, so much so that this technique demands serious consideration as a valuable treatment option, and quite possibly the treatment of choice in elderly or infirm

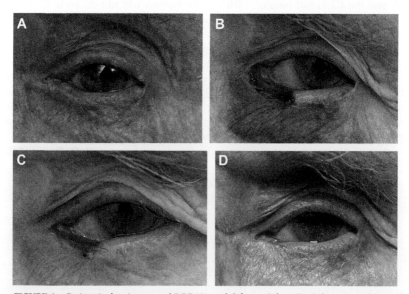

FIGURE 1.—Patient 1, showing punctal BCC (A), and defect at 2 days (B), 9 days (C), and 8 months (D). Note that in image B, at 48 h, the cut apex of the lid margin is seen falling away from the globe. (Reprinted from Morton J. Secondary intention healing in lower eyelid reconstruction – a valuable treatment option. *J Plast Reconstr Aesthet Surg.* 2010;63:1921-1925, copyright 2010, with permission from British Association of Plastic, Reconstructive and Aesthetic Surgeons.)

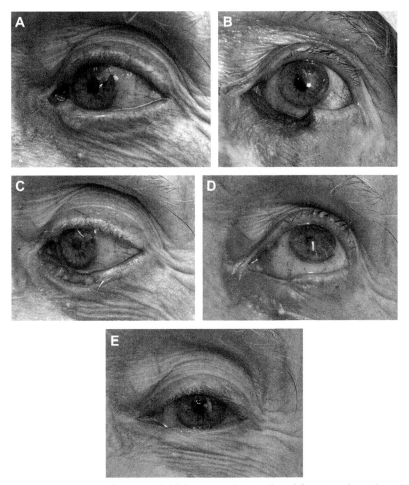

FIGURE 2.—Patient 2, showing medial lid BCC (A), the immediate defect (B), and at 6 days (C), 15 days (D), and 2 months (E). (Reprinted from Morton J. Secondary intention healing in lower eyelid reconstruction – a valuable treatment option. *J Plast Reconstr Aesthet Surg.* 2010;63:1921-1925, copyright 2010, with permission from British Association of Plastic, Reconstructive and Aesthetic Surgeons.)

patients whose tolerance of more complicated procedures may be limited (Figs 1-4).

▶ This article demonstrates 4 patients (Figs 1—4) with large defects that are left to heal by secondary intention. This was either because of patient preference or because of a medical condition that prevented safe surgical reconstruction. These patients had excellent cosmetic results after these large defects were allowed to heal without reconstruction.

This is a technique that is often forgotten with the rush to reconstruct all eyelid defects after tumor excision. The only concern I have is that if no

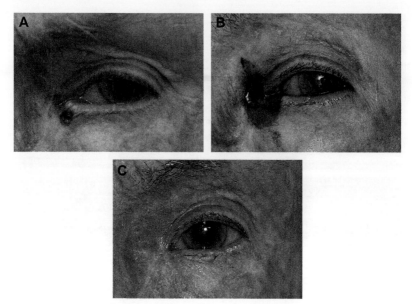

FIGURE 3.—Patient 3, showing the lesion (A), the immediate defect (B), and the result at 6 weeks (C). (Reprinted from Morton J. Secondary intention healing in lower eyelid reconstruction — a valuable treatment option. *J Plast Reconstr Aesthet Surg*. 2010;63:1921-1925, copyright 2010, with permission from British Association of Plastic, Reconstructive and Aesthetic Surgeons.)

reconstruction is attempted and the results are not ideal, the patient may always wonder what might have been if the defect was reconstructed. With careful and proper preoperative discussion, this technique should certainly be considered in select patients.

R. B. Penne, MD

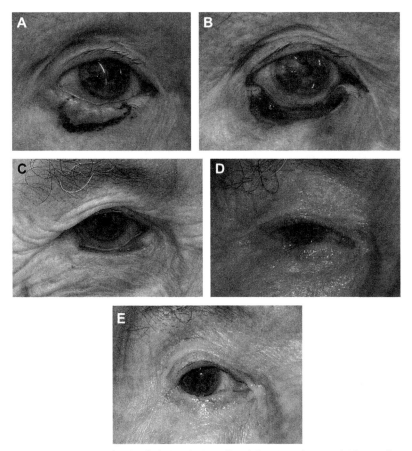

FIGURE 4.—Patient 4, showing the lesion (A), immediate defect (B), and at 1 week (C), 5 weeks (D) and 6 months (E). (Reprinted from Morton J. Secondary intention healing in lower eyelid reconstruction — a valuable treatment option. *J Plast Reconstr Aesthet Surg*. 2010;63:1921-1925, copyright 2010, with permission from British Association of Plastic, Reconstructive and Aesthetic Surgeons.)

Evaluation of homeopathic Arnica montana for ecchymosis after upper blepharoplasty: a placebo-controlled, randomized, double-blind study

Kotlus BS, Heringer DM, Dryden RM (Univ of Arizona Health Science Ctr, Tucson)
Ophthal Plast Reconstr Surg 26:395-397, 2010

Purpose.—Ecchymosis is commonly encountered after upper eyelid blepharoplasty. The use of homeopathic preparations of Arnica montana, a flowering herb, has been advocated by physicians, patients, and manufacturers for reduction of postsurgical ecchymosis. The authors evaluate its efficacy after upper eyelid blepharoplasty.

Methods.—A prospective, placebo-controlled, double-blind study was performed in which patients were randomly assigned to the administration of homeopathic A. montana or placebo concurrent with unilateral upper eyelid blepharoplasty followed by contralateral treatment at least 1 month later. Ecchymosis was evaluated at days 3 and 7 by rank order of severity and measurement of surface area of observable ecchymosis.

Results.—There was no statistically significant difference in area of ecchymosis or rank order of ecchymosis severity for days 3 and 7 after treatment with A. montana versus placebo. Additionally, there was no difference in ease of recovery per patient report, and there was no difference in the rate of ecchymosis resolution.

Conclusions.—The authors find no evidence that homeopathic A. montana, as used in this study, is beneficial in the reduction or the resolution of ecchymosis after upper eyelid blepharoplasty.

▶ The use of *Arnica montana* to lessen postoperative bruising is common, especially in cosmetic surgery. This prospective, placebo-controlled, double-blinded study showed no evidence that *A montana* lessens bruising after an upper lid blepharoplasty.

This study looked at 30 patients, each undergoing upper eyelid blepharoplasty, one lid at a time. The patients received *A montana* or placebo on the day of surgery and for 3 days after. A month later, the other eyelid was done, and the patient received arnica if they had received placebo, or vice versa. The patient was then evaluated with photos at day 3 and 7. The patient was also asked to rank which side was easier.

There was no statistical difference in the amount of ecchymosis, nor was there a difference in the rate of patient recovery as per the patients' report. Thus, there was no objective or subjective difference in the use of *A montana*. One interesting thing about this study is that all 30 patients were male. I am not sure why that was because more females than males undergo cosmetic surgery.

This is a simple, well-designed study that shows no value in the use of *A montana* in decreasing the post-operative bruising from upper eyelid blepharoplasty. Although this is a medication with low incidence of side effects, if it has no value, I will no longer be recommending this to any of my surgical patients.

R. B. Penne, MD

Eyelash Growth from Application of Bimatoprost in Gel Suspension to the Base of the Eyelashes
Wester ST, Lee WW, Shi W (Univ of Miami Miller School of Medicine, FL)
Ophthalmology 117:1024-1031, 2010

Objective.—To determine whether bimatoprost (Lumigan, Allergan Inc., Irvine, CA) causes increased lash length when used in gel suspension applied to the base of the eyelashes.

Design.—Randomized controlled trial.

Participants.—Nineteen subjects were enrolled.

Methods.—Subjects recruited from the Bascom Palmer Eye Institute were screened, and those who met inclusion criteria were enrolled. Each participant received 2 vials of gel suspension, which contained bimatoprost and normal saline, respectively, each mixed 1:1 with Gonak gel (Akorn Inc., Lake Forest, IL) and labeled "right eye" and "left eye" according to randomization. The suspension was applied to the upper eyelid eyelashes every evening on the designated eye for 6 weeks.

Main Outcome Measures.—Lash length was measured with a caliper at enrollment, at weekly intervals during the application of the gel, and at 1 and 3 months after discontinuation of its use. Visual acuity, ocular symptoms, intraocular pressure, and photographs were documented at these same intervals.

Results.—The mean eyelash growth from baseline in the bimatoprost group was 2.0 mm versus a mean of 1.1 mm in the placebo group, which was a statistically significant difference ($P = 0.009$). The average intraocular pressure decreased equally in both groups (2 mmHg). No change in visual acuity or iris discoloration was noted in any of the subjects.

Conclusions.—Our data showed an increase in eyelash length with the use of bimatoprost in gel suspension, suggesting the product's eyelash-lengthening properties (Fig 2, Table 2).

► This is a prospective, randomized, controlled, double-blinded study to evaluate bimatoprost effect on eyelash growth. This study had subjects apply Gonak with saline daily on the eyelashes of one eye and Gonak with bimatoprost to the eyelashes of the other eye. The patient and physician were blinded to which eye was receiving the medication. The lashes receiving bimatoprost grew an average of 2 mm over 6 weeks. Just as interesting, however, is the fact that the lashes receiving Gonak and saline grew an average of 1.1 mm over 6 weeks. Finally, the improvement in lash length did not change 6 weeks after stopping the treatment.

There were 2 remarkable findings in this simple well-done study. The expected was that bimatoprost applied to eyelashes daily results in eyelash growth. This is the first study done with one eye receiving the drug and the other a placebo to demonstrate this. What was not expected is that the control eyes showed eyelash growth of 1.1 mm over 6 weeks as well. It is not clear why the application of Gonak and saline would result in eyelash growth. The authors speculate this could be because of eyelash hydration.

Latisse, the commercially available drug to lengthen eyelashes, is a solution. This study used this solution (they used Lumigan) mixed with Gonak, which is 2.5% hydroxypropyl methylcellulose. In Allergan's study of Latisse, they found a 1.4 mm growth of eyelashes from baseline and only 0.1 mm growth in the controls. Remember, these controls were receiving as solution and not as gel as in this study.

This study confirms that bimatoprost, commercially available as Latisse, when applied daily to eyelashes causes growth of eyelashes. It appears that applying

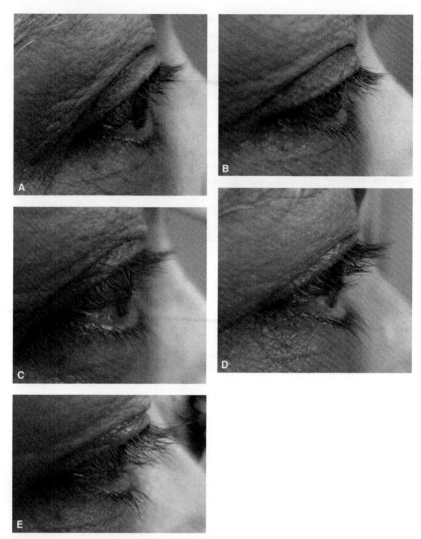

FIGURE 2.—Pictures demonstrating lash growth in subject 6 at several study intervals. A, Pre-study photograph. B, Two weeks after treatment. C, Three weeks after treatment. D, Five weeks after treatment. E, Three months after cessation of treatment. (Reprinted from Wester ST, Lee WW, Shi W. Eyelash Growth from Application of Bimatoprost in Gel Suspension to the Base of the Eyelashes. *Ophthalmology.* 2010;117:1024-1031, Copyright 2010, with permission from the American Academy of Ophthalmology.)

just 2.5% hydroxypropyl methylcellulose results in moderate eyelash growth. Although the gel containing bimatoprost was not compared with the solution containing bimatoprost (Latisse), the study suggests that a gel containing bimatoprost, which is not commercially available, would give additional eyelash growth over the solution. Finally, 6 weeks after stopping the medication, the

TABLE 2.—Change in Eyelash Length

| | Bimatoprost Group | | | Control Group | | | | |
	N	Changes (Mean ± SD)	P Value	N	Changes (Mean ± SD)	P Value	Mean Difference ± SD	P Value*
Changes from baseline to cessation of gel application (6 wks)	15	2.0±1.5	<0.001	15	1.1±1.1	0.001	0.9±1.1	0.009
Changes from baseline to 1 mo after cessation	13	1.9±1.3	<0.001	13	1.0±1.1	0.009	0.9±1.2	0.013
Changes from baseline to 3 mos after cessation	15	1.9±1.2	<0.001	15	0.8±1.2	0.017	1.1±0.7	<0.001
Changes from cessation of gel application to 3 mos after cessation	15	−0.1±0.6	0.58	15	−0.3±0.7	0.09	0.2±1.0	0.39

SD = standard deviation.
*Paired *t* test.

eyelashes were still long. How long it takes for them to return to pretreatment length is not answered in this article.

R. B. Penne, MD

Factors prompting sneezing In intravenously sedated patients receiving local anesthetic injections to the eyelids

Morley AM, Jazayeri F, Ali S, et al (Queen Victoria Hosp, East Grinstead, UK)
Ophthalmology 117:1032-1036, 2010

Purpose.—To investigate the frequency of sneezing among patients receiving intravenous sedation and periocular local anesthetic for oculoplastic procedures in a single center. To identify potential risk factors involved.

Design.—Prospective, consecutive, interventional case series in a single tertiary-referral oculoplastic unit.

Participants.—A total of 294 patients undergoing 314 isolated oculoplastic procedures, performed under intravenous sedation with periocular local anesthetic from November 2007 to November 2008.

Methods.—Prospective data collection on patient demographics, history of photic sneezing, intravenous sedative, depth of sedation, nasal oxygen, and periocular infiltration site. Standard local anesthetic was used in all cases, but the intravenous sedation was at the discretion of the attending anesthesiologist (7 in total).

Main Outcome Measures.—Sneezing or attempted sneezing within 5 minutes of injection of the local anesthetic, as determined by agreed observation between attending staff.

Results.—Sneezing was observed in 16% of cases. No association was found between sneezing and patient age or presence of nasal oxygen. A weakly positive association was observed with male gender (55% sneezers vs. 37% non-sneezers, P = 0.03, relative risk [RR] = 1.5, confidence interval [CI], 1.1-2.0), bilateral infiltration (65% vs. 40%, P = 0.005, RR = 1.6, CI, 1.2-2.1), and upper eyelid infiltration (73% vs. 54%, P = 0.01, RR = 1.4, CI, 1.1-1.7). Photic sneezing was described in 47% of sneezers and 19% of non-sneezers (P = 0.0004, RR = 2.6, CI, 1.6-4.0). Because propofol was given to 95% of patients, no association with sneezing could be ascertained. However, opioid derivatives were found to be protective (12% vs. 43%, P<0.0001, RR = 0.3, CI, 0.1-0.6), whereas midazolam doubled the risk of sneezing (45% vs. 22%, P = 0.0008, RR = 2.1, CI, 1.4-3.0). Deep sedation (Ramsay score 5-6) also strongly increased the sneeze risk (65% vs. 23%, P<0.0001, RR = 2.8, CI, 2.1-3.8).

Conclusions.—Propofol-based intravenous sedation, in combination with periocular local anesthetic injections, induces sneezing in approximately one sixth of general oculoplastic cases. Male gender, a history of photic sneezing, bilateral or upper eyelid infiltration, deep sedation, and the concurrent administration of midazolam all increased the risk, whereas adjunctive opioid use reduced the risk.

▶ This is a prospective, consecutive, interventional case study looking at the incidence of and factors promoting sneezing in patients undergoing oculoplastic surgical procedures under sedation. The article is interesting, but its big value is to raise awareness of this sneezing reflex associated with local eyelid injection and sedation. Despite previous articles about this phenomenon, it still does not seem to be commonly recognized in the anesthesia world and even among non-oculoplastic ophthalmologists. I was surprised it was found in 16% of the 314 procedures that were included in the study. This percentage seemed high to me from my experience.

The factors that seem to be associated with sneezing are the use of propofol for sedation, bilateral eyelid injections and upper lid injections, and a deeper level of sedation. As other articles have suggested, a narcotic such as fentanyl being given with the sedation decreased the chance the patient would sneeze during the injection of local anesthesia.

For me, this has never been a big problem. When you are aware this can happen you can recognize the patient is about to sneeze. This generally happens soon after sedation is given and when the local is being injected. The patient will make a few brief inhalational sniffs, move their head slightly, and then will sneeze. Simply stopping the injection, holding pressure on the injection site while the patient sneezes is all that needs to be done. It is rare that the patient sneezes more than 2 to 3 times.

R. B. Penne, MD

Utilization patterns for the diagnostic imaging in the evaluation of epiphora due to lacrimal obstruction: a national survey
Nagi KS, Meyer DR (Albany Med College, NY)
Ophthal Plast Reconstr Surg 26:168-171, 2010

Purpose.—To evaluate current physician patterns for diagnostic lacrimal imaging in patients with epiphora related to lacrimal obstruction. *Methods.*—An invitation was sent to members of the American Society of Ophthalmic Plastic and Reconstruction Surgeons in September 2008 to participate in a short web-based questionnaire. The survey focused on basic demographic information and the use and indications for various types of diagnostic imaging modalities in the evaluation of epiphora. Specific imaging modalities queried included facial x-ray, lacrimal ultrasound, CT, MRI, contrast dacryocystography, and radionuclide dacryoscintigraphy. Responses were analyzed using standard statistical methods. *Results.*—Less than 5% of respondents use lacrimal imaging of any type for the majority of their patients with epiphora thought due to lacrimal obstruction. When lacrimal imaging was used, CT was the most common type overall. CT was the preferred modality for all indications surveyed when an imaging modality was elected, except when confirming the site or type of obstruction in which case dacryocystography was preferred. Excluding CT, a majority of respondents indicated that they "never" (0%) used any of the specific lacrimal imaging studies surveyed, including dacryoscintigraphy, which was never used by over 75% of respondents. *Conclusions.*—The low overall imaging rate suggests that most lacrimal problems are diagnosed with office testing alone. For most specific indications, respondents indicated a preference for CT. No difference in imaging frequency was found for the majority of our respondents when considering external versus endonasal dacryocystorhinostomy. Most respondents favored external approach dacryocystorhinostomy.

▶ This article is a survey of oculoplastic surgeons regarding how they evaluate lacrimal obstruction. This specifically looked at the use of x-ray, CT, MRI, dacryocystography (DCG), dacryoscintigraphy (DSG), and lacrimal ultrasound. It is important to realize that this is not a guide for how to treat individual cases, but the survey does seem to indicate that some of the traditional tests that are still being taught as part of evaluating a patient with tearing may rarely be used by the average busy oculoplastic surgeon.

The survey found that less than 5% of responding physicians routinely use lacrimal imaging of any type on a routine basis. DCG and DSG were rarely used. Eighty-six percent of respondents said they never or rarely used DCG, and 91% never or rarely used DSG. These tests that are taught to our residents as part of lacrimal testing are very seldom used in practice. CT scan is the most common imaging used if there is concern about a mass or when the obstruction is associated with trauma.

I know in my practice I have not done a DCG for 8 or 9 years and have never used a DSG. This is partially because it is not readily available, and with time I have found very little information was gained, in my hands, from these tests. Others may practice differently, but it appears that most lacrimal obstructions are diagnosed based on lacrimal irrigation. In patients with blood from the lacrimal system or other reasons to suspect a lacrimal sac malignancy, then a CT or MRI is the imaging of choice to evaluate the lacrimal sac.

R. B. Penne, MD

A Modified Schirmer Test in Dry Eye and Normal Subjects: Open Versus Closed Eye and 1-Minute Versus 5-Minute Tests
Kashkouli MB, Pakdel F, Amani A, et al (Iran Univ of Med Sciences, Tehran)
Cornea 29:384-387, 2010

Objective.—To assess the results of 1-minute and 5-minute Schirmer test (ST) when eyes are open (STo) and closed (STc) in normal subjects and patients with dry eye disease.

Methods.—In a comparative, observational case series study, 34 normal volunteers (group 1) and 34 patients with dry eye disease (DED) associated with Sjogren syndrome (group 2) were included in the study. STo and STc for 1 minute and 5 minutes were performed separately for all subjects with an interval of at least 24 hours using Whatman No. 41 (5×60 mm) with bended end of the paper inserted into the lateral side of the lower conjunctival fornix.

Results.—In group 1, there were 19 females and 15 males with a mean age of 20.8 years (range 18 to 23 years). In group 2, there were 29 females and 5 males with a mean age of 53.7 years (range 35 to 75 years). Mean value of STc was significantly less than STo in both 1 minute and 5 minutes in both groups. One-minute STo and STc showed significantly less wetting than the 5-minute test in both healthy and patients with DED. Normal distribution was observed for all the values. A significant correlation between 1-minute and 5-minute tests in both STo and STc were found in the two groups. Therefore, two equations were proposed to calculate the 5-minute from 1-minute ST in each group. Statistical analysis did not provide a reliable equation for calculating the standard ST (5-minute STo) from the most comfortable state (1-minute STc).

Conclusion.—Faster and more comfortable ST (1-minute) is a reliable test to calculate the 5-minute ST in both open and closed eyes, using the provided equations. The 1-minute STc is not a reliable test to calculate the 5-minute STo.

▶ The value of Schirmer testing for the evaluation of tear function remains debatable. This study looks at the correlation between 5-minute and 1-minute Schirmer tests with the eyes open and closed. Previously, studies had suggested that a 1-minute Schirmer test multiplied by 3 was equal to the 5-minute Schirmer test. The results showed good correlation between the 1-minute and 5-minute Schirmer tests with eyes open or closed, but there was no good correlation between the 5-minute Schirmer test with opened eye and 1-minute Schirmer test with closed eye.

I believe that Schirmer testing is one objective measurement of tear function, and I do perform it prior to eyelid surgery. Not all oculoplastic surgeons use this or find it of value prior to eyelid surgery. I use a 1-minute Schirmer test with the eyelids open and multiply that number by 3. Even though this study does not find this conversion to be accurate and offers a more complicated formula, it seems to work in my practice. As has been seen in other studies of tear function, Schirmer testing is only one part of evaluating lacrimal function.

R. B. Penne, MD

Blink Lagophthalmos and Dry Eye Keratopathy in Patients with Non-Facial Palsy: Clinical Features and Management with Upper Eyelid Loading
Patel V, Daya SM, Lake D, et al (Queen Victoria Hosp, East Grinstead, UK)
Ophthalmology 118:197-202, 2011

Purpose.—To evaluate the outcome of using upper eyelid gold weight implantation for patients with non-paralytic lagophthalmos on blink (LOB) only. We highlight the features of incomplete blink and reduced blink rate in patients with non-facial palsy as an exacerbating factor in dry eye keratopathy.

Design.—Retrospective, noncomparative case series.

Participants.—Twelve patients (21 procedures) who underwent upper eyelid gold weight implantation for non-paralytic LOB only.

Methods.—Retrospective case note review of patients who underwent upper eyelid loading for non-paralytic LOB only over a 5-year period at a single institution.

Main Outcome Measures.—Improvement in LOB, gentle and forced closure, increased frequency of blinking (FOB), degree of corneal staining, incidence of epithelial defects or corneal ulcer, improvement in vision, and subjective improvement in ocular discomfort.

Results.—Twenty-one procedures in 12 patients. Nine patients underwent bilateral surgery. Mean age was 56 (range, 8—80) years. Median postoperative follow-up was 15 months, and mean follow-up was 20.38 ± 16.61 (6—58) months. Eleven of 12 patients had an improvement in LOB and increased FOB, resulting in improvement of keratopathy and reduced ocular discomfort. One patient developed superior corneal thinning and descemetocele, requiring removal of the gold weight; 1 patient required ptosis surgery; and 1 patient developed a gold allergy and underwent platinum chain exchange.

Conclusions—We highlight the need to consider incomplete blink and reduced FOB as exacerbating factors for corneal-related disorders, including dry eye. Upper eyelid loading with gold weight implantation is

TABLE 1.—Patient Demographics and Preoperative Morbidity

Patient	Case	Age (yrs)	Disease	Side	Previous Ocular Surface Surgery	Previous Adnexal Surgery	Best-corrected Preoperative Visual Acuity	Corneal-related Complications (Other than Punctate Keratopathy)	Further Surgery after Upper Eyelid Loading (Months after Surgery)
1	1a	8	Chromosomal abnormality 46XY	R	Tectonic graft	Lateral tarsorrhaphy	U	Perforation, MK	Upper lid pretarsal skin graft (6)
	1b			L			U		
2	2a	71	Dry eye	R	n	Lateral tarsorrhaphy	U		Platinum chain exchange for gold allergy (6)
	2b			L		Plug	6/9		
3	3a	80	Dry eye	R	n	Plug	6/9		
	3b			L	n	Plug	U		
4	4	47	SJS	R	EVSCALT	Cautery, dacryocystectomy	U / CF	PED, MK	Upper fornix reconstruction with inferior turbinate mucosal graft (3)
5	5	11	Congenital glaucoma with nodular keratopathy	R	Epithelial keratectomy with AMT	n	CF		
6	6a	77	Bullous keratopathy	R	PK	n	6/19	MK	
	6b			L	n		6/12		
7	7	50	SJS	R	PK; PK + KEP; LRCLAL, DLK; phaco/IOL, DLK + AMT, EVSCALT + AMT	n	Multiple lid procedures for trichiasis, including cryotherapy and resection > 200; entropion (Weis) and cryotherapy 120; lateral tarsorrhaphy, upper lid mm graft 60	HM	PED, MK	Removal of weight because of superior thinning (2)
8	8a	39	SJS	R	n	Cautery	6/12		
	8b			L	n	Cautery	6/7.5		
9	9a	73	OCP	R	n	Cautery	6/60	PED/MK	
	9b			L	n	Cautery	6/9		Ptosis repair (6)

10	10a	60	Dry eye	R	n	n	6/7.5	
	10b			L	n	n	6/6	
11	11a	78	Dry eye	R	n	Plugs	6/9	
	11b			L	n	Plugs	6/6	
12	12a	76	OCP	R	n	Plugs	HM	Corneal melt
	12b			L	n	Plugs	6/9.5	Corneal melt

AMT = amniotic membrane transplant; cautery = punctal cautery; CF = counting fingers; DLK = deep lamellar keratoplasty; EVSCALT = ex vivo expanded corneal allograft; HM = hand movements; IOL = intraocular lens; KEP = keratoepithelioplasty; KLAL = keratolimbal allograft; L = left; LRCLAL = living-related conjunctival limbal allograft; MK = microbial keratitis; mm = mucous membrane; n = no previous surgery; OCP = ocular cicatricial pemphigoid; PED = persistent epithelial defect; plugs = punctal plugs; PK = penetrating keratoplasty; R = right; SJS = Stevens–Johnson Syndrome; U = unable to record visual acuity.

TABLE 2.—Outcome Measures at 3-Month Follow-up

	Before Gold Weight Implantation N = 21 Cases	After Gold Weight Implantation at 3-Month Follow-up
Mean logMAR VA	0.79	0.77
Mean LOB (mm)	3.47 (1–7)	0.57 (1–3)
Mean lagophthalmos on gentle closure (mm)	0.76 (0–5)	0.095 (0–1)
Mean lagophthalmos on forced closure (mm)	0.19 (0–2)	0.14 (0–2)
Upper MRD	3.42 (2–5)	3.29 (1–4)

LOB = lagophthalmos on blink; logMAR = logarithm of the minimum angle of resolution; MRD = marginal reflex distance; VA = visual acuity.

a useful and predictive method of improving exposure-related keratopathy due to LOB in the absence of facial palsy (Tables 1 and 2).

▶ This article offers a potential treatment for a difficult subset of patients with dry eyes and corneal exposure secondary to an incomplete blink. These patients generally have dry eye and/or other ocular surface issues, but these issues are made worse by a blink that only covers the superior part of the cornea and at a less frequent blink rate. In this article, the implantation of gold weights in the upper eyelids resulted in an improvement in all patients in lagophthalmos on blinking, frequency of blink, keratopathy, and a subjective improvement in vision and ocular discomfort.

This is a promising treatment for these difficult patients. It is important to emphasize that all medical treatments for this problem should be tried first. For those patients who continue to have significant exposure, this is a treatment that offers hope for improvement.

R. B. Penne, MD

A Randomized Controlled Trial Comparing Everting Sutures with Everting Sutures and a Lateral Tarsal Strip for Involutional Entropion

Scheepers MA, Singh R, Ng J, et al (Charing Cross and Western Eye Hosp, London, UK)
Ophthalmology 117:352-355, 2010

Objective.—To determine whether there is a statistically significant difference in the surgical outcome of everting sutures (ES) alone versus everting sutures with a lateral tarsal strip (ES+LTS) in the treatment of involutional entropion.

Design.—Prospective randomized comparative trial.

Participants.—Sixty-three patients with primary involutional lower eyelid entropion were enrolled in the study. The age range was 54 to 94 years, with a mean age of 77 years. Baseline characteristics of the comparative groups were similar.

Methods.—Patients requiring primary surgical repair for involutional entropion were selected, and those providing informed consent were randomized for surgery. Thirty-six patients were randomized to ES alone, and 27 patients were randomized to ES+LTS. Patients were evaluated at 3 weeks and 6, 12, and 18 months postoperatively.

Main Outcome Measures.—Successful surgery was defined as a normal eyelid position at rest and inability to induce entropion on tetracaine provocation testing at or before the 18-month follow-up visit.

Results.—Eight patients were lost to follow-up (7 had ES alone). Of the 55 patients with complete follow-up data, there were 6 failed procedures in the patients who underwent ES alone and no failed procedures in the patients who underwent ES+LTS ($P = 0.02$).

Conclusions.—These data provide strong evidence that success rates at 18 months are higher in patients treated with ES+LTS procedure compared with ES alone.

▶ This is a randomized trial comparing everting sutures (ES) alone versus everting sutures plus a lateral tarsal strip (ES + LT) for correction of involutional entropion. This is a simple well-done study that confirms what is generally taught about entropion surgery. ES are a temporary way to address an involutional entropion, and ES + LT is a treatment that is more likely to be permanent.

It was slightly surprising that there were no cases where the entropion recurred using ES + LT, but the follow-up was 18 months, which is not a long time when looking for entropion recurrence. The recurrence for ES alone was 21%, which is generally what is taught. That number will likely be higher with longer follow-up.

This is a nice study that provides a basis for our clinical approach to an entropion. If at all possible, ES + LT is preferred as the chance of recurrence is lower. If medical conditions and the use of anticoagulation prevent this, then the use of ES provides a short-term surgical treatment, and it will last longer in a moderate number of patients.

R. B. Penne, MD

Long-term Outcomes of Surgical Approaches to the Treatment of Floppy Eyelid Syndrome

Ezra DG, Beaconsfield M, Sira M, et al (Moorfields Eye Hosp and UCL Inst of Ophthalmology, London, UK; Moorfields Eye Hosp NHS Foundation Trust, London, UK; Western Eye Hosp, London, UK)
Ophthalmology 117:839-846, 2010

Objective.—To identify and describe the different procedures used in the treatment of floppy eyelid syndrome (FES) at Moorfields Eye Hospital and to evaluate their effectiveness.

Design.—Cross-sectional study.

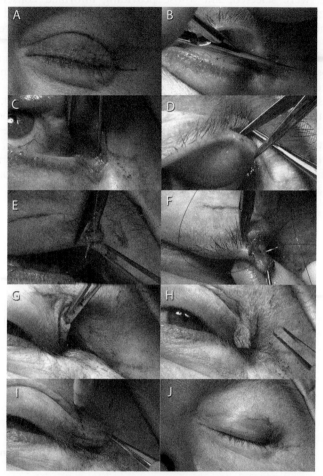

FIGURE 1.—Upper lid LTS procedure. **A,** Upper lid skin crease is marked. "Crows feet" are also marked to guide the incision and allow it to be disguised in one of these preexisting skin creases. The degree of laxity is assessed, and a vertical mark is placed perpendicular to the lid margin, indicating the extent to which the tarsus is to be shortened. **B,** Lateral cantholysis of the upper limb of the LC tendon is performed by cutting down onto the lateral orbital rim periosteum. **C,** Lateral orbital wall periosteum is exposed, and the tarsus is mobilized from its LC attachment. **D,** Upper lid is shortened, and the remaining lateral aspect of the upper lid tarsal plate (posterior lamella) is separated from the orbicularis and skin (anterior lamella). **E,** Eyelid margin together with its resident pilosebaceous components are excised. **F,** Lateral tarsal strip is fashioned and secured with a 6-0 nonabsorbable suture. **G,** Tarsal strip is then sutured down onto the periosteum of the lateral orbital wall at the level of Whitnall's tubercle. **H,** Tarsal strip is secured. Note how the unshortened anterior lamella is now "dog eared." **I,** Redundant skin is marked to allow the scar to run into the upper lid skin crease to minimize any disfiguring incision scars. **J,** Final result with a secured upper lid and skin incision disguised in the skin creases. LTS = lateral tarsal strip. (Reprinted from Ezra DG, Beaconsfield M, Sira M, et al. Long-term outcomes of surgical approaches to the treatment of Floppy eyelid syndrome. *Ophthalmology.* 2010;117:839-846, copyright © 2010, with permission from the American Academy of Ophthalmology.)

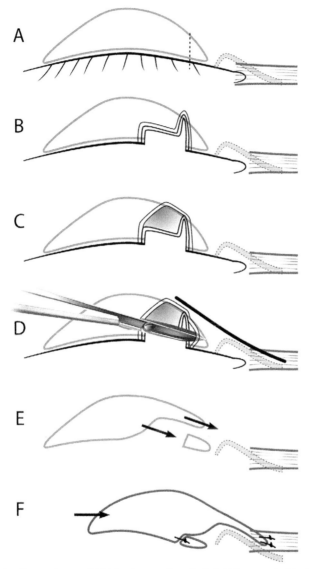

FIGURE 2.—Illustrated upper lid MC strip procedure. **A,** Full-thickness vertical incision is made lateral to the lacrimal punctum. **B,** Assessment of the amount of shortening required is made. A 3-mm high full-thickness strip of required length is then excised from the lid margin, creating a strip of tarsus superiorly. **C,** Anterior lamellar pentagon is fashioned around the defect. **D,** Lacrimal probe is placed to protect and identify the canaliculus. The anterior and posterior lamellae of the medial lid remnant are divided, and a medial skin crease incision is made extending over the MC tendon. **E,** Superior strip of tarsus is advanced into the incision toward the MC tendon, and the medial tarsal remnant is approximated to the lateral end. **F,** Medial strip apex is sutured to the MC tendon. The approximated tarsal ends are also sutured together. MC = medial canthus. (Reprinted from Ezra DG, Beaconsfield M, Sira M, et al. Long-term outcomes of surgical approaches to the treatment of Floppy eyelid syndrome. *Ophthalmology.* 2010;117:839-846, copyright © 2010, with permission from the American Academy of Ophthalmology.)

TABLE 1.—Details of Failures and Follow-up Time by Surgical Procedure

Procedure	Cases	Failures	Mean Time to Failure/mos (SD)	Resolved	Resolved Cases Mean Follow-up Time/mos (SD)	Mean Follow-up Time of All Cases/mos (SD)
FTWE N = 26						
Total cases	33	20	8.1 (4.9)	13	9.8 (9.4)	8.7 (6.9)
		60.6%	Range 0–17		Range 2–29	Range 0–29
Unilateral cases	19	12	6.4 (4.7)	7	13.6 (11.1)	9.1 (8.1)
			Range 0–14		Range 2–29	0–29
Bilateral cases	14	8	10.5 (4.6)	6	5.3 (4.4)	8.3 (5.1)
			Range 4–17		Range 2–12	Range 2–17
LTS N = 31						
Total cases	43	11	15.8 (9.6)	32	34.2 (32.6)	29.5 (29.5)
		25.6%	Range 1–26		Range 2–131	Range 1–131
Unilateral cases	19	6	19.7 (8.4)	13	50.3 (41.3)	40.6 (37.1)
			Range 3–26		Range 4–131	Range 3–131
Bilateral cases	24	5	11.2 (19.7)	19	23.2 (19.3)	20.6 (18.2)
			Range 1–23		Range 2–55	Range 1–55
MC/LC plication N = 15						
Total cases	19	9	18.4 (14.6)	10	87.6 (49.6)	54.8 (50.8)
		47%	Range 2–42		Range 30–136	Range 2–136
Unilateral cases	11	5	16 (13.1)	6	90.6 (46.3)	56.7 (49.6)
			Range 2–36		Range 2–135	Range 2–135
Bilateral cases	8	4	21.5 (17.9)	4	83 (61.2)	52.3 (53.1)
			Range 2–42		Range 30–136	Range 2–136
MC strip N = 6						
Unilateral only	6	2	7 (9.9)	4	25.5 (24.4)	19.3 (21.6)
		33.3%	Range 0–14		Range 1–57	Range 0–57

LC = lateral canthus; LTS = lateral tarsal strip; FTWE = full-thickness wedge excision; MC = medial canthus; SD = standard deviation.

Participants.—A total of 71 patients who had undergone surgery for FES over a 13-year period since 1995 at Moorfields Eye Hospital were recruited. Retrospective data from 7 patients were also included, providing data for 78 patients.

Methods.—Patients underwent a full ocular examination. A survival analysis was determined by plotting Kaplan–Meier curves for each type of procedure encountered. Comparison of survival trends was made using a log-rank test. The possible effects of bias arising from bilaterality of the condition were investigated using a sensitivity analysis and a Cox regression analysis allowing for clusters. Tests for surgeon bias were made using the Fisher exact test.

Main Outcome Measures.—Recurrence of the condition. An assessment of recurrence was made clinically by 2 independent observers who were masked to the type of surgery the patient had undergone.

Results.—Four different forms of surgical treatment were encountered: (1) Full-thickness wedge excision (FTWE) (26 patients, 33 procedures); (2) Upper lid lateral tarsal strip (LTS) (31 patients, 43 procedures); (3) Medial canthal (MC) and lateral canthal (LC) plication (15 patients, 19 procedures); (4) Medial tarsal strip (6 patients, 6 procedures). A total of 44 of 101 procedures had failed. Superior long-term survival outcomes of both LC/MC plication ($P = 0.003$) and upper lid LTS ($P = 0.001$)

procedures over FTWE was demonstrated. However, survival comparison between the LC/MC plication and LTS groups did not achieve significance ($P = 0.37$). No significant difference in outcome between surgeon groups of equivalent experience was demonstrated ($P = 0.18$). No bias arising from bilaterality of the condition was identified.

Conclusions.—These data provide strong evidence of better survival outcomes in FES using the MC/LC plication and LTS procedures in comparison with the FTWE procedure. On the basis of experience from our unit, we recommend that the FTWE procedure be avoided as a form of treatment for FES in favor of the MC/LC plication, LTS, or medial tarsal strip procedure (Figs 1 and 2, Table 1).

▶ Floppy eyelid syndrome (FES) is generally a surgical disease that requires shortening of the upper eyelid(s) to improve the symptoms. There are a number of ways to tighten the upper eyelid including full-thickness wedge excision (FTWE) (26 patients, 33 procedures), upper lid lateral tarsal strip (31 patients, 43 procedures) (Fig 1), medial canthal (Fig 2) and lateral canthal plication (15 patients, 19 procedures), and medial tarsal strip (6 patients, 6 procedures). This article shows that FTWE has a higher failure rate (Table 1) and one of the other 3 procedures should be used. I have traditionally used FTWE for FES, but this article will change that, and I will try one of the other 3 procedures.

R. B. Penne, MD

Orbital solitary fibrous tumor: encompassing terminology for hemangiopericytoma, giant cell angiofibroma, and fibrous histiocytoma of the orbit: reappraisal of 41 cases

Furusato E, Valenzuela IA, Fanburg-Smith JC, et al (Armed Forces Inst of Pathology, Washington, DC; Armed Forces Inst of Pathology/Inova Fairfax Hosp, Falls Church, VA; et al)
Hum Pathol 42:120-128, 2011

Hemangiopericytomas and solitary fibrous tumors are uncommon neoplasms found in many locations, including the orbit. Both mesenchymal neoplasms share several clinicopathologic features, thus prompting intense debate as to whether they are variants of the same entity or merit separate designations in the orbit. These 2 entities, with the addition of giant cell angiofibroma of orbit, are of benign- to uncertain-behavior, CD34-positive, collagen-rich, specialized fibroblastic tumors, which may have overlapping or histologically identical features. In addition, so-called fibrous histiocytoma of orbit, a previous designation, has overlapping morphologic features with these tumors. To date, a large series of these collagen-rich fibroblastic tumors of the orbit has not been fully explored. Forty-one fibroblastic orbital tumors, originally diagnosed as hemangiopericytomas (n = 16), fibrous histiocytomas (n = 9), mixed tumors (hemangiopericytomas/fibrous histiocytoma) (n = 14), and giant cell angiofibromas of orbit (n = 2) between 1970 and 2009, were retrieved from our consultation files, the Ophthalmic Registry, at the Armed Forces Institute of Pathology. Slides and clinical records were reviewed, analyzed, and compared. Immunochemistry was performed for CD34, CD99, Bcl-2, Ki-67, and p53. Upon histologic review, all cases were reclassified as solitary fibrous tumor (41/41). The patients included 23 (56%) males, 17 (41%) females, and 1 unknown, with a mean age at presentation of 40.7 years (range, 16-70 years). The sites of involvement were the right orbit in 18 (44%) cases and the left in 16 (39%) cases. Tumors ranged in size from 0.4 to 5.0 cm (mean, 2.2 cm). Seventeen (41%) patients presented with an orbital mass, 8 (20%) with proptosis, 2 (5%) with painful mass, and 2 (5%) with painless mass. Duration of symptoms ranged from 3 to 96 months, with a mean of 23 months (median, 9 months). Microscopically, all lesions showed considerable similarity, varying in degree of cellularity, stromal collagen, and the presence of giant cells. Overlapping features with soft tissue giant cell fibroblastoma were observed. Immunochemistry revealed positivity for CD34 in all cases (100%), p53 in 85%, CD99 in 67.5%, and Bcl-2 in 47.5%. Although Ki-67 labeling was seen in all cases, it ranged from less than 1% in 54.3% of cases to 5% to 10% in 20% of cases. Taken together, the findings of this study suggest that orbital hemangiopericytoma and some cases previously designated as fibrous histiocytoma, giant cell angiofibroma of orbit, and solitary fibrous tumor have overlapping morphologic and immunohistochemical features and should be designated as solitary fibrous tumor. Adipocytes and unusual multivacuolated adipocytic cells may be present in these tumors, as well stromal myxoid change; and even stromal intramembranous ossification can be observed. There are overlapping features of orbital solitary fibrous tumor with another CD34-positive specialized fibroblastic tumor of soft tissue, giant cell fibroblastoma. Morphologic criteria for uncertain behavior to low-grade malignant ocular solitary fibrous tumors can be made by cytologic atypia and increased mitotic activity, but overall outcome for malignant solitary fibrous tumors of the eye should be further explored.

▶ All the tumors looked at in this study are rare tumors. This article is significant because much of the clinical information we have about hemangiopericytoma, giant cell angiofibroma, and fibrous histiocytoma of the orbit may be misleading, as the pathologic diagnosis was not correct. Now that we have special stains, we are better able to categorize these tumors. Many of these tumors may have been solitary fibrous tumors. This already very confusing group of tumors has become easier to diagnose pathologically, but this has put into question all the clinical information we have about these tumors and about solitary fibrous tumors. Over time, this improved ability to make the correct pathologic diagnosis will make our knowledge about these tumors more accurate. However, for now we need to realize clinical information about these individual tumors and how they act may not be entirely accurate.

R. B. Penne, MD

The efficacy, sensitivity, and specificity of in vivo laser confocal microscopy in the diagnosis of meibomian gland dysfunction
Ibrahim OM, Matsumoto Y, Dogru M, et al (Keio Univ School of Medicine, Tokyo, Japan)
Ophthalmology 117:665-672, 2010

Purpose.—To evaluate the efficacy, sensitivity and specificity of confocal microscopy (CM) parameters: meibomian gland (MG) acinar longest diameter (MGALD), MG acinar shortest diameter (MGASD), inflammatory cell density (ICD), and MG acinar unit density (MGAUD) in the diagnosis of MG dysfunction (MGD).

Design.—Prospective, controlled, single-center study.

Participants.—Twenty MGD patients (9 males, 11 females; mean age, 63.5 ± 16.5 years) and 26 age- and gender-matched control subjects (13 males, 13 females; mean age, 53.2 ± 15.7 years) were recruited.

Methods.—All subjects underwent slit-lamp examinations, tear film break-up time (BUT) measurements, assessment of tear evaporation rate from the ocular surface (TEROS), vital stainings, Schirmer test, meibography, MG expressibility, and CM of the MG. Data were compared between the 2 groups using the Mann-Whitney and chi-square tests.

Main Outcome Measures.—The correlation between the clinical findings of tear functions, vital staining scores, and the 4 CM parameters were tested by Spearman's correlation coefficient by rank test. Receiver operating characteristic curve technique was used to evaluate the sensitivity, specificity, and cutoff values of CM parameters.

Results.—The mean tear film BUT, vital staining scores, TEROS values, MG expressibility, and MG dropout grades by meibography were significantly worse in MGD patients compared with controls ($P<0.001$). The mean values of the MGALD, MGASD, ICD, and MGAUD in MGD patients were significantly worse than those observed in the controls with CM. All CM parameters showed a strong, significant correlation with tear functions, ocular surface vital stainings, MG expressibility, and MG dropout grades. The cutoff values for MGALD, MGASD, ICD, and MGAUD in the diagnosis of MGD were 65 microm, 25 microm, 300 cells/mm2, and 70 glands/mm2, respectively. The sensitivity and specificity values of these parameters under these cutoff values were 90% and 81% for MGALD, 86% and 96% for MGASD, 100% and 100% for ICD, 81% and 81% for MGAUD.

Conclusions.—Confocal microscopy has the potential to diagnose the simple MGD with high sensitivity and specificity. The CM-based diagnostic parameters correlated significantly and strongly with the status of the ocular surface disease.

▶ This article is an important foundation for objective evaluation of meibomian gland dysfunction (MGD) and blepharitis. In the past, there has been very little science behind the treatment of blepharitis. Blepharitis is a common disease, and more and more we find that it not only causes redness and irritation of the eyelids but also affects vision. We have multiple potential treatments, none of which work for everyone. For as common a disease as blepharitis is, there has never been a high degree of science behind its diagnosis or treatment. We have very little information about how to evaluate treatment at a tissue level. We don't even have good information about how improving meibomian gland (MG) function affects the ocular surface.

Laser confocal microscopy is a technique for obtaining high-resolution optical images with depth selectivity. It has been used to evaluate the cornea for years. The unique feature of confocal microscopy is its ability to acquire in-focus images from selected depths, a process known as optical sectioning.

The information in this article demonstrates measurable in vivo laser confocal microscopy parameters (MG size, density, and inflammatory cell density) in MGD that appear to correlate with traditional measurements of ocular surface disease (tear film break-up time, vital staining scores, tear evaporation rate, MG expressibility, and MG dropout). I doubt laser confocal microscopy will ever become a practical clinical tool, but it may become a standard in the research into effective treatment for MGD. It hopefully is one of many future advances that can be made in the science of blepharitis. The next step will be to see if clinically successful treatment will reverse the tissue changes that have been identified.[1] That will then set the stage for treatment trial of various medications we use for blepharitis to evaluate their effectiveness.

There is a lot to be learned not only about the cause of blepharitis and MGD but also about its treatment. I don't think confocal microscopy will be the only or last objective way to evaluate MGD. It is encouraging to see real science becoming a part of this common disease, which can be very frustrating to treat. I believe that is the greatest aspect of this article. Hopefully in the future, this will lead to better understanding of blepharitis as well as better and more specific ways to treat this disease.

R. B. Penne, MD

Reference

1. Matsumoto Y, Shigeno Y, Sato EA, et al. The evaluation of the treatment response in obstructive meibomian gland disease by in vivo laser confocal microscopy. *Graefes Arch Clin Exp Ophthalmol.* 2009;247:821-829.

Effectiveness of Low-Voltage Radiofrequency in the Treatment of Xanthelasma Palpebrarum: A Pilot Study of 15 Cases
Dincer D, Koc E, Erbil AH, et al (Gulhane School of Medicine, Keçiören, Ankara, Turkey)
Dermatol Surg 36:1973-1978, 2010

Background.—Xanthelasma palpebrarum (XP) is the most common form of xanthoma, which is mostly located on the eyelids. Various treatment options are available, with certain limitations, and none of them is satisfactory.

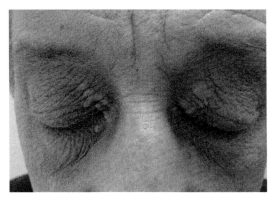

FIGURE 1.—Before treatment. (Reprinted from Dincer D, Koc E, Erbil AH, et al. Effectiveness of low-voltage radiofrequency in the treatment of xanthelasma palpebrarum: a pilot study of 15 cases. *Dermatol Surg.* 2010;36:1973-1978, with acknowledgement of Blackwell Publishing.)

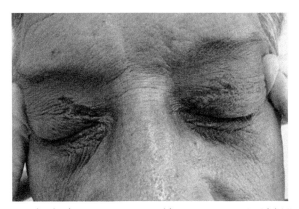

FIGURE 2.—Immediately after treatment. (Reprinted from Dincer D, Koc E, Erbil AH, et al. Effectiveness of low-voltage radiofrequency in the treatment of xanthelasma palpebrarum: a pilot study of 15 cases. *Dermatol Surg.* 2010;36:1973-1978, with acknowledgement of Blackwell Publishing.)

Objectives.—To offer another treatment option (low-voltage radiofrequency (RF)) and to evaluate its efficacy in XP.

Methods.—Fifteen patients were included in the study. The patients were examined before treatment, at the end of treatment, and 5 months later at a follow-up visit. Improvement was judged according to clinical examination by comparing before and after photographs. Electrodes from a dual-frequency 4.0-MHz RF machine were applied superficially to the lesions. The clinical scores were calculated using a 5-point scale (0 — no result, 0–25% = mild, 26–50% = moderate, 51–75% = good, 76–100% = excellent).

Results.—All participants completed the study. Of these, scores of nine patients were excellent, scores of five were good, and the score of one was

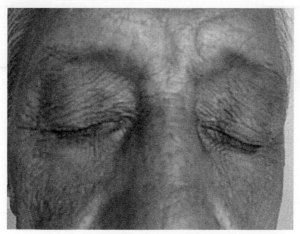

FIGURE 3.—Five months after treatment. (Reprinted from Dincer D, Koc E, Erbil AH, et al. Effectiveness of low-voltage radiofrequency in the treatment of xanthelasma palpebrarum: a pilot study of 15 cases. *Dermatol Surg.* 2010;36:1973-1978, with acknowledgement of Blackwell Publishing.)

moderate. Statistically significant percentage improvement of the clinical scores from baseline was seen at the end ($p < .05$).

Conclusion.—Low-voltage RF treatment of XP is effective. If the lesions are too close to the eyes or are multiple or patched with indistinct borders, low-voltage RF can be used (Figs 1-3).

▶ Xanthomas are fairly common lesions that have had many different modalities suggested for treatment, including surgical excision, chemical peels, and laser. I have always advocated that because of the depth of these lesions, surgical excision is best. This article presents a simple alternative that can be done under topical anesthesia using the Ellman radiofrequency unit. The results were generally good (Figs 1 and 3). Three of the 15 patients required retreatment because the lesion was not completely gone. Two patients had hyperpigmentation after treatment and 1 had hypopigmentation.

This treatment leaves a skin defect where the lesion was, which will take some time to heal (Fig 2). I believe surgical excision, if possible, is still the treatment of choice. This does offer an alternative for patients with lesions that are too large to excise or are on anticoagulants that cannot be stopped. There still is a chance of skin contraction and an ectropion as these areas heal.

R. B. Penne, MD

7 Pediatric Ophthalmology

Exotropic drift and ocular alignment after surgical correction for intermittent exotropia
Leow PL, Ko ST, Wu PK, et al (Hong Kong Island Cluster Ophthalmology Service, The People's Republic of China)
J Pediatr Ophthalmol Strabismus 47:12-16, 2010

Purpose.—To evaluate changes in the angle of deviation over time and compare the motor success rate with different initial postoperative deviation in patients undergoing surgical correction for intermittent exotropia.

Methods.—Forty-eight patients aged between 1 and 10 years who underwent bilateral lateral rectus recession for intermittent exotropia were retrospectively evaluated. Preoperative and postoperative ocular deviations at 1 week, 1 month, and 6 months were analyzed. Full surgical correction was attempted in all patients. Motor success was defined as ocular deviation within 10 prism diopters of orthophoria at 6 months postoperatively.

Results.—The follow-up period ranged from 6 months to 3 years. Although most patients had exotropic drift, this drift was greater in patients with initial esotropia (86.7%) and orthophoria (70.0%) compared to patients with exotropia (26.1%). Motor success was achieved in 29 (60.4%) patients. There was no statistical difference between ocular alignment at 1 week postoperatively and final motor success (P = .782). There was good correlation between ocular alignment at 1 week and 6 months postoperatively (rho = 0.585, P < .001). Age and preoperative deviation were not found to be associated with motor success.

Conclusions.—The success rate appears to be unaffected by initial ocular alignment, suggesting that deliberate initial overcorrection may be unnecessary. Future studies are warranted to evaluate the long-term stability of this alignment.

► Many pediatric ophthalmologists have been trained with the understanding that an initial postoperative exotropia of 10 to 20 prism diopters following surgical correction for intermittent exotropia is a desirable initial outcome. This recommendation was suggested to apparently reduce the possibility of subsequent recurrence of exotropia. However, pediatric ophthalmologists who do unilateral recession for exotropia with a successful long-term outcome may not always find an initial esotropia. Therefore, the success rate for surgery for intermittent exotropia appears to be unaffected by the initial postoperative alignment. Further studies need to be performed to evaluate what, if any, desirable initial postoperative alignment following surgical correction for intermittent exotropia results in the best long-term stability of the alignment.

L. B. Nelson, MD, MBA

An analysis of neonatal risk factors associated with the development of ophthalmologic problems at infancy and early childhood: a study of premature infants born at or before 32 weeks of gestation
Saldir M, Sarici SU, Mutlu FM, et al
J Pediatr Ophthalmol Strabismus 47:331-337, 2010

Background.—To determine the frequency of ophthalmologic problems and the risk factors that affect the occurrence of these problems in premature newborns with a gestational age of 32 weeks or less.

Methods.—Premature newborns observed at a neonatal intensive care unit between January 2002 and March 2006 were included. A control visit including an ophthalmologic examination was performed at 10 months of age or later. Primary ocular morbidities were studied, and the association between these parameters and prenatal, perinatal, and neonatal characteristics were evaluated.

Results.—A total of 169 premature newborns were included in the study, and they were examined at a mean age of 25.85 ± 11.79 months (range: 10 to 42 months). There was complete vision loss (blindness) in 1 (0.6%) case, strabismus in 15 (8.9%) cases, and refractive errors in 10 (5.9%) cases. Twenty (77%) cases with any abnormality and 50 (35%) cases with a normal examination at follow-up had a history of retinopathy of prematurity (ROP) at any stage during the neonatal period (P = .001). Short gestational age (P = .018), low birth weight (P = .002), and the presence of ROP requiring retinal surgery during the neonatal period (P = .007) were determined to be significant risk factors for the development of vision loss, strabismus, and refractive errors.

Conclusion.—Neonates with a gestational age of 32 weeks or less, especially those younger than 30 weeks, should not only be screened for ROP in the neonatal period, but should also have regular follow-up examinations to check for the development of other ophthalmologic problems during infancy and early childhood.

▶ The authors emphasize the importance of regular follow-up of premature infants for the ophthalmologic problems during early childhood. Retinopathy of prematurity is the primary ocular disorder that the ophthalmologist must screen for in the neonatal period. However, it seems that there is a higher incidence of strabismus and refractive errors that develop in premature infants during early childhood. These ocular disorders are more commonly found in neonates with a gestational age of younger than 30 weeks. Both strabismus and refractive errors can have a profound effect on the visual outcome of these premature infants. Therefore, regular and careful ophthalmologic follow-up in these infants is a necessity. It is also important that the parents or guardians of these premature infants are advised of the possibility of these ocular disorders that may develop so that they realize the importance of follow-up ocular examinations for their children.

L. B. Nelson, MD, MBA

Outpatient treatment of periocular infantile hemangiomas with oral propranolol
Haider KM, Plager DA, Neely DE, et al (Indiana Univ School of Medicine, Indianapolis)
J AAPOS 14:251-256, 2010

Background.—Propranolol has recently been reported to be useful in the treatment of infantile hemangiomas. However, there are still many questions regarding the dosage, duration, and method of delivery.

Methods.—In this retrospective, observational case series, all patients had complete eye examinations and were found to have vision-threatening hemangiomas. All patients had a baseline electrocardiogram. Outpatient, oral propranolol therapy was initiated between 3 weeks and 12 months of age. The dosage was slowly increased to 2 mg/kg daily over the course of 1-2 weeks. Response to therapy was deemed "excellent" (>50% reduction in size), "good" (decreased size but <50%), "fair" (no further growth), or "poor" (continued growth or intolerable adverse effects).

Results.—A total of 17 patients were treated with oral therapy. Of these, 10 had excellent results, 6 had a good response, 1 fair, and none poor. Mild adverse effects were noted in 6 of the 17 patients and included the following: increased gastric reflux lasting 1 week, intermittent fatigue during the first 2 weeks, gastrointestinal upset, and slight "shakiness" with a missed dose. No symptoms were severe enough to discontinue treatment. All families were satisfied with the treatment.

Conclusions.—Outpatient propranolol treatment reduced the size or stopped the growth of all hemangiomas treated, with excellent response in more than half of all patients treated and only minor side effects. Although this is a small initial series, we are encouraged with the efficacy of this treatment modality in comparison with other currently available treatment options.

▶ The number of reports using oral propranolol for the treatment of capillary hemangiomas in infancy has escalated since the initial report. Propranolol treatment should be administered by pediatric ophthalmologists in consultation with primary care physicians to ensure safe and effective treatment. Although the authors provided a protocol for treatment with propranolol, they do not define care standards, so it remains unclear when to initiate therapy, assess therapy, adjust dosage, and stop or discontinue the treatment. Further studies using propranolol to successfully treat capillary hemangiomas will elucidate these questions that remain in the treatment.

L. B. Nelson, MD, MBA

Outcome study of unilateral lateral rectus recession for small to moderate angle intermittent exotropia in children
Wang L, Nelson LB (Wills Eye Inst, Philadelphia, PA)
J Pediatr Ophthalmol Strabismus 47:242-247, 2010

Purpose.—To report an outcome study of 100 consecutive children with intermittent exotropia treated by unilateral rectus recession for small to moderate angle exodeviation with a minimum follow-up of 6 months.

Methods.—The records of patients with intermittent exotropia younger than 15 years who underwent 7-to-10-mm unilateral lateral rectus recession for exodeviation measuring 15 to 35 prism diopters (PD) from January 2000 to July 2008 were retrospectively reviewed. The surgery were performed accordingly to the amount of distance deviation. A successful alignment was defined as an exodeviation of 5 PD or less and absence of any esotropia in primary and lateral gaze while viewing distant or near targets.

Results.—Successful alignment was achieved in 99%, 88%, and 76% of patients at early postoperative, 6-month, and final follow-up, respectively. One overcorrected patient had an esodeviation of 20 PD at 6 months. The results of the final follow-up did not depend on age or refraction at the level of 0.05, whereas the amount of initial exodeviation was found to be significantly correlated with success at the final examination (P = .041). There was a positive significant relationship between results at 6 months and final follow-up (P = .000, r = 0.449). Eleven of the 13 patients who had a second surgery and were observed more than 6 months had successful alignment. Eighty-nine percent of the patients achieved a successful outcome with the combined primary and secondary surgery at the final follow-up.

Conclusion.—Unilateral lateral rectus recession is a safe and effective treatment for small to moderate angle intermittent exotropia in children.

▶ Unilateral lateral rectus muscle recession is a safe and effective method of treating small to moderate angle of exotropia. This technique avoids the necessity of operating on both eyes, leaves other muscles available if further surgery is necessary, and shortens the anesthesia time for the patient. Larger recessions on the lateral rectus that have been performed in the past will need to be done. Clinically significant lateral incomitance has not been demonstrated when the patients are followed long term.

L. B. Nelson, MD, MBA

Prevalence of Eye Disease in Early Childhood and Associated Factors: Findings from the Millennium Cohort Study

Cumberland PM, for the Millennium Cohort Study Child Health Group (Univ College London (UCL), UK)
Ophthalmology 117:2184-2190, 2010

Purpose.—To report the prevalence and distribution of eye conditions and visual impairment and associations with early social and biological factors using parental report of diagnosed eye conditions and additional chronic illnesses.

Design.—Population-based, cross-sectional study.

Participants.—We included 14 981 children, aged 3 years, participating in the United Kingdom Millennium Cohort Study.

Methods.—Data on demographic, socioeconomic, and maternal and child health factors were obtained by maternal report through structured interview and verbatim reports of diagnosed eye problems and additional chronic illnesses were recorded. Multinomial regression analyses were used to calculate risk ratios of the association of eye disease (with or without associated visual impairment), with socioeconomic and early life factors.

Main Outcome Measures.—Parental report of diagnosed eye conditions and other chronic illnesses.

Results.—Overall, at 3 years, 5.7% (95% confidence interval, 5.2–6.3%; n = 881) of children had ≥1 eye condition with 0.24% (0.15–0.3%; n = 45) reported to have associated visual impairment. In the majority, time of onset was reported to be the first year of life. Eye disorders without report of visual impairment were independently associated with lower socioeconomic status, decreasing birth weight, and prematurity. Visual impairment was more likely in those of low birthweight for gestational age and from an ethnic minority group. Maternal illnesses during pregnancy were associated with eye disease without reported visual impairment, as was white ethnicity.

Conclusions.—Good research opportunities exist within the context of population-based general health surveys to use parental report to estimate minimum prevalence, investigate associations of eye disease with a broad range of environmental factors, and as a mechanism for "flagging" individuals with eye disease in a population sample for further study. Our findings regarding the association of parentally reported childhood eye disease with early life factors such as modest degrees of prematurity, ethnicity and maternal ill-health warrant further investigation.

▶ Eye diseases, many with associated visual impairment, are common in children and make it a necessity to have adequate vision screening programs. For instance, amblyopia occurs in approximately 2% of the general population and because it is asymptomatic warrants appropriate testing of vision in young children. While low birth weight and prematurity increase the incidence of ocular disorders in children, the authors do not adequately explain why lower socioeconomic status produces similar results. I was also surprised that parents who were surveyed were able to report a broad range of ocular disorders with accurate medical terminology.

L. B. Nelson, MD, MBA

Termination of amblyopia treatment: when to stop follow-up visits and risk factors for recurrence
De Weger C, Van Den Brom HJ, Lindeboom R
J Pediatr Ophthalmol Strabismus 47:338-346, 2010

Background.—This study estimated when it is safe to stop follow-up visits after cessation of amblyopia treatment and to identify factors associated with deterioration of visual acuity.

Methods.—Study patients included 282 patients aged 7 to 13 years who were monitored for deterioration after cessation of amblyopia treatment (median follow-up: 3.9 years).

Results.—Six (2.1%) patients lost 2 or more logarithm of the minimum angle of resolution levels of visual acuity and 77 (27.3%) patients lost 1 or more Snellen lines of visual acuity. Good compliance with re-treatment stopped further deterioration and lost visual acuity was regained (average follow-up after re-treatment: 3.3 years). Life table analysis indicated that 95% of the cases that deteriorated occurred within 24 months after cessation of treatment. Multivariable analysis corrected for duration of treatment uncovered factors independently associated with deterioration.

Conclusion.—A clinically important risk of deterioration of visual acuity was found during the first 2 years after cessation of amblyopia treatment. Follow-up time longer than 2 years is recommended in the presence of a developing risk factor such as increasing anisometropia. With prompt re-treatment and good compliance, deterioration can be stopped and visual acuity can be restored.

▶ Most pediatric ophthalmologists consider the sensitive period of visual development to end at approximately 9 years of age. It is at that time that amblyopia treatment is usually discontinued. Some pediatric ophthalmologists will temporarily discontinue amblyopia treatment prior to age 9 if the visual acuity in the amblyopic eye improves significantly. In patients whose amblyopia treatment was discontinued at age 9, commonly, the visual acuity decreases a line or perhaps two subsequently. This is similar to the authors' findings. The drop-off in the visual acuity in the amblyopic eye also typically decreases when treatment is discontinued prior to age 9. Most of the time, the visual acuity will improve again once treatment is reinstated. It may be better to maintain some form of patching prior to age 9, as it often becomes a difficult compliance issue to reinstate patching. Ultimately, children with amblyopia whose patching is discontinued need to have a careful follow-up.

L. B. Nelson, MD, MBA

Long-term Changes in Refractive Error in Patients with Accommodative Esotropia

Park K-A, Kim S-A, Oh SY (Sungkyunkwan Univ School of Medicine, Seoul, Korea; Sungmo Eye Hosp, Pusan, Korea)
Ophthalmology 117:2196-2207, 2010

Purpose.—To evaluate changes in the spherical equivalent (SE) refractive error and astigmatism in Korean patients with accommodative esotropia.

Design.—Retrospective cases series.

Participants.—A total of 111 patients with accommodative esotropia who received at least 2 years of follow-up after receiving prescription spectacles.

Methods.—Patients were divided into groups according to the age at which spectacles were prescribed (youngest, middle, and oldest age groups), initial degree of SE refractive error (lowest, moderate, and highest SE group), initial degree of astigmatism (least, moderate, and most astigmatic group), and presence of amblyopia (amblyopic or nonamblyopic). Changes in SE refractive error and astigmatism were compared between groups. Factors that significantly influenced changes in refractive error were analyzed using mixed linear models.

Main Outcome Measures.—Changes in SE refractive error and changes in astigmatism according to the duration of time after the initiation of wearing spectacles.

Results.—Patients were followed up for a mean of 7.55 ± 3.59 years. Although an initial increase in SE was noted in the youngest-age group, an overall decreasing tendency in SE refractive error during the follow-up period was noted in the youngest ($P < 0.01$, mixed linear model), the middle ($P < 0.01$), and the oldest ($P < 0.01$) age groups. Amblyopic eyes showed greater decreases in SE compared with nonamblyopic eyes ($P=0.01$). The most hyperopic group showed the greatest decrease in hyperopia over time ($P=0.01$). The initial degree of hyperopia ($P < 0.01$) and amblyopia ($P < 0.01$) showed significant associations with changes in SE refractive error. The initial degree of astigmatism ($P < 0.01$) showed a significant association with changes in astigmatism.

Conclusions.—Patients with accommodative esotropia showed a continuous decrease in SE refractive error over time. Changes in refractive error in patients with accommodative esotropia may be influenced by both spectacle wearing and amblyopia.

▶ Children with accommodative esotropia usually have a hyperopic refractive error that averages $+4.75D$. The hyperopic correction typically remains relatively stable until adolescence approaches when the refractive error tends to decrease. Many of these children whose hyperopic correction begins to decrease don't complain but will often begin looking over their glasses to improve their vision. The authors' finding that there was a greater decrease in hyperopia in amblyopic eyes compared with nonamblyopic eyes further supports the premise that careful attention to the possible changes in refractive error in these children needs to be documented. Parents of children with accommodative esotropia often find it puzzling when the ophthalmologist decreases the hyperopic correction to improve the vision.

L. B. Nelson, MD, MBA

Surgery for Esotropia Under Topical Anesthesia
Tejedor J, Ogallar C, Rodríguez JM (Hosp Ramón y Cajal, Madrid, Spain)
Ophthalmology 117:1883-1888, 2010

Purpose.—To compare a surgically adjusted dose of strabismus surgery using topical anesthesia in cooperative patients with dosage guidelines adapted to the surgeon's personal technique using sub-Tenon's anesthesia.

Design.—Randomized, controlled, single-site clinical trial.

Participants.—Sixty patients with nonparalytic, nonrestrictive esotropia who were cooperative for surgery under topical anesthesia.

Methods.—Twenty-eight patients were assigned to topical anesthesia, and 32 patients were assigned to sub-Tenon's anesthesia. Visual acuity, refraction, and deviation angle were determined in all patients preoperatively and postoperatively, and stereoacuity was measured postoperatively. Deviation angle was measured by simultaneous and alternate prism and cover test, and stereoacuity was measured using Randot circles (Stereo Optical Co., Chicago, IL). The amount of surgery under topical anesthesia was adjusted intraoperatively.

Main Outcome Measures.—The amount of surgery used in the 2 treatment groups (measured in millimeters and millimeter/degree of deviation angle) and 6-month motor and stereoacuity outcomes.

Results.—Patients in the topical group required 3.2 mm less surgery on average than those in the sub-Tenon's group (5.9 and 9.1 mm, respectively; 0.4 and 0.6 mm of recession/degree, respectively) ($P < 0.01$). Motor success (84% and 75%, respectively, $P=0.38$) and stereoacuity (339.6 and 323.9 arc seconds, respectively, $P=0.87$) at 6 months were similar in the 2 groups.

Conclusions.—Topical anesthesia requires a smaller amount of surgery and number of operated muscles to correct esotropia compared with classic surgery guidelines adapted to the surgeon's personal technique.

▶ Regardless of whether topical or sub-Tenon's infusion is used, using adjustable sutures technique in the operating room has its limitation. The main issue is that the alignment that is obtained after adjustment does not necessarily result in the final outcome. Often the anesthesia alters the extraocular muscles temporarily, which can impact the final result. It is unclear to me how the patients were assigned to each group. Were they randomized appropriately or was there a different process that could have introduced bias into the study? Why were the examiners masked in 84% of the topical group and 89% of the sub-Tenon's group and not 100%? Again an element of bias could have been introduced in the study.

L. B. Nelson, MD, MBA

Neonatal Dacryostenosis as a Risk Factor for Anisometropia
Piotrowski JT, Diehl NN, Mohney BG (Mayo Clinic and Mayo Foundation, Rochester, MN)
Arch Ophthalmol 128:1166-1169, 2010

Objective.—To determine whether there is a relationship between congenital nasolacrimal duct obstruction (CNLDO) and subsequent refractive error disorders in children.

Methods.—The medical records of children 5 years and younger diagnosed as having CNLDO between January 1, 2000, and December 31, 2007, were retrospectively reviewed.

Results.—Three hundred five consecutive children were diagnosed as having CNLDO at a median age of 12.3 months (range, 0.8 months to 4.8 years). Thirty children (9.8%) were diagnosed as having anisometropia with (n = 16) or without (n = 14) amblyopia at a median age of 19.2 months (range, 3.6 months to 7.4 years). Twentysix of the 30 patients had hyperopic anisometropia; more severe hyperopia occurred in the eye with CNLDO in 23 patients (88.5%), 2 patients had more severe hyperopia in the fellow eye, and 1 patient had bilateral CNLDO. The median initial ($P = .005$) and final ($P < .001$) refractive error was significantly more hyperopic in those with both CNLDO and anisometropia compared with those with CNLDO alone.

Conclusions.—The development of anisometropia with or without amblyopia seems to be more frequent in children examined by an ophthalmologist for CNLDO compared with that reported for the general public. The laterality of more severe hyperopia and amblyopia is generally on the side of the previous dacryostenosis.

▶ This article further supports the premise that children who present with the classic clinical symptoms or signs of a congenital nasolacrimal duct obstruction (NLDO) should be refracted. Because NLDO is such a common ocular condition, it is not surprising that other ophthalmic findings can and do occur. Because 13% of the children in this study were premature, it would have been interesting to know what percent of these children had anisometropia. Premature infants, especially those that are of a very low birth weight, tend to have a higher percentage of myopia than nonpremature infants. If many of the children who had anisometropia and NLDO were premature, then there may have been a biased slant to the study.

L. B. Nelson, MD, MBA

Simultaneous vs Sequential Bilateral Cataract Surgery for Infants With Congenital Cataracts: Visual Outcomes, Adverse Events, and Economic Costs

Dave H, Phoenix V, Becker ER, et al (Emory Univ, Atlanta, GA)

Arch Ophthalmol 128:1050-1054, 2010

Objectives.—To compare the incidence of adverse events and visual outcomes and to compare the economic costs of sequential vs simultaneous bilateral cataract surgery for infants with congenital cataracts.

Methods.—Retrospective review of simultaneous vs sequential bilateral cataract surgery for infants with congenital cataracts who underwent cataract surgery when 6 months or younger at our institution.

Results.—Records were available for 10 children who underwent sequential surgery at a mean age of 49 days for the first eye and 17 children who underwent simultaneous surgery at a mean age of 68 days ($P = .25$). We found a similar incidence of adverse events between the 2 treatment groups. Intraoperative or postoperative complications occurred in 14 eyes. The most common postoperative complication was glaucoma. No eyes developed endophthalmitis. The mean (SD) absolute interocular difference in logMAR visual acuities between the 2 treatment groups was 0.47 (0.76) for the sequential group and 0.44 (0.40) for the simultaneous group ($P = .92$). Payments for the hospital, drugs, supplies, and professional services were on average 21.9% lower per patient in the simultaneous group.

Conclusions.—Simultaneous bilateral cataract surgery for infants with congenital cataracts is associated with a 21.9% reduction in medical payments and no discernible difference in the incidence of adverse events or visual outcomes. However, our small sample size limits our ability to make meaningful comparisons of the relative risks and visual benefits of the 2 procedures.

▶ In this relatively small series, the authors found no cases of endophthalmitis or a difference in other serious ocular or systemic complications in either group. The incidence of these complications is relatively small, so it is not surprising that the authors did not find these complications to be present. The authors suggested that the increased risk of general anesthesia is an important reason to perform simultaneous versus sequential surgery. However, the authors did not discuss the fact that longer anesthetic procedures in infants can increase anesthetic mortality. Therefore, the authors need to address the anesthetic risk of 1 longer procedure versus 2 shorter procedures. The use of different equipment and rescrubbing between eyes does not totally eliminate the risk of endophthalmitis that, while rare, could happen in simultaneous surgery and overshadow any long-term cost saving from this surgical approach.

L. B. Nelson, MD, MBA

Dietary Factors, Myopia, and Axial Dimensions in Children

Lim LS, Gazzard G, Low Y-L, et al (Singapore Eye Res Inst, Republic of Singapore; Singapore Inst for Clinical Sciences, Republic of Singapore)
Ophthalmology 117:993-997, 2010

Purpose.—To evaluate the possible associations between dietary factors and myopia.

Design.—Cross-sectional study.

Participants.—Eight hundred fifty-one Chinese schoolchildren from the Singapore Cohort Study of Risk Factors for Myopia.

Methods.—Diet was assessed using a semiquantitative food-frequency questionnaire. Spherical equivalent (SE) refraction was assessed with an autorefractometer, and axial length (AL) by contact ultrasound A-scan biometry.

Main Outcome Measures.—Myopia was defined as SE$\leq$−0.5 diopters (D). Spherical equivalent and AL were analyzed by quartile groups.

Results.—The mean age (± standard deviation) was 12.81 ± 0.83 years, approximately half were male (422 children [49.6%]), and 653 (73.8%) children had myopia. In multivariate models, AL was longest in the highest quartile group of total cholesterol intake compared with the lowest (adjusted mean [95% confidence interval], 24.66 [24.62−24.71] mm vs. 24.32 [24.27−24.36] mm; $P = 0.026$, for trend) and was longest in the highest quartile group of saturated fat intake compared with the lowest (24.65 [24.60−24.70] vs. 24.36 [24.32−24.41] mm; $P = 0.039$, for trend). None of the nutrients was associated with SE or a diagnosis of myopia.

Conclusions.—Higher saturated fat and cholesterol intake are associated with longer AL in otherwise healthy Singapore Chinese school children.

▶ Besides the lifetime financial costs of myopia and common childhood avoidance of wearing glasses, there are potential ocular pathologic consequences of myopia. While many pediatric ophthalmologists continue to believe that genetics play the dominant role in the development of myopia, whether environmental factors such as diet influence myopia progression remains unclear. One of the main limitations of this study is the authors' reliance on a questionnaire administered to children. Not only are questionnaires to children often unreliable, but to base the conclusion that the foods consumed by these children over the past month in which they were interviewed as a representation of this long-term diet is questionable. The authors also point out that the type of questionnaire used in this study has not been validated for children.

L. B. Nelson, MD, MBA

Longitudinal Postnatal Weight Measurements for the Prediction of Retinopathy of Prematurity

Wu C, VanderVeen DK, Hellström A, et al (Children's Hosp Boston, MA; Sahlgrenska Academy at Univ of Gothenburg, Göteborg, Sweden)
Arch Ophthalmol 128:443-447, 2010

Objective.—To validate longitudinal postnatal weight gain as a method for predicting severe retinopathy of prematurity (ROP) in a US cohort.

Methods.—Both ROP evaluations and weekly weight measurements from birth to postmenstrual week 36 for 318 infants were entered into a computer-based surveillance system, WINROP. This system signaled an alarm when the rate of weight gain decreased compared with control subjects. Infants were classified into 3 groups: (1) no alarm, (2) low-risk alarm, or (3) high-risk alarm. Maximum ROP for each infant was categorized as (1) no ROP (immature or mature vascularization), (2) mild ROP (stage 1 or 2 ROP in zone II or III, without plus disease), or (3) severe ROP (any prethreshold, any stage 3, or threshold ROP). A high-risk alarm identified infants at risk for developing severe ROP.

Results.—A high-risk alarm occurred in 81 infants (25.5%) and detected all infants who developed severe ROP a median of 9 weeks before diagnosis. The remaining infants received no alarm or a low-risk alarm. None of these infants developed more than mild ROP.

Conclusions.—Longitudinal postnatal weight gain may help predict ROP. In a US cohort, the WINROP system had a sensitivity of 100% and identified infants early who developed severe ROP. With further validation, WINROP has the potential to safely reduce the number of ROP examinations.

▶ Appropriate screening and timely detection and treatment of retinopathy of prematurity (ROP) give the premature infant the best chance of successful visual and structural outcome. Those premature infants with the earliest gestational age have a higher evidence of systemic complications. These infants tend to be the ones that have a greater chance of developing ROP. Morbidity may accompany the examination process of some of the younger more at-risk premature infants. The development of new approaches using postnatal risk factors may provide a protocol for determining which premature infants require more selective examinations and target those infants who may be at a greater risk of developing ROP that requires treatment. Whether the weight, insulin-like growth factor, neonatal ROP algorithm will be the approach that can provide these criteria remains unclear. Further studies using this method are necessary.

L. B. Nelson, MD, MBA

Incidence and clinical characteristics of childhood glaucoma: a population-based study

Aponte EP, Diehl N, Mohney BG (Mayo Clinic College of Medicine, Rochester, MN)

Arch Ophthalmol 128:478-482, 2010

Objective.—To describe the incidence and clinical characteristics of childhood glaucoma in a defined population of the United States.

Methods.—The medical records of all pediatric patients younger than 20 years living in Olmstead County, Minnesota, from January 1, 1965, through December 31, 2004, who met diagnostic criteria for glaucoma or glaucoma suspect were reviewed.

Results.—Thirty children were diagnosed as having glaucoma during the 40-year study period. The incidence of childhood glaucoma was 2.29 (95% confidence interval, 1.47-3.12) per 100,000 residents younger than 20 years, with the following types and incidences: 19 acquired (1.46/100,000; 0.80-2.12), 6 secondary (0.45/100,000; 0.08-0.82), and 5 primary glaucoma (0.38/100,000; 0.05-0.72). The birth prevalence of primary congenital glaucoma during the 40-year period was 1 per 68 254 residents younger than 20 years or 1.46 per 100,000 (95% confidence interval, 0.03-8.16). Twenty-four individuals with glaucoma suspect were also identified, yielding an incidence of 1.9 per 100,000 residents younger than 20 years (95% confidence interval, 1.14-2.66).

Conclusion.—The incidence of childhood glaucoma in this population was 2.29 per 100,000 residents younger than 20 years or 1 per 43 575 residents younger than 20 years. Acquired and secondary forms of glaucoma were the most common, whereas congenital and juvenile glaucoma were rare.

▶ Childhood glaucoma is an uncommon ocular condition that is rarely encountered by many pediatricians or general ophthalmologists. Unfortunately, this condition can cause significant visual impairment. The actual incidence of childhood glaucoma within the United States is not known. While the authors clearly documented the rarity of childhood glaucoma, it may be difficult to extrapolate their findings to the general population. The study was performed in a defined population of Olmsted County, a relatively homogenous semiurban white population. This population study does not represent the heterogeneity of the United States and may not accurately reflect the true incidence of childhood glaucoma.

L. B. Nelson, MD, MBA

Randomized Evaluation of Spectacles Plus Alternate-Day Occlusion to Treat Amblyopia

Agervi P, Kugelberg U, Kugelberg M, et al (Karolinska Institutet, Stockholm, Sweden; et al)
Ophthalmology 117:381-387, 2010

Purpose.—To compare spectacles plus patching ≥8 hours daily 6 days a week with spectacles plus patching ≥8 hours on alternate days to treat amblyopia in children 4 to 5 years of age.

Design.—Prospective, randomized clinical trial.

Participants.—Forty children (median age, 4.3 years) with untreated amblyopia and a median best-corrected visual acuity (BCVA) in the amblyopic eye of 0.9 (range, 0.3–1.5) logarithm of the minimum angle of resolution.

Methods.—Refractive correction was provided, and the children were randomized to patching ≥8 hours daily 6 days a week or patching ≥8 hours on alternate days. The BCVA, binocular function, and refractive errors were measured repeatedly during the study.

Main Outcome Measure.—Median change in BCVA of the amblyopic eye after 1 year.

Results.—The median change in BCVA of the amblyopic eye did not differ significantly between the 2 groups (0.6 log units for daily occlusion; 0.8 log unit for alternate-day occlusion). The final median BCVA in the amblyopic eyes was 0.1 logarithm of the minimum angle of resolution in both groups. Binocular function improved in both groups with no significant differences between the groups at 1 year. The median spherical equivalent refractive error did not change significantly during the study period in the amblyopic eyes in either group; however, a significant increase was found in the fellow eyes in both groups (daily occlusion, $P<0.05$; alternate-day occlusion, $P<0.001$).

Conclusions.—The magnitude of change in the BCVA 1 year after spectacles plus prescribed alternate-day patching was not significantly different than that after spectacles plus prescribed daily patching to treat amblyopia in children 4 to 5 years old. The effect of patching was not separate from that of optical correction with a period of refractive adaptation. Thus, the improvement in visual acuity is a combined effect of spectacle wear and occlusion therapy.

▶ Any study evaluating different patching regimens in treating amblyopia suffers the same fundamental problem of assuming that the prescribed patching for each group was actually carried out. Even if the number of hours was instituted, was there someone always present with the child to monitor whether any peeking was done by the child? Another concern in this study is when the design protocol for alternate-day patching is one of the options. It is often difficult to maintain consistency in any type of alternate-day treatment plan. Patients often find it confusing over a period of time to follow alternate-day treatment programs accurately.

L. B. Nelson, MD, MBA

8 Neuro-ophthalmology

A novel mitochondrial tRNA^{IIe} point mutation associated with chronic progressive external ophthalmoplegia and hyperCKemia

Souilem S, Chebel S, Mancuso M, et al (Natl Inst of Neurology, Tunis, Tunsia; Univ Hosp of Monastir, Tunsia; Univ of Pisa, Italy)
J Neurol Sci 300:187-190, 2011

We have sequenced the entire mitochondrial DNA (mtDNA) from a 54-year-old man with chronic progressive external ophthalmoplegia (PEO) and hyperCKemia. Muscle biopsy showed ragged red and SDH positive/COX negative fibres, and the biochemistry was suggestive mitochondrial respiratory chain dysfunction. Analysis of mtDNA revealed a heteroplasmic m. 4308G>A mutation in the transfer RNA isoleucine gene (MT-TI gene). Our report expands the genetic heterogeneity of PEO.

▶ This article reports a new mitochondrial DNA mutation for the clinical syndrome of chronic progressive external ophthalmoplegia. While the specific mutation is not critical for practicing ophthalmologists to recall, what is important is for us to realize how mitochondrial disease may present to ophthalmologists. There are basically 3 ways: (1) bilateral ophthalmoplegia and ptosis, like this case; (2) bilateral optic neuropathies, like Leber hereditary optic neuropathy; and (3) bilateral pigmentary retinopathies. As this research moves forward, the question is not if we will eventually treat these patients with gene therapy but WHEN. Remember to include mitochondrial disease in the differential diagnosis of any patient with a chronically progressive neuro-ophthalmic syndrome.

R. C. Sergott, MD

Acquired myelinated nerve fibers in association with optic disk drusen

Duval R, Hammamji K, Aroichane M, et al (Univ of Montreal, Canada; British Columbia's Children's Hosp, Vancouver, Canada)
J AAPOS 14:544-547, 2010

Myelinated retinal nerve fibers are a well-recognized anomaly of the ocular fundus associated with many ocular and systemic conditions. Myelination is almost always congenital and stable, but progression has been documented in rare cases. Optic disk drusen are the result of a degenerative

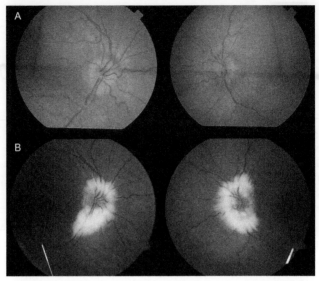

FIGURE 1.—Fundus photographs, Case 1. A, Elevated optic disks at age 6 years. B, Myelinated retinal nerve fibers at age 18 years. (Reprinted from Duval R, Hammamji K, Aroichane M, et al. Acquired myelinated nerve fibers in association with optic disk drusen. *J AAPOS.* 2010;14:544-547, Copyright 2010, with permission from the American Association for Pediatric Ophthalmology and Strabismus.)

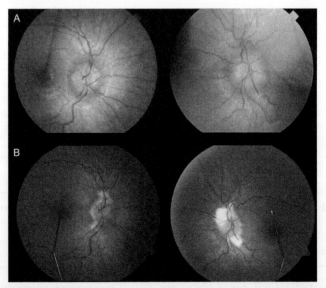

FIGURE 2.—Fundus photographs, Case 2. A, Elevated disks secondary to buried optic nerve drusen are visible at age 5 years, as well as a patch of myelinated retinal nerve fibers inferiorly in the left eye. B, Progression of myelinated retinal nerve fibers at age 10 years, with newly myelinated retinal nerve fibers in the right eye. (Reprinted from Duval R, Hammamji K, Aroichane M, et al. Acquired myelinated nerve fibers in association with optic disk drusen. *J AAPOS.* 2010;14:544-547, Copyright 2010, with permission from the American Association for Pediatric Ophthalmology and Strabismus.)

process at the optic nerve head and are often found incidentally on ophthalmologic examination. To our knowledge, optic disk drusen have only been reported once in association with acquired and progressive myelinated retinal nerve fibers. We present 2 such cases and consider the implications for the pathogenesis of myelinated nerve fibers (Figs 1 and 2).

▶ Myelinated retinal nerve fibers have often been viewed as a passing curiosity of ophthalmoscopy. However, this fascinating report of 2 cases of acquired myelinated fibers (Figs 1 and 2) suggests that understanding this phenomenon could lead to a greater understanding of the process of myelination and lead the way to develop treatments for demyelinating diseases such as multiple sclerosis, neuromyelitis optica, and hereditary defects in myelination. In these 2 cases, the development of myelinated retinal nerve fibers is associated with optic disc drusen, another poorly understood optic disc anomaly for which no treatment exists when the drusen compromise peripheral visual field.

R. C. Sergott, MD

Acute Transient Cortical Blindness Due to Seizure Following Cerebral Angiography
Newman CB, Schusse C, Hu YC, et al (St Joseph's Hosp and Med Ctr, Phoenix, AZ)
World Neurosurg 75:83-86, 2011

Objective.—Transient cortical blindness (TCB) is reported as a rare complication of coronary and cerebral angiography. Angiography of the vertebral arteries carries the highest incidence of causing TCB. The etiology of this phenomenon is unknown.

Clinical Presentation.—A 42-year-old woman underwent treatment for an enlarging pseudoaneurysm of her vertebral artery. The patient had a brief complex seizure during angiography. Following the procedure, she experienced TCB. During this time, an electroencephalogram (EEG) showed seizure activity. This case represents the first recorded instance of abnormal EEG during angiography-associated TCB.

Intervention.—The patient was immediately given intravenous lorazepam and phenytoin sodium. Her EEG returned to normal in the ensuing hours and subsequently her vision returned to normal.

Conclusion.—We present the first reported case of abnormal EEG activity during angiography-associated TCB. We hypothesize that seizure activity is a possible underlying cause of angiography-induced TCB (Fig 1A and B).

▶ This single case report serves as a reminder to clinicians about the fortunately rare, but important, development of cortical blindness after cerebral angiography. The authors describe perfectly the differential diagnosis and the basis for considering this event a complex seizure as follows: "Proposed mechanisms include an

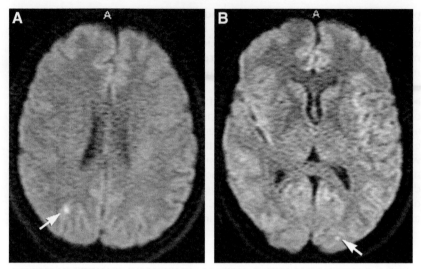

FIGURE 1.—**A**, Emergency MRI showing punctate focus of diffusion restriction in the right parietal lobe. **B**, MRI showing punctate diffusion restriction (arrow) in the left occipital lobe. *Used with permission from Barrow Neurological Institute.* (Reprinted from Newman CB, Schusse C, Hu YC, et al. Acute transient cortical blindness due to seizure following cerebral angiography. *World Neurosurg.* 2011;75:83-86, with permission from Elsevier.)

embolic phenomenon, contrast-induced posterior reversible leukoencephalopathy syndrome, or blood—brain barrier disruption followed by direct neural toxicity. Given the lack of T2-weighted signal prolongation or small foci of diffusion restriction in the posterior circulation, our patient's MRI findings are incompatible with the first two mechanisms. The postulated mechanism of direct neurotoxicity related to a local breakdown of the blood—brain barrier is not mutually exclusive in our case."

Please see Fig 1A and B for the important MRI findings. Therefore, in these cases, after clinical evaluation, a patient with this syndrome needs to have an urgent MRI with diffusion-weighted images. If the MRI does not show an acute stroke, then treatment with antiepileptic medications may be beneficial.

R. C. Sergott, MD

An unusual case of optic neuritis

Doegel D, Mueller W, Deckert M, et al (Univ Hosp, Heidelberg, Germany; Univ Hosp, Cologne, Germany)
J Neurol Sci 304:138-141, 2011

Optic neuritis is a frequent disease with well established tests and therapeutic strategies. However, possible differential diagnoses cover a broad spectrum. Therefore, clinical work-up can be challenging and routine testing and therapies may not be sufficient.

In this case, a 26 year old female is described who presented with clinical features of optic neuritis, yet failed to respond to common therapeutic strategies and lost vision on the affected eye. Diagnostic nerve transection was performed, histopathology suggested inflammation. As the second nerve became affected, immunosuppressive therapy with cyclophosphamide was started and stopped further deterioration. Although additional molecular work-up of the transected nerve revealed clonal rearrangement of the B-cell-receptor-locus IgH, overall histopathologic features and the absence of systemic disease suggested an aggressive inflammatory process rather than lymphoma. Additional B-cell depletion with rituximab prompted significant and sustained visual improvement. This case emphasizes the necessity to consider rare differential diagnoses of optic neuritis, when uncommon features arise during the course of disease. Aggressive immunosuppression might be required to achieve stable improvement of vision (Fig 2).

▶ Because of its high rate of spontaneous recovery, optic neuritis is often considered a benign disease, but 15% of patients will not regain vision better than the 20/30 to 20/40 range, and in rare cases like this one, the first eye becomes blind and then the second eye becomes involved.

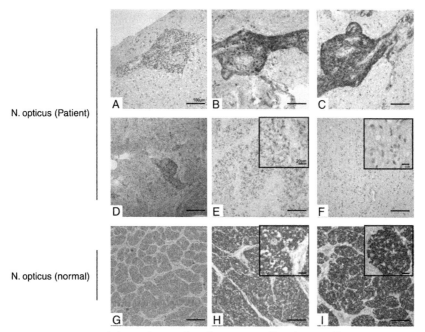

FIGURE 2.—Histopathology and Immunohistochemistry. Mixed lymphocytic infiltration, (A, H & E), with T- (B, CD3) and B-cells (C, CD20). Note extensive loss of myelin (D, Luxol/PAS & E, MBP) and axons (F, NF). Normal density of myelin (G—H) and axons (I) in the unaffected human optic nerve. (Reprinted from Doegel D, Mueller W, Deckert M, et al. An unusual case of optic neuritis. *J Neurol Sci.* 2011;304:138-141, with permission from Elsevier B.V.)

The authors are to be congratulated not only for an excellent publication but also for the expertise of their clinical care for this patient. Performing the optic nerve transectional biopsy and then processing the tissue with elegant immunological techniques (Fig 2) enabled the clinicians to make a logical decision to proceed not only with cyclophosphamide therapy but also with B-cell-specific rituximab. The clinical improvement in vision speaks for itself.

One has to wonder whether or not such a brilliant intervention and moving to new areas of innovative care that saved this patient's vision will be allowed under alleged health care reform now confronting American medicine.

R. C. Sergott, MD

Comparison of the Correlations Between Optic Disc Rim Area and Retinal Nerve Fiber Layer Thickness in Glaucoma and Nonarteritic Anterior Ischemic Optic Neuropathy
Suh MH, Kim SH, Park KH, et al (Kwandong Univ Myongji Hosp, Koyang, Korea; Seoul Natl Univ College of Medicine, Seoul; et al)
Am J Ophthalmol 151:277-286, 2011

Purpose.—To test whether comparison of the correlation between optic disc rim area and retinal nerve fiber layer thickness (rim-RNFL correlation) can differentiate eyes with nonarteritic anterior ischemic optic neuropathy (NAION) from eyes with open-angle glaucoma (OAG).

Design.—Prospective cross-sectional study.

Methods.—One hundred and thirteen eyes with OAG and 22 with NAION were included in this study. The rim-RNFL correlation in OAG eyes was analyzed in global and 12-clock-hour parameters using rim areas determined by Heidelberg retina tomography (HRT II) and RNFL thicknesses determined by optical coherence tomography (Cirrus OCT). The eyes with NAION were determined whether to be out of the 95% prediction interval (PI) for the rim-RNFL correlation of OAG in global and clock-hour parameters.

Results.—A significant linear rim-RNFL correlation was observed in global and all clock-hour sectors, except the 3-, 4-, and 9-o'clock sectors, in OAG ($0.045 < r^2 < 0.64$, $P < .05$, respectively). All eyes with NAION were outside the 95% PI of the rim-RNFL correlation of OAG in at least 1 clock-hour sector in terms of clock-hour parameters, as compared with 63.6% of eyes in terms of global parameter. All NAION eyes (n = 21) with 7- or 11-o'clock involvement had a rim-RNFL correlation outside the 95% PI of OAG for corresponding clock-hour sectors.

Conclusions.—By comparison of the rim-RNFL correlation, eyes with NAION were found to be well differentiated from OAG eyes, especially in clock-hour sectors. It might be an objective approach to discriminate NAION from OAG.

▶ While this study is very well done scientifically, I believe its greater value is in confirming the small disc at risk for nonarteritic anterior ischemic optic neuropathy

(NAION) compared with glaucoma and how this anatomic substrate contributes to the pathogenesis of this disorder. Establishing the diagnosis of NAION versus primary chronic open-angle glaucoma depends on taking a detailed history about an acute onset, which is classic for NAION, but in some cases optic disc pallor from NAION will be found incidentally. In those cases, the clinicians must reexamine the patient with specific attention to intraocular pressures, visual fields, and now optical coherence tomography (OCT). In my opinion, spectral-domain OCT is the best way to look for progression of retinal nerve fiber layer loss. There is too much variability of visual field testing in many patients, especially elderly individuals with other ophthalmic problems such as keratitis sicca, cataract, and macular disease, to rely solely on visual fields.

R. C. Sergott, MD

Diagnostic pitfalls: Posterior ischemic optic neuropathy mimicking optic neuritis
Lysandropoulos AP, Carota A (CHUV, Lausanne, Switzerland; Hildebrand Clinic, Brissago, Switzerland)
Clin Neurol Neurosurg 113:162-163, 2011

In young people, the most frequent cause of isolated monocular visual loss due to an optic neuropathy is optic neuritis. We present the case of a 27 year old woman who presented monocular visual loss, excruciating orbital pain and unusual temporal headache. The initial diagnosis of optic neuritis revealed later to be a posterior ischemic optic neuropathy (PION). In this case, PION was the first unique presentation of a non-traumatic carotid dissection, and it was followed 24 h later by an ischemic stroke.

Sudden monocular visual loss associated with a new-onset headache are clinical symptoms that should immediately prompt to a carotid dissection.

▶ Dissection of the internal carotid artery is one of the most difficult diagnostic situations faced by ophthalmologists. Patients may present with an acute or subacute Horner syndrome with or without the classic accompanying jaw pain. The patients may also have sensory changes in the distribution of the first and second division of the trigeminal nerve. Previously, the only reported involvement in the afferent visual system was a central retinal artery occlusion. This article now adds the syndrome of posterior ischemic optic neuropathy to the possible presentations. The authors are to be congratulated on a very important addition to the literature and on their clinical expertise, given that the only clues to the diagnosis were the sudden loss of vision (too rapid for optic neuritis) and the excruciating pain (again too severe for optic neuritis).

R. C. Sergott, MD

Directional diffusivity changes in the optic nerve and optic radiation in optic neuritis

Li M, Li J, He H, et al (Chinese Academy of Sciences, China; Capital Med Univ, China; et al)
Br J Radiol 84:304-314, 2011

Objective.—Optic neuritis (ON) is defined as an inflammation of the optic nerve and provides a useful model for studying the effects of inflammatory demyelination of white matter. The aim of this study was to assess the diffusion changes in both the optic nerve and optic radiation in patients with acute and chronic ON using diffusion tensor (DT) MRI.

Methods.—33 patients with idiopathic demyelinating optic neuritis (IDON) and 33 gender- and age-matched healthy controls were examined with DT-MRI and with T_1 and T_2 weighted MRI.

Results.—Compared with controls, both first-episode and recurrent patients with IDON in the acute stage showed significantly increased radial diffusivity ($\lambda_\perp$) and decreased mean fractional anisotropy (FA) in the affected nerves. Reduced FA, increased $\lambda_\perp$, mean diffusivity (MD) and axial diffusivity ($\lambda_\parallel$) were determined in patients with subacute IDON. We found no significant difference in the directional diffusivity of optic radiation in patients whose disease had lasted less than 1 year compared with healthy controls. However, significant changes in the FA and $\lambda_\perp$ of the optic radiation were detected in patients with disease duration of more than 1 year.

Conclusion.—These results show the great potential and capacity of DT-MRI measures as useful biomarkers and indicators for the evaluation of myelin injury in the visual pathway.

▶ The authors provide elegant data about the differences in diffusion tensor (DT) MRI in patients with optic neuritis of less than 1 year compared with patients who have had optic neuritis greater than a year and to normal controls. "DT-MRI uses water diffusion characteristics to reconstruct white matter structure through diffusion direction and amplitude. Altered diffusion parameters were found in patients with chronic ON compared with healthy controls." The authors provide a clear and concise interpretation of the importance of their findings: "Our study found no significant changes in diffusion parameters in patients with ON of less than 1 year in duration, but a significantly decreased FA and higher $\lambda_\perp$ if the disease duration exceeded 1 year. This difference indicates more serious atrophy of the optic radiation after the recurrence of symptoms. The most likely pathogenesis of abnormal diffusion in the optic radiation would appear to be secondary lesions induced by axonal degeneration after ON. We also observed an increased MD value in the optic radiation in chronic ON patients when compared with control subjects." These findings further emphasize that optic neuritis is not a benign disease and is associated with long-term damage to the afferent visual system.

R. C. Sergott, MD

Interferon Alfa-associated Anterior Ischemic Optic Neuropathy
Fraunfelder FW, Fraunfelder FT (Oregon Health & Science Univ, Portland)
Ophthalmology 118:408-411, 2011

Purpose.—To report a possible association between interferon alfa therapy and anterior ischemic optic neuropathy (AION).
Design.—Database study and review of the literature.
Participants.—Thirty-six case reports from spontaneous reporting systems and the literature.
Methods.—Case reports from a review of the literature were combined with spontaneous reports from the National Registry of Drug-Induced Ocular Side Effects, the World Health Organization, and the Food and Drug Administration looking for reports on interferon therapy associated with optic neuropathy.
Main Outcome Measures.—Data from the spontaneous reports include the type of interferon, age, gender, adverse drug reaction (ADR), dosage, duration of therapy until onset of ADR, concomitant drugs, systemic disease, and dechallenge and rechallenge data.
Results.—Thirty-six case reports of AION are described in association with interferon alfa therapy. The average age of subjects was 54.5 years; 26 were male and 10 were female. The median duration of therapy to onset of AION was 4.5 months, with 50% of subjects having some form of permanent vision loss. Anterior ischemic optic neuropathy was bilateral in 67% of subjects. There are 3 positive rechallenge case reports.
Conclusions.—Interferon alfas association with AION can be classified as "possible" using the World Health Organization classification system. If optic neuropathy is suspected, rapid cessation of interferon therapy may portend a better prognosis because multiple case reports indicate visual defects may be permanent if this possible ADR remains unrecognized.

▶ I was the lead discussant for this article at the American Ophthalmological Society meeting in 2010. I believe that the association is a valid one because of the high percentage of cases with bilateral involvement—67%. I raised the question as to whether the optic nerve ischemia in these cases might be the effect of 2 medications, interferon alfa and ribavirin that is often used in combination with interferon alfa for increased rate of viral clearance. The issue becomes whether the combination of interferon alfa and ribavirin produced a significant anemia in these patients and the resulting anemia, a known risk factor for anterior ischemic optic neuropathy, was the inciting factor. Ribavirin causes dose-dependent hemolytic anemia, and interferon suppresses bone marrow production of red blood cells. Anemia developed in 9% to 23% of 1192 patients in 3 pivotal controlled clinical trials with dual therapy. Sixteen patients (50%) in this report were also taking ribavirin. Therefore, the question arises as to whether the optic nerve ischemia is the result of the interaction of these 2 medications. A larger retrospective review of the reported cases of this syndrome might confirm or refute this hypothesis.

R. C. Sergott, MD

Ischemic Optic Neuropathy and Implications for Plastic Surgeons: Report of a New Case and Review of the Literature

Agostini T, Lazzeri D, Agostini V, et al (Univ of Florence, Italy; Hosp of Pisa, Italy; et al)

Ann Plast Surg 66:416-420, 2011

Background.—Postoperative visual loss is a rare and devastating complication after nonocular as well as ocular surgery. A case of such a complication arising as a consequence of nonocular surgery prompted a review of the literature, and an appraisal of current theories on etiology, risk factors, and potential treatment options, as well as implications for informed consent. It is clear from our review that all patients undergoing both reconstructive and cosmetic surgery are at risk.

Methods.—A literature review was performed to identify all cases of ischemic optic neuropathy (both anterior and posterior subtypes) subsequent to any type of plastic, reconstructive, and aesthetic surgery procedures. An analysis of current knowledge regarding risk factors, etiology, prevention, and treatment options was undertaken.

Results.—A total of 38 patients aged between 16 and 76 years affected by ischemic optic neuropathy were identified, many as a consequence of routine and sometimes minor operative procedures.

Conclusions.—Ischemic optic neuropathy can be a devastating complication of surgery. Plastic surgeons need to be aware of the risks, as well as the signs and symptoms, and counsel at-risk patients accordingly because of the potentially devastating nature of this complication. There are significant implications in relation to informed consent, underscored by the legal case of *Rogers v Whitaker*, 67 ALJR 47 (Aust 1992), which highlights

TABLE 1.—Risk Factors for Ischemic Optic Neuropathy Can Be Divided Into Predisposing and Precipitating

Predisposing	Precipitating
Systemic	Prolonged hypotension
Hypertension	Nocturnal arterial hypotension
Diabetes mellitus	Anemia
Arteriosclerosis	Surgery
Hyperlipidemia	Trauma
Sleep apnea	Gastrointestinal bleeding (average, 44.7%; range, 10%−200%)
Ischemic cardiac disease	Facial edema
Nocturnal hypotension	Increate venous pressure
Arterial hypotension	
Ocular	Hemorrhage
Absent/small cap	Shock
Angle closure glaucoma	Prone position
Optic disk edema	Direct pressure
Vascular disorders in nutrient vessels	Long operative times (average, 6.5 h; ranging, 2−12)
	Phosphodiesterase type-5 inhibitors

the importance within the consent process of complications threatening sight, no matter how small (Table 1).

▶ This syndrome of perioperative and postoperative bilateral ischemic optic neuropathy is one of the most devastating events in surgery and neuro-ophthalmology. This article provides a comprehensive review of the subject and highlights its potential development following plastic surgical procedures. Table 1 is a helpful outline of the predisposing and precipitating factors for this syndrome.

R. C. Sergott, MD

Mapping the visual brain: how and why
Bridge H (Univ of Oxford, UK)
Eye 25:291-296, 2011

Over the past 15 years, techniques for identifying visual areas using magnetic resonance imaging (MRI) in human subjects have been applied widely to multiple populations. This review will cover the basic techniques of using functional MRI and very high-resolution structural MRI to determine boundaries between different areas of the visual cortex. Recent applications of these methods to ophthalmological patient populations are discussed, and the future potential applications of very high field strength MRI are considered.

▶ Various self-proclaimed prophets, oracles, soothsayers, politicians, and palm readers have all claimed to be able to see and predict the future. This diverse group could gain a significant measure of credibility if they were to gaze into the future and hold forth that mapping of the visual system in the brain will someday have clinical application. While we are not at that day yet, this superb review article beautifully identifies where we are and where we are going. This article is a must-read for all residents, fellows, and neuroscientists with an interest in the visual system.

R. C. Sergott, MD

Narrowing of Meckel's Cave and Cavernous Sinus and Enlargement of the Optic Nerve Sheath in Pseudotumor Cerebri
Degnan AJ, Levy LM (George Washington Univ Med Ctr, DC)
J Comput Assist Tomogr 35:308-312, 2011

Objective.—Pseudotumor cerebri (PTC) is a clinical entity of uncertain etiology associated with several subtle findings on magnetic resonance imaging (MRI) including posterior flattening of the globes, enlargement of the optic nerve sheath (ONS), empty sella sign. We aimed to characterize the incidence of and significance of 2 novel MRI findings: narrowing of Meckel's cave and of cavernous sinus.

Methods.—Forty-six patients with a condition diagnosed as PTC based on clinical history were retrospectively reviewed, and their MRI studies were assessed for previously reported imaging findings associated with PTC. The maximal diameters of the cavernous sinuses, Meckel's caves, and ONSs were measured along with those of age-matched controls on axial T2-weighted images.

Results.—The Meckel's caves and cavernous sinuses are significantly ($P < 0.01$) narrowed in patients (mean diameters: 0.41 and 0.25 cm) versus controls (0.54 and 0.36 cm), respectively. The ONS was enlarged in patients with a mean diameter of 0.65 cm versus 0.54 cm ($P < 0.01$). Meckel's cave narrowing and ONS enlargement seem to be better indicators of PTC than cavernous sinus narrowing, with sensitivities of 78.3% and 86.9% and specificities of 84.8% and 76.1% versus 60.9% and 76.1%, respectively.

Conclusions.—This finding of narrowed Meckel's caves in PTC may be clinically useful as a novel imaging finding seen on routine MRI studies. Optic nerve sheath enlargement is also confirmed as an important finding in PTC (Figs 1 and 2).

▶ The authors extend the increasing array of abnormalities found in the cerebral venous system in pseudotumor cerebri. This article illustrates 2 important points

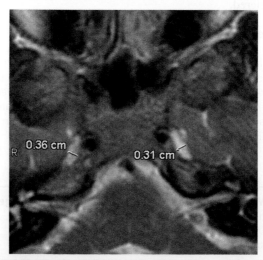

FIGURE 1.—Measurement of the Meckel's caves in a patient with PTC. Depicted here is the standard measurement used for determining the maximal diameter of the Meckel's caves on axial T2-weighted images taken of a 36-year-old woman who presented with headache, found to have an opening CSF pressure of 32 cm H$_2$O. The Meckel's caves measure 0.36 and 0.31 cm, considered narrow in our study. Also noted on imaging were empty sella sign and narrowed venous sinuses in addition to quantitatively narrowed cavernous sinuses as well. (Reprinted from Degnan AJ, Levy LM. Narrowing of Meckel's cave and cavernous sinus and enlargement of the optic nerve sheath in pseudotumor cerebri. *J Comput Assist Tomogr.* 2011;35:308-312, with permission from Lippincott Williams & Wilkins.)

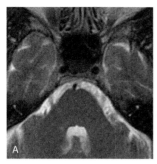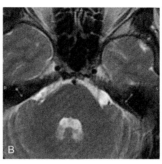

FIGURE 2.—A, Bilateral narrowing of Meckel's cave. Bilateral narrowing of the Meckel's caves and cavernous sinuses are additional signs seen on axial T2-weighted MRI proposed as indicators of elevated intracranial pressure. This 58-year-old woman presented with visual disturbances and was found to have papilledema. B, Normal Meckel's caves. This age-matched 58-year-old female patient with vasculitis demonstrates normal-sized Meckel's caves measuring 0.63 cm bilaterally. (Reprinted from Degnan AJ, Levy LM. Narrowing of Meckel's cave and cavernous sinus and enlargement of the optic nerve sheath in pseudotumor cerebri. *J Comput Assist Tomogr.* 2011;35:308-312, with permission from Lippincott Williams & Wilkins.)

in clinical research: (1) there is still value in retrospective studies and (2) we only see and identify abnormalities that we look for. With this background and methodology, the authors have discovered 2 potentially novel findings of narrowed Meckel caves and cavernous sinuses as the result of intracranial hypertension. Further studies are required to determine if these changes occur with obstructive hydrocephalus or if they can be used to monitor patients with increased intracranial pressure as a gauge to the effectiveness of therapy. Figs 1 and 2 very nicely illustrate this new finding.

R. C. Sergott, MD

Optic Disc Evaluation in Optic Neuropathies: The Optic Disc Assessment Project

O'Neill EC, on behalf of the Optic Nerve Study Group (Univ of Melbourne, Australia; et al)
Ophthalmology 118:964-970, 2011

Objective.—Optic nerve morphology is affected by genetic and acquired disease. Glaucoma is the most common optic neuropathy; autosomal-dominant optic atrophy (ADOA) and Leber's hereditary optic neuropathy (LHON) are the most prevalent hereditary optic neuropathies. These 3 entities can exhibit similar topographical changes at the optic nerve head. Both ADOA and LHON have been reported to be misdiagnosed as glaucoma. Our aim was to determine whether glaucoma subspecialists and neuro-ophthalmologists can distinguish these diagnoses on optic disc assessment alone.

Design.—Observational study.

Participants.—Twenty-three optic nerve experts.

Methods.—We randomized and masked 60 high-resolution stereoscopic optic disc photographs (15 ADOA images, 15 LHON, 15 glaucoma, and 15 normal controls). Experts were asked to assess the discs on 12 conventional topographic features and assign a presumptive diagnosis. Intra- and interanalysis was performed using the index of qualitative variation and absolute deviation.

Main Outcome Measures.—Can glaucoma specialists and neuro-ophthalmologists distinguish among the disease entities by optic nerve head phenotype.

Results.—The correct diagnosis was identified in 85%, 75%, 27%, and 16% of the normal, glaucoma, ADOA, and LHON disc groups, respectively. The proportion of correct diagnoses within the ADOA and LHON groups was significantly lower than both normal and glaucomatous ($P<0.001$). Where glaucoma was chosen as the most likely diagnosis, 61% were glaucomatous, 34% were pathologic but nonglaucomatous discs, and 5% were normal. There was greater agreement for individual parameters assessed within the normal disc set when compared with pathologic discs ($P<0.05$). The only parameter to have a significantly greater agreement within the glaucomatous disc set when compared with ADOA or LHON disc sets was pallor, whereby experts agreed on is absence in the glaucomatous discs but were not in agreement on its presence or its absence in the ADOA and LHON discs ($P<0.01$).

Conclusions.—Optic neuropathies can result in similar topographic changes at the optic disc, particularly in late-stage disease, making it difficult to differentiate ADOA and LHON from glaucoma based on disc assessment alone. Other clinical parameters such as acuity, color vision, history of visual loss, and family history are required to make an accurate diagnosis.

▶ Somewhere in the history and evolution of ophthalmology and ophthalmoscopy, the perception began that we can make a diagnosis based on the appearance of the optic disc. Trying to practice ophthalmology this way will result in major problems for patients and clinicians. Nothing in this world is pathognomonic, no matter how hard we try to envision that simple world. Diagnosis depends on a thorough meticulous history, detailed and focused physical examination, and integration of the credible facts from these 2 exercises with laboratory, imaging, and other diagnostic procedures. This article very nicely illustrates that disc appearance alone is useless to make an accurate diagnosis. Hopefully, this article will put an end to any future studies in which investigators try to make any diagnosis based solely on the appearance of the optic disc.

R. C. Sergott, MD

The Basal Temporal Approach for Mesial Temporal Surgery: Sparing the Meyer Loop With Navigated Diffusion Tensor Tractography

Thudium MO, Campos AR, Urbach H, et al (Univ of Bonn Med Ctr, Germany)
Neurosurgery 67:ons385-ons390, 2010

Background.—Visual field defects are a common side effect after mesial temporal resections such as selective amygdalohippocampectomy (SelAH).

Objective.—To present a method of diffusion tensor tractography (DTT) of the Meyer loop for preoperative planning of the surgical approach for SelAH and for intraoperative visualization on a navigation-guided operating microscope.

Methods.—Twelve patients were selected for SelAH to treat mesial temporal lobe epilepsy. All received preoperative MRI with diffusion tensor imaging sequences. The Meyer loop was determined and reconstructed as an object with DTT. Images were utilized for preoperative planning in which a safe approach not affecting the Meyer loop was specified. A navigation-guided operating microscope was used for image-guided surgery.

Results.—DTT was a reliable method for visualization of the Meyer loop. Reconstruction of the Meyer loop had a direct impact on the approach planning. In all 12 cases, the optic tract could only be spared using a basal approach. Ten patients underwent SelAH by the subtemporal approach, and 2 underwent SelAH by the transcortical approach through the inferior temporal gyrus. During the critical early phase of the operation image guidance remained accurate until entry into the ventricle. Nine of 12 patients had no postoperative field deficits (75%). Three patients (25%) experienced peripheral incomplete quadrantanopia.

Conclusion.—DTT and intraoperative visualization of the Meyer loop is a helpful tool for preoperative planning and during surgery to find a safe trajectory to mesial temporal structures while avoiding the optic radiation. This technique in combination with a basal approach seems to be a promising

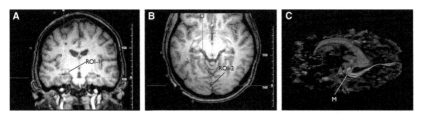

FIGURE 1.—Diffusion tensor tractography of the Meyer loop. A, coronal view, positioning of the first region of interest covering the roof of the temporal horn. B, axial view, positioning of the second region of interest retaining only the fibers passing to the primary visual cortex. C, resulting fiber pattern: Meyer loop. M, Meyer loop; ROI, region of interest. (Reprinted from Thudium MO, Campos AR, Urbach H, et al. The basal temporal approach for mesial temporal surgery: sparing the Meyer loop with navigated diffusion tensor tractography. *Neurosurgery.* 2010;67:ons385-ons390, with permission from the Congress of Neurological Surgeons.)

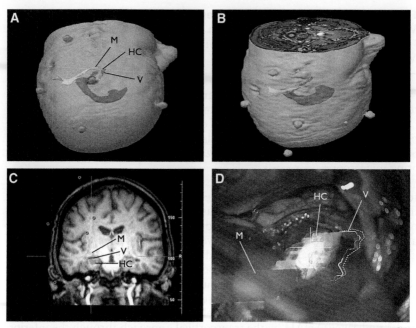

FIGURE 2.—A, B, simulated surgeon's view in preoperative 3D reconstructed images after fiber tracking and object creation of the Meyer loop. A, view mimicking a transsylvian approach. No safe trajectory to the temporal horn can be identified because of the position of the Meyer loop. B, view from a direction as used for a subtemporal approach. Note that hippocampus and the temporal horn are exposed so that the temporal horn can easily be accessed without injury of the Meyer loop. C, coronal view after fiber tracking. In this coronal slice, the temporal horn is superiorly covered completely by the Meyer loop; interference can only be avoided by a basal approach. D, intraoperative view after ventricle entry with image injection on the head-up display of the navigation-bound operating microscope. HC, hippocampus; M, Meyer loop; V, ventricle. (Reprinted from Thudium MO, Campos AR, Urbach H, et al. The basal temporal approach for mesial temporal surgery: sparing the Meyer loop with navigated diffusion tensor tractography. *Neurosurgery.* 2010;67:ons385-ons390, with permission from the Congress of Neurological Surgeons.)

strategy to prevent postoperative visual field deficits in most patients (Figs 1 and 2).

▶ In the commentary for *Mapping the visual brain: how and why,*[1] we recommended that clinicians become familiar with brain mapping radiological techniques because they will become clinically useful in the future. Well, the future is now, as this article illustrates. Epilepsy surgery can be the most successful treatment for intractable seizures if a single locus of brain abnormality can be identified. A major risk of the surgery is damage to Meyer loop causing a homonymous hemianopsia or quadrantanopia. In this series of patients, diffusion tensor tractography was a reliable method for visualization of the Meyer loop. Reconstruction of the Meyer loop had a direct impact on the approach planning. In all 12 cases, the optic tract could only be spared using a basal approach, which is beautifully illustrated in Figs 1 and 2. In my opinion, this advanced imaging technique will decrease the visual morbidity of epilepsy surgery.

R. C. Sergott, MD

Reference

1. Bridge H. Mapping the visual brain: how and why. *Eye*. 2011;25:291-296.

Toluene optic neurotoxicity: magnetic resonance imaging and pathologic features
Gupta SR, Palmer CA, Curé JK, et al (Univ of Alabama at Birmingham; et al)
Hum Pathol 42:295-298, 2011

Toluene, a colorless liquid found in glues, paints, and industrial products, is lipid soluble and rapidly absorbed by the lipid-rich central nervous system. Prolonged exposure through occupation or purposeful inhalation may lead to neurologic abnormalities. Two men presented with multifocal central nervous system defects and bilateral optic neuropathy of unclear etiology. After numerous diagnostic tests, including brain magnetic resonance imaging, lumbar puncture, hematologic studies, and in one patient a brain biopsy, chronic inhalation of toluene was found to be the cause. Timely diagnosis is important because patients may experience improvement in neurologic and ocular manifestations with cessation of exposure, whereas continued inhalant abuse or exposure can result in permanent loss of neurologic function.

▶ Excessive exposure to toluene can occur during occupational exposure in the painting industry or because of intentional substance abuse, huffing. This very informative report of 2 cases demonstrates both the MRI and pathological features of this condition (reference Figs 1 and 3 in the original article for the MRI studies). Any time a patient presents with bilateral optic nerve involvement as well as multifocal central nervous system findings, toxic chemical or drug-induced changes must be considered in the differential diagnosis. Stopping exposure may result in visual and neurological improvement.

R. C. Sergott, MD

Vigabatrin-induced peripheral visual field defects in patients with refractory partial epilepsy

Sergott RC, Bittman RM, Christen EM, et al (Thomas Jefferson Univ Med College, Philadelphia, PA; Bittman Biostat, Inc, Glencoe, IL; AYW Consulting, Knoxville, TN; et al)
Epilepsy Res 92:170-176, 2010

Purpose.—Vigabatrin can cause retinopathy, resulting in bilateral visual field constriction. Previous analyses of results from a prospective, observational study assessing vigabatrin-induced visual field constriction (described below) employed a partially subjective interpretation of static perimetery. To affirm these previous findings through more objective, quantitative methodology, we now report data from a subset analysis of refractory partial epilepsy patients in the study who underwent Goldmann kinetic perimetry.

Methods.—Patients aged ≥ 8 years with refractory partial seizures were enrolled and grouped: those receiving vigabatrin for ≥ 6 months (Group I); those who had received vigabatrin for ≥ 6 months and then had discontinued for ≥ 6 months (Group II); and those naïve to vigabatrin (Group III). Patients underwent static or kinetic perimetry, or both, every 4−6 months for ≤ 3 years. For kinetic perimetry, the temporal and nasal visual fields were measured along the horizontal meridian with the largest (V4e, IV4e) and smallest (I2e, I1e) isopters, respectively.

Results.—Of 735 patients enrolled, 341 had Goldmann perimetry data. Of these, 258 received vigabatrin. Sixteen percent of vigabatrin-exposed patients had moderate visual field defects (30-60° retained temporal vision), and 3% had severe defects (<30° retained temporal vision). Visual function questionnaire results indicated a weak correlation between visual field constriction severity and visual symptoms.

Conclusions.—These results affirm both an analysis of the same study based primarily on static perimetry and findings from cross-sectional studies. The present analysis verifies that visual field constriction, when it occurs, is most often mild or moderate and is not associated with symptoms of abnormal visual function. The clinical decision to prescribe vigabatrin should be based on a benefit-risk analysis for each individual patient (Fig 3).

▶ Vigabatrin (Sabril) is a powerful medication approved by the Food and Drug Administration approximately 18 months ago for infantile spasms and refractory complex epilepsy, both very severe life-threatening seizure disorders. Vigabatrin's use has been limited by its unpredictable effect on the retina in 30% to 40% of patients, which produces bilateral constricted visual field. This article and another by Gonzalez and coworkers from Scotland report that patients with refractory seizures may have visual field defects at baseline without ever having been exposed to vigabatrin. The current risk evaluation mitigation strategy program and two phase 4 studies will gather some prospective

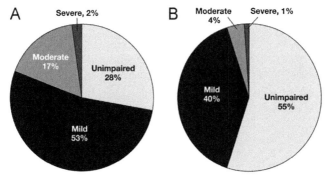

FIGURE 3.—Severity of visual field defect at last kinetic perimetry in (A) vigabatrin-exposed and (B) vigabatrin-naïve patients. Unimpaired: >80° monocular temporal field retained; mild: 60—80° monocular temporal field retained; moderate: 30—60° monocular temporal field retained; severe: <30° monocular temporal field retained. Measurements are of largest isopter tested at final Goldmann perimetry. (Reprinted from Sergott RC, Bittman RM, Christen EM, et al. Vigabatrin-induced peripheral visual field defects in patients with refractory partial epilepsy. *Epilepsy Res.* 2010;92:170-176, with permission from Elsevier B.V.)

information about this critical question. Carefully defining the onset of the visual field problem, its severity, progression, and prevalence will enhance the safe use of this medication. Fig 3 illustrates the percentage of patients taking vigabatrin and those never exposed who demonstrated visual field defects.

R. C. Sergott, MD

9 Imaging

Cerebral, Facial, and Orbital Involvement in Erdheim-Chester Disease: CT and MR Imaging Findings
Drier A, Haroche J, Savatovsky J, et al (Pitié-Salpêtrière Hosp, Paris, France; Rothschild Foundation, Paris, France; et al)
Radiology 255:586-594, 2010

Purpose.—To retrospectively review the brain magnetic resonance (MR) imaging and computed tomographic (CT) findings in patients with Erdheim-Chester disease (ECD).

Materials and Methods.—The ethics committee required neither institutional review board approval nor informed patient consent for retrospective analyses of the patients' medical records and imaging data. The patients' medical files were retrospectively reviewed in accordance with human subject research protocols. Three neuroradiologists in consensus analyzed the signal intensity, location, size, number, and gadolinium uptake of lesions detected on brain MR images obtained in 33 patients with biopsy-proved ECD.

Results.—Thirty patients had intracranial, facial bone, and/or orbital involvement, and three had normal neurologic imaging findings. The hypothalamic-pituitary axis was involved in 16 (53%) of the 30 patients, with six (20%) cases of micronodular or nodular masses of the infundibular stalk. Meningeal lesions were observed in seven (23%) patients. Three (10%) patients had bilateral symmetric T2 high signal intensity in the dentate nucleus areas, and five (17%) had multiple intraaxial enhancing masses. Striking intracranial periarterial infiltration was observed in three (10%) patients. Another patient (3%) had a lesion in the lumen of the superior sagittal sinus. Nine (30%) patients had orbital involvement. Twenty-four (80%) patients had osteosclerosis of the facial and/or skull bones. At least two anatomic sites were involved in two-thirds ($n = 20$) of the patients. Osteosclerosis of the facial bones associated with orbital masses and either meningeal or infundibular stalk masses was seen in eight (27%) patients.

Conclusion.—Lesions of the brain, meninges, facial bones, and orbits are frequently observed and should be systematically sought on the brain MR and CT images obtained in patients with ECD, even if these patients are asymptomatic. Careful attention should be directed to the periarterial environment.

▶ Erdheim-Chester disease (ECD) is a rare non-Langerhans cell type of histiocytosis that is diagnosed based on radiologic finding of osteosclerosis typically in the long bones of lower extremities and histological characteristics of the

209

abnormal histiocytes (including immunohistology). About 50% cases have extraskeletal manifestations.[1]

In this retrospective study, the authors have reviewed the MRI and CT findings in head and neck in histologically diagnosed cases of ECD. The authors have shown that lesions of brain, meninges, facial bones, and orbits are frequently found in ECD and should be systematically sought on MRI and CT irrespective of corresponding clinical manifestations. The most common intracranial lesion is 1 or more dural-based masses that mimic meningiomas or diffuse pachymeningeal thickening that mimics pachymeningitis. The imaging hallmark of ECD is the combination of the typical dural lesions and osteosclerosis of the facial bone (the most common manifestation on head and neck imaging) and/or orbital lesions. Intraorbital lesions were found in 9 of 30 patients consisting primarily of bilateral and intraconal masses, enhancing well-defined retro-ocular masses that ensheathed the optic nerves or diffusely infiltrated the orbital fat. Despite the large size of the orbital masses, in some cases, there was no visual impairment; only exophthalmos was present. Additionally, a small number of cases have been shown to have periarterial involvement that may potentially result in stroke. The hypothalamic-pituitary axis was a common intracranial location for this disease process with lack of posterior pituitary T1-bright signal being the commonly documented abnormality in this study. Although lack of posterior pituitary T1-bright signal can be a normal physiological occurrence, especially in the elderly, a majority of their patients had endocrine abnormalities related to the pituitary (like diabetes insipidus) suggesting that this may in fact be pathological. A constellation of facial bone osteosclerosis, the typical intracranial lesions, and/or orbital lesions may point to the diagnosis of ECD in cases with uncertain etiology. Although ECD disease is relatively rare, it and its related diseases (ie, Langerhans cell histiocytosis and Wegener granulomatosis) should be included in the differential diagnosis of any bilateral infiltrative retro-orbital process.

K. Talekar, MD

A. E. Flanders, MD

Reference

1. Veyssier-Belot C, Cacoub P, Caparros-Lefebvre D, et al. Erdheim-Chester disease. Clinical and radiologic characteristics of 59 cases. *Medicine (Baltimore)*. 1996;75: 157-169.

Indeterminate Orbital Masses: Restricted Diffusion at MR Imaging with Echo-planar Diffusion-weighted Imaging Predicts Malignancy
Sepahdari AR, Aakalu VK, Setabutr P, et al (Massachusetts General Hosp, Boston; Univ of Illinois at Chicago; et al)
Radiology 256:554-564, 2010

Purpose.—To determine whether magnetic resonance (MR) imaging with diffusion-weighted (DW) imaging can help discriminate between radiologically indeterminate benign and malignant orbital masses and to identify optimal apparent diffusion coefficient (ADC) thresholds for such discrimination.

Materials and Methods.—Informed consent was waived for this HIPAA-compliant institutional review board—approved retrospective study. Forty-seven orbital masses imaged with echo-planar DW imaging were identified in 47 patients (25 female patients, 22 male patients; average age, 35 years). A fellowship-trained orbital surgeon determined reference-standard diagnoses on the basis of chart review, and a neuroradiology fellow and senior neuroradiologist who were blinded to the diagnoses selected a region of interest for each lesion by consensus. ADC was calculated from signal intensity on DW images obtained with $b = 1000$ and $b = 0$ sec/mm^2. Lesion ADC was also compared with that of normal-appearing white matter (ADC ratio). The Student t test was used to compare groups. Receiver operating characteristic analysis was performed. Intraobserver agreement was assessed with a repeat data collection.

Results.—Malignant lesions had lower ADCs than benign lesions, irrespective of patient age $(P < .02)$ and in adults specifically $(P < .05)$. Lymphomas had lower ADCs than pseudotumors $(P < .001)$. An ADC of less than 1.0×10^{-3} mm^2/sec and an ADC ratio of less than 1.2 were optimal for predicting malignancy (sensitivity, 63% for both; specificity, 84% and 90%, respectively; and accuracy, 77% and 81%, respectively). Lymphoma was differentiated from pseudotumor with 100% accuracy (in 16 of 16 cases) by using these values. Infiltrative lesions that were hypointense on T2-weighted images were better characterized with DW imaging than lesions that were hyperintense or well defined.

Conclusion.—Echo-planar DW MR imaging can help characterize indeterminate orbital masses.

▶ This retrospective study evaluated the role of diffusion-weighted MRI techniques to discriminate malignant orbital lesions from benign or inflammatory processes using apparent diffusion coefficient (ADC) threshold values. The technique was applied to 47 patients, with 31 patients with benign lesions and 16 patients with malignant processes.

In this study, they have found significantly lower ADC and ADC ratios (ADC of the lesion divided by ADC of ipsilateral normal-appearing white matter) in malignant lesions compared with benign lesions irrespective of age but with a higher statistical significance in adult population. The difference was even more significant when comparing lymphomas with inflammatory pseudotumor. They identified an ADC threshold of 1.0×10^{-3} mm^2/s that was 63% sensitive, 84% specific, and 77% accurate in differentiating malignant from benign lesion, while the same threshold proved 100% sensitive and 100% specific in differentiating lymphoma from pseudotumor. Although the study cohort included only 6 lymphoma and 10 pseudotumor cases, the statistical power of this threshold was quite significant.

The authors also grouped the lesions in 4 different categories based on T2 signal and tumor margins and found that ADC values were most useful in predicting malignancy in infiltrative T2-dark lesions. An infiltrative T2-dark lesion is most likely to represent either an inflammatory lesion with fibrosis (like orbital pseudotumor), which is likely to be hypocellular and demonstrate high ADC, or an aggressive tumor, which is likely to be hypercellular with low ADC. This is reflected in the 100% sensitivity and specificity they have demonstrated in differentiating lymphoma and orbital pseudotumor.

Although restricted diffusion correlates well with increased cellularity, not all hypercellular lesions are malignant, for example, meningiomas can demonstrate low ADC. As such, meningiomas were the more common cause of false positives in this study, which, however, can often be reasonably diagnosed based on clinical criteria and routine MRI features, including location. Metastasis, which represents a heterogeneous category with a wide range of cellularity depending on the nature of primary tumor and presence of necrosis, contributed most to the false negatives in this study. This is an important consideration if this method is to be considered for general clinical use.

While the authors provide a compelling new metric to aid in the discrimination of benign to malignant orbital pathologies, there are practical considerations that could prove to be somewhat problematic in the clinical setting. While diffusion techniques are ubiquitous in most neuroimaging protocols in use today, methods to process the diffusion data to produce actual diffusion metrics (eg. ADC values) are less available and the time commitment to measure and analyze the imaging data may be out of scope for many busy clinical practices. Therefore, although the technique is within reach for most clinical practices, whether it would be implemented as a routine decision support tool for orbital neoplasia remains to be determined.

K. Talekar, MD

A. E. Flanders, MD

Ocular Adnexal Lymphoma: Diffusion-weighted MR Imaging for Differential Diagnosis and Therapeutic Monitoring
Politi LS, Forghani R, Godi C, et al (San Raffaele Scientific Inst, Via Olgettina, Milan, Italy; Massachusetts General Hosp, Boston; et al)
Radiology 256:565-574, 2010

Purpose.—To describe the magnetic resonance (MR) imaging and diffusion-weighted (DW) imaging features of ocular adnexal lymphomas (OALs), to determine the diagnostic accuracy of apparent diffusion coefficient (ADC) for discriminating OALs from other orbital mass lesions, and to assess whether variations in ADC constitute a reliable biomarker of OAL response to therapy.

Materials and Methods.—Institutional ethical committee approval and informed consent were obtained. In this prospective study, 114 white subjects (65 females and 49 males) were enrolled. Thirty-eight patients with histopathologically proved OAL underwent serial MR and DW imaging examination of the orbits. ADCs of OALs were compared with those of normal orbital structures, obtained in 18 healthy volunteers, and other orbital mass lesions, prospectively acquired in 58 patients (20 primary non-OAL neoplasms, 15 vascular benign lesions, 12 inflammatory lesions, 11 metastases). Interval change in ADC of OALs before and after treatment was analyzed in 29 patients. Analysis of covariance and a paired t test were used for statistical analysis.

Results.—Baseline ADCs in OALs were lower than those in normal structures and other orbital diseases $(P < .001)$. An ADC threshold of 775×10^{-6} mm^2/sec resulted in 96% sensitivity, 93% specificity, 88% positive predictive value, 98.2% negative predictive value, and 94.4% accuracy in OAL diagnosis. Following appropriate treatment, 10 (34%) of 29 patients showed OAL volumetric reduction, accompanied $(n = 7)$ or preceded $(n = 3)$ by an increase in ADC $(P = .005)$. Conversely, a further reduction of ADC was observed in the seven patients who experienced disease progression $(P < .05)$.

Conclusion.—ADC permits accurate diagnosis of OALs. Interval change in ADC after therapy represents a helpful tool for predicting therapeutic response.

▶ Ocular adnexal lymphoma (OAL) is the most common orbital malignancy in adults, yet it is potentially curable; therefore, early diagnosis is imperative. Although MRI is the optimal imaging study for characterizing orbital tumors, distinction between different tumor types and differentiating tumor from non-neoplastic processes like inflammatory orbital pseudotumor is not frequently possible and biopsy is usually required. Biopsies of less accessible retrobulbar lesions can be technically challenging, and in view of the additional risk a reliable noninvasive predictor of lesion histology could prove valuable.

In this prospective study, which is one of the largest of its nature, the authors have showed that values of free water diffusion, the apparent diffusion coefficients (ADCs), provide an accurate noninvasive quantitative index for differentiating OALs from the other orbital mass lesions investigated. Diffusion-weighted (DW) imaging is one of the most clinically useful pulse sequences that is based on the physiologic process of molecular diffusion. Diffusion simply refers to translation that particles and molecules experience because of random collision. Pathologies that obstruct free diffusion (such as acute cerebral infarction, abscesses, and certain tumors including lymphoma) lead to what is widely referred to as restricted diffusion, which is seen as hyperintense signal on the DW sequence and more importantly appears dark on the ADC maps that can be measured.

ADC values have been previously shown to be of value in distinguishing tumors in head and neck.[1,2] Among the various pathological correlates demonstrated for low ADC values in literature, tumor cellularity is the most widely accepted correlate.[1,2] Other correlates include high nuclear-cytoplasmic ratio, nuclear angulations, and low extracellular space volume.[2] This helps us understand the false positives in this study. The 4 non-OAL lesions that had ADC values below their suggested threshold of 775×10^{-6} mm^2/s were all malignant tumors, presumably with very high cellularity. However, it should be noted that all malignancies are not hypercellular and, therefore, can demonstrate high ADC values; for example, metastasis (which is a broad category) can demonstrate a wide range of ADC values. Benign processes, especially pseudotumor and benign vascular lesions, were noted to have distinctly high ADC values.

Fig 3 in the original article shows that OAL (a), inflammatory orbital pseudotumor (b), monolateral thyroid-associated orbitopathy (c), and metastasis (d) have similar appearance on conventional postcontrast fat-suppressed images, but only OAL is hyperintense on the DW images with a corresponding low ADC value. Lymphomas have been consistently shown to exhibit very low ADC values when compared with other malignant lesions in the head and neck.[2,3] In this study, the authors found that lesions whose ADCs measured below a threshold of 775×10^{-6} mm^2/s were 96% sensitive, 93% specific, and 94.4% accurate in diagnosing OAL. They concluded that this threshold had a positive predictive value of 88% and negative predictive value of 98.2% for diagnosing OALs.

The authors also showed that OALs have lower ADC than normal orbital structures, making it possible to distinguish tumor from normal structures like lacrimal gland and extraocular muscles that can have similar signal characteristics on conventional sequences.

Additionally, the investigators found that temporal changes in the ADC values on serial MRI examinations coincide with or precede tumor volume changes following treatment, suggesting that diffusion MRI may have a role as a noninvasive biomarker to predict therapeutic response. While larger studies are required to confirm its role as an early biomarker of response to therapy, this prognostic role might be of great value in therapeutic planning.

K. Talekar, MD
A. E. Flanders, MD

References

1. Kono K, Inoue Y, Nakayama K, et al. The role of diffusion-weighted imaging in patients with brain tumors. *AJNR Am J Neuroradiol.* 2001;22:1081-1088.
2. Wang J, Takashima S, Takayama F, et al. Head and neck lesions: characterization with diffusion-weighted echo-planar MR imaging. *Radiology.* 2001;220:621-630.
3. Yamasaki F, Kurisu K, Satoh K, et al. Apparent diffusion coefficient of human brain tumors at MR imaging. *Radiology.* 2005;235:985-991.

Radial diffusivity in remote optic neuritis discriminates visual outcomes
Naismith RT, Xu J, Tutlam NT, et al (Washington Univ, St Louis, MO)
Neurology 74:1702-1710, 2010

Objective.—Diffusion tensor imaging (DTI) quantifies Brownian motion of water within tissue. The goal of this study was to test whether, following a remote episode of optic neuritis (ON), breakdown of myelin and axons within the optic nerve could be detected by alterations in

DTI parameters, and whether these alterations would correlate with visual loss.

Methods.—Seventy subjects with a history of ON ≥6 months prior underwent DTI of the optic nerves, assessment of visual acuities (VA) and contrast sensitivities (CS), and laboratory measures of visual evoked potentials (VEP) and optical coherence tomography (OCT).

Results.—Radial diffusivity (RD) correlated with visual acuity ($r = -0.61$), Pelli-Robson CS ($r = -0.60$), 5%CS ($r = 0.61$), OCT ($r = -0.78$), VEP latency ($r = 0.61$), and VEP amplitude ($r = -0.46$). RD differentiated the unaffected fellow nerves from affected nerves in all visual outcome categories. RD also discriminated nerves with recovery to normal from mild visual impairment, and those with mild impairment from profound visual loss. RD differentiated healthy controls from both clinically affected nerves and unaffected fellow nerves after ON. RD differentiated all categories of 5%CS outcomes, and all categories of Pelli-Robson CS with the exception of normal recovery from mildly affected.

Conclusions.—Increased optic nerve radial diffusivity (RD) detected by diffusion tensor imaging (DTI) was associated with a proportional decline in vision after optic neuritis. RD can differentiate healthy control nerves from both affected and unaffected fellow nerves. RD can discriminate among categories of visual recovery within affected eyes. Optic nerve injury as assessed by DTI was corroborated by both optical coherence tomography and visual evoked potentials.

▶ The association between clinical findings and radiological extent of involvement in multiple sclerosis is generally poor.[1] Although conventional MR imaging provides valuable information about location and volume of white matter lesions, its inability to quantify the underlying tissue destruction may contribute to this clinicoradiological paradox.

In this cohort study, the authors have demonstrated the role of quantitative diffusion tensor imaging (DTI) in differentiating severity of myelin and axonal injury within the optic nerve following a remote episode of optic neuritis. DTI, an advancement of diffusion MRI technique, is based on estimation of diffusion anisotropy. The free random motion of water molecules, for example in cerebrospinal fluid, is called isotropic diffusion. However, diffusion in brain parenchyma is not isotropic, especially in white matter, where the presence of natural barriers to diffusion such as cell membrane, myelin sheath, and parallel arrangement of axons restricts diffusion across them and facilitates diffusion preferentially along main direction of the axons and the fiber tracts. Such preferentially oriented diffusion is called anisotropic diffusion. Chronic injury because of loss of myelin and axons leads to reduced anisotropy. This results in increased diffusion perpendicular to the white matter tract (analogous to radial diffusivity), increased overall diffusivity (mean diffusivity), and reduced diffusion directionality (fractional anisotropy). Optic nerve, a relatively straight white matter tract whose clinical function is readily measured, offers a special advantage to study the relationship between DTI and function/disease. DTI has also been shown to detect early degeneration of visual pathway in glaucoma before the clinical manifestations become evident.[2] DTI also has application in white matter of the brain and spinal cord. DTI has been shown to be useful for detecting Wallerian degeneration of optic radiation even in the early stages after temporal lobe surgery for temporal lobectomy.[3]

The authors have demonstrated that optic nerve injury as assessed by DTI is corroborated by both optical coherence tomography and visual evoked potentials, and thus DTI could serve as a surrogate of myelin and axon integrity. DTI could be used to quantify the severity of myelin and axon injury and thereby supplement routine MRI sequences in better quantification of disease burden in demyelinating diseases like multiple sclerosis.

K. Talekar, MD

A. E. Flanders, MD

References

1. Barkhof F. The clinico-radiological paradox in multiple sclerosis revisited. *Curr Opin Neurol.* 2002;15:239-245.
2. Garaci FG, Bolacchi F, Cerulli A, et al. Optic nerve and optic radiation neurodegeneration in patients with glaucoma: in vivo analysis with 3-T diffusion-tensor MR imaging. *Radiology.* 2009;252:496-501.
3. Taoka T, Sakamoto M, Iwasaki S, et al. Diffusion tensor imaging in cases with visual field defect after anterior temporal lobectomy. *AJNR Am J Neuroradiol.* 2005;26:797-803.

10 Ocular Oncology

A prospective comparison of fine-needle aspiration cytopathology and histopathology in the diagnosis of orbital mass lesions
Karcioglu ZA, Fleming JC, Haik BG (Hamilton Eye Inst Univ of Tennessee, Memphis)
Br J Ophthalmol 94:128-130, 2010

Aim.—To assess the diagnostic value of the orbital fine needle aspiration biopsy (FNAB) with an in vitro technique, eliminating the sampling error.

Design.—Prospective, non-randomised, interventional case series.

Methods.—Sixty-eight patients were studied prospectively in institutional clinical practices. Immediately after excision of orbital mass lesions, the removed tissue was stabilised under the hand of the surgeon and biopsied with a 23- or 25-gauge needle. The samples were processed for cytopathological examination with Cytospin®. The excised specimens were then submitted for routine histological examination. The cytopathological diagnoses were compared with the final histopathological diagnoses.

Results.—Six out of 68 lesions were excluded and the remaining 62 cases were divided into four groups as primary malignant, primary benign, secondary malignant and inflammatory lesions, based on histopathological diagnoses. In 43 cases the cytopathological and histopathological diagnoses were the same, with a concordance rate of 69%. Among the malignant tumours, the cytopathological diagnoses correlated with the histopathological diagnoses in 14/14 and 17/27 cases of metastatic/secondary and primary orbital malignancies, respectively. Of 11 primary benign tumours, two cytopathological diagnoses correlated with histopathology. In inflammatory lesions, the cytopathological diagnoses were matched with the histopathological diagnoses in 10/10 biopsies.

Conclusion.—Even when the sampling error is eliminated with an "in vitro FNAB" technique, the concordance rates between histopathological and cytopathological diagnoses varied considerably among different types of orbital mass lesions. FNAB diagnoses were most reliable in metastatic and secondary malignancies and inflammatory lesions, and least reliable in benign orbital neoplasms and cysts.

▶ Fine-needle aspiration biopsy (FNAB) has been long studied for intraocular tumors and, to some extent, for orbital diseases. A recent publication has shown that FNAB yields cells adequate for cytogenetic testing in 97% of cases if the trans pars plana technique is used.[1] Little has been written on this technique for orbital tumors. In this report, the authors evaluated FNAB after the tumor is removed from the orbit and sitting on the surgical tray. In this way, they maximize their tumor yield and hopefully their accuracy. Of 62 FNAB-tested specimens, there was agreement between cytopathology and histopathology in only 69% of cases. They conclude that even in the most ideal situation with direct visualization of the FNAB site, tissue concordance is not perfect.

The authors found that the main discordant lesion was orbital lymphoma. In these cases, cytopathology showed lymphoproliferative lesion, atypical lymphocyte–dominated lesion, or lymphoid proliferation, but the term lymphoma was not often used based on cytopathology. They admit that the diagnosis of lymphoma is based on a series of tests, including flow cytometry and immunophenotyping, which usually requires a larger volume of tumor tissue. Perhaps FNAB could be used in these circumstances to confirm involvement in the ocular region after the diagnosis is already established.

C. L. Shields, MD

Reference

1. Shields CL, Ganguly A, Bianciotto CG, Turaka K, Tavalalli A, Shields JA. Prognosis of uveal melanoma in 500 consecutive cases using genetic testing of fine needle aspiration biopsy. *Arch Ophthalmol.*

Choroidal Vitiligo Masquerading as Large Choroidal Nevus: A Report of Four Cases

Shields CL, Ramasubramanian A, Kunz WB, et al (Thomas Jefferson Univ, Philadelphia, PA)
Ophthalmology 117:109-113, 2010

Purpose.—To describe 4 patients with choroidal vitiligo masquerading as large choroidal nevus.

Design.—Retrospective chart review.

Participants.—Observational case series of 4 patients.

Methods.—Retrospective chart review.

Main Outcome Measures.—Clinical features.

Results.—Four patients referred with the diagnosis of large choroidal nevus were found to have unilateral (n = 1) or bilateral (n = 3) extensive patchy choroidal depigmentation classified as choroidal vitiligo. There was no evidence of choroidal nevus, and the pigmented "lesion" proved to be normal choroidal pigment surrounded by a region of pigment absence (vitiligo). There was no evidence of ocular inflammation or related retinal or retinal pigment epithelial changes. The choroidal vitiligo was clinically flat and measured 12 to 24 mm diameter, involving the postequatorial fundus in all cases. There were no related anterior segment abnormalities. Cutaneous vitiligo was present in all cases. There was no documented progression of the choroidal or cutaneous vitiligo over a maximum 2-year follow-up.

Conclusions.—Choroidal vitiligo is an idiopathic benign process that can involve large segments of the posterior choroid, leaving only patches of residual choroidal pigment, simulating, in reverse, a large choroidal nevus.

▶ Vitiligo is a cutaneous disorder attributed to autoimmune dysfunction, viral infection, chemical exposure, or other mechanisms. It can be found with other autoimmune disorders such as Graves disease, Addison disease, and hypothyroidism. It is a notable feature of Vogt-Koyanagi-Harada (VKH) syndrome. In some instances, vitiligo can affect the eye following inflammation as a secondary process, leaving depigmented areas within the choroid. These are often associated with extensive retinal pigment epithelial changes as seen with VKH. In this report, the authors describe choroidal vitiligo as a primary process whereby the choroidal pigment is absent and there are no retinal pigment epithelial alterations.

They described 4 patients with cutaneous vitiligo who also manifested choroidal vitiligo as a unilateral or bilateral condition. In these cases, the depigmented choroid was the pathologic feature, but each patient was referred for suspicion of large choroidal nevus, which proved to be the normal pigment contrasted against the vitiligo sections. The vitiligo was patchy and extensive over the entire fundus, in each case leaving dark and light spots in a dalmatian-like pattern. There was no related vision loss in any case. Only short follow-up was provided. The long-term implications of primary choroidal vitiligo have yet to be determined.

C. L. Shields, MD

Conjunctival Nevi: Clinical Features and Therapeutic Outcomes

Levecq L, De Potter P, Jamart J (Cliniques Universitaires St-Luc, Brussels, Belgium; Cliniques Universitaires de Mont-Godinne, Yvoir, Belgium)
Ophthalmology 117:35-40, 2010

Objective.—To determine the epidemiology and the clinical and therapeutic outcomes of conjunctival nevi and to identify the clinical variables statistically associated with operative excision.

Design.—Prospective, observational, noncomparative case series.

Participants.—Two hundred fifty-five patients with the clinical diagnosis of conjunctival nevus.

Methods.—Consecutive cases of conjunctival nevi managed at a single institution were studied to identify the clinical risk factors for operative excision.

Main Outcome Measures.—Reasons for operative excision.

Results.—Of the 255 patients who were periodically observed for a mean of 5.3 years (range, 1–11), nevi were clinically diagnosed in 140 females and 115 males and modified operative excision was performed in 75 patients (29%). The decision of operative excision was made by the surgeon in 13 cases (17%) and by the patient in 62 cases (83%). In those 13 patients, the operative decision was prompted by our concern for possible malignant transformation based on suspicious biomicroscopic features in 10 patients (13%) and photographically documented tumor growth in 3 patients (4%). For the other 62 patients who elected to undergo surgery, their reasons for excision included patient's concern for cancer in 34 cases (45%), cosmetic arguments in 9 cases (12%), and patient's request owing to lesion-induced ocular surface irritation in 19 cases (25%). Comparison between groups showed that the clinical factors at initial visit that were statistically predictive of surgical excision were the older age of the patient ($P = 0.001$), the largest basal tumor diameter ($P<0.001$), tumor location ($P = 0.023$), and presence of clear cysts ($P = 0.013$), of intrinsic vasculature ($P<0.001$), of prominent feeder vessels ($P<0.001$), and of corneal involvement ($P = 0.008$). None of the excised lesions showed histopathologically malignant features.

Conclusions.—In our series, documented tumor growth of conjunctival nevus remained relatively a uncommon event with a incidence of 4%. Conjunctival nevi in older patients, associated with dilated feeder vessels, prominent intrinsic vasculature, and corneal involvement were more likely to be treated with operative excision.

▶ Conjunctival nevi represent the most common lesion of the conjunctiva. In a large series of 1643 conjunctival tumors in all age groups, the nevus represented 28% of all tumors and 52% of melanocytic tumors.[1] The nevus is diagnosed by clinical examination, often without biopsy. This lesion is initially recognized in children, and hesitancy toward surgery for a benign condition often leads to observation of the lesion. In the report by Levecq and associates, they explored reasons for removal of conjunctival nevi.

Of 255 patients with conjunctival nevus observed for a period of time, 75 ultimately underwent surgical excision. The reason for surgery stemmed from surgeons' concerns (17%) and patients' concerns (83%). The surgeons' concerns were for fear of melanoma in all cases. The patients'/parents' concerns were for fear of cancer (55%), cosmetic improvement (15%), and ocular surface irritation (31%). Fortunately, there proved to be no melanoma in the excised lesions, as all proved to be nevi.

Previous studies of conjunctival nevi have shown that transformation is low at 1% or less over time.[2] However, studies of conjunctival melanoma show that approximately 7% arise from a longstanding nevus. Conjunctival nevi should be monitored annually, and increase in size during adulthood or relationship to primary acquired melanosis could suggest melanoma.

C. L. Shields, MD

References

1. Shields CL, Demirci H, Karatza E, Shields JA. Clinical survey of 1643 melanocytic and nonmelanocytic conjunctival tumors. *Ophthalmology.* 2004;111:1747-1754.
2. Shields CL, Fasiudden A, Mashayekhi A, Shields JA. Conjunctival nevi: clinical features and natural course in 410 consecutive patients. *Arch Ophthalmol.* 2004;122:167-175.

Cyclophosphamide for Ocular Inflammatory Diseases

Pujari SS, Kempen JH, Newcomb CW, et al (The Massachusetts Eye Res and Surgery Inst, Cambridge; Univ of Pennsylvania, Philadelphia; et al)
Ophthalmology 117:356-365, 2010

Purpose.—To evaluate the outcomes of cyclophosphamide therapy for noninfectious ocular inflammation.

Design.—Retrospective cohort study.

Participants.—Two hundred fifteen patients with noninfectious ocular inflammation observed from initiation of cyclophosphamide.

Methods.—Patients initiating cyclophosphamide, without other immunosuppressive drugs (other than corticosteroids), were identified at 4 centers. Dose of cyclophosphamide, response to therapy, corticosteroid-sparing effects, frequency of discontinuation, and reasons for discontinuation were obtained by medical record review of every visit.

Main Outcome Measures.—Control of inflammation, corticosteroid-sparing effects, and discontinuation of therapy.

Results.—The 215 patients (381 involved eyes) meeting eligibility criteria carried diagnoses of uveitis (20.4%), scleritis (22.3%), ocular mucous membrane pemphigoid (45.6%), or other forms of ocular inflammation (11.6%). Overall, approximately 49.2% (95% confidence interval [CI], 41.7%−57.2%) gained sustained control of inflammation (for at least 28 days) within 6 months, and 76% (95% CI, 68.3%−83.7%) gained sustained control of inflammation within 12 months. Corticosteroid-sparing success (sustained control of inflammation while tapering prednisone to 10 mg or less among those not meeting success criteria initially) was gained by 30.0% and 61.2% by 6 and 12 months, respectively. Disease remission leading to discontinuation of cyclophosphamide occurred at the rate of 0.32/person-year (95% CI, 0.24−0.41), and the estimated proportion with remission at or before 2 years was 63.1% (95% CI, 51.5%−74.8%). Cyclophosphamide was discontinued by 33.5% of patients within 1 year because of side effects, usually of a reversible nature.

Conclusions.—The data suggest that cyclophosphamide is effective for most patients for controlling inflammation and allowing tapering of systemic corticosteroids to 10 mg prednisone or less, although 1 year of therapy may be needed to achieve these goals. Unlike with most other immunosuppressive drugs, disease remission was induced by treatment in most patients who were able to tolerate therapy. To titrate therapy properly and to minimize the risk of serious potential side effects, a systematic program of laboratory monitoring is required. Judicious use of cyclophosphamide seems to be beneficial for severe ocular inflammation cases where the potentially vision-saving benefits outweigh the substantial potential side effects of therapy, or when indicated for associated systemic inflammatory diseases.

▶ The mainstay of treatment for ocular inflammatory conditions is the use of corticosteroids. First introduced in 1951 for ocular inflammation, this therapy has lasted as a reliable cost-effective treatment but with occasional unwanted side effects. The dose-dependent chronic side effects of oral corticosteroids include induction or worsening of diabetes mellitus or hypertension, weight gain, water gain, peptic ulcer disease, psychiatric imbalance, myopathy, bone fracture, infection, shock, and death. Hence, oral corticosteroids are often used to acutely control ocular inflammation, but switch to noncorticosteroid therapies, like immunosuppressive agents, is considered for long-term control. One agent is cyclophosphamide.

Cyclophosphamide is an alkylating agent originally used for systemic cancers and was introduced for uveitis treatment in 1952. Its method of action is to exert a direct cytotoxic effect on rapidly proliferating cells by alkylating nucleophilic groups on DNA bases, particularly on guanine. This causes cross-linking and leads to cell death during mitosis. This is particularly effective for T and B cells and causes profound immune suppression. This medication is used for Wegener granulomatosis, rheumatoid vasculitis, polyarteritis nodosa, lupus, mucous membrane pemphigoid, and other ocular conditions.

In this report, the community of ocular inflammation scientists collaborated to study the pattern of inflammation control with cyclophosphamide for various conditions, including uveitis (20%), scleritis (22%), pemphigoid (45%), and others (12%). They noted that this medication acted slowly and was only tolerated for up to 1 year in < 70% cases. By 6 months, nearly 50% showed inflammation control and by 1 year, 76% showed control. The good news is that inflammatory remission allowing discontinuance of cyclophosphamide occurred in 63% by 2 years. This medication must be carefully titrated by experienced medical personnel.

C. L. Shields, MD

Giant Choroidal Nevus: Clinical Features and Natural Course in 322 Cases
Li HK, Shields CL, Mashayekhi A, et al (Thomas Jefferson Univ, Philadelphia, PA)
Ophthalmology 117:324-333, 2010

Purpose.—Evaluation of clinical features and natural course of giant choroidal nevi (diameter ≥10 mm).
Design.—Retrospective observational case series.
Participants.—We included 322 eyes of 322 patients.
Methods.—Clinic-based study of tumor features, tumor outcome, and vision outcome. Kaplan–Meier analysis was used to assess time to transformation into melanoma. Cox proportional hazards regressions evaluated clinical factors predictive of nevus transformation into melanoma and nevus-related decreased vision (defined as <20/20 and unrelated to other eye pathology).
Main Outcome Measures.—Transformation of giant choroidal nevus into melanoma and nevus-related decreased vision.
Results.—A medical record review of 4100 patients diagnosed with choroidal nevus identified 322 (8%) giant choroidal nevi. Median nevus

basal diameter was 11 mm (range, 10—24). Median thickness was 1.9 mm (range, 0—4.4). Related retinal findings included drusen overlying nevus (n = 261 [81%]), subretinal fluid (n = 26 [8%]), orange pigment (n = 4 [1%]), retinal pigment epithelial (RPE) detachment (n = 6 [2%]), hyperplasia (n = 48 [15%]), fibrous metaplasia (n = 48 [15%]), atrophy (n = 63 [20%]), or trough (n = 6 [2%]). Kaplan—Meier analysis estimated transformation into melanoma in 13% at 5 years and 18% at 10 years. Multivariate analyses revealed factors predictive of transformation into melanoma including involvement or close proximity to the foveola ($P = 0.017$) and acoustic hollowness ($P = 0.052$). Nevus-related decreased vision was found in 2.2% of eyes at initial visit and 3.7% at final visit (median 41 and mean 61 months follow-up). Factors associated with nevus-related decreased vision at initial visit included subretinal fluid ($P = 0.001$), involvement or close proximity to foveola ($P = 0.005$), RPE detachment ($P = 0.033$), and nevus-related choroidal neovascular membrane ($P = 0.044$). Factors predictive of nevus-related decreased vision at final visit included involvement or close proximity to the foveola ($P = 0.001$) and presence of symptoms at the initial visit ($P = 0.032$).

Conclusions.—Giant choroidal nevi can clinically resemble choroidal melanoma but show features of chronicity, such as overlying drusen and RPE alterations. Over time, 18% transformed into melanoma, underscoring the importance of life-long surveillance.

▶ Choroidal nevus is a benign melanocytic lesion that appears deep to the retina as a pigmented or nonpigmented mass. The main concern with choroidal nevus is its risk to cause poor visual acuity and to evolve into melanoma. The average size of choroidal nevus by population screening is approximately 1.5-mm diameter. The average size of choroidal nevus from an oncology clinic screening is naturally larger as more suspicious lesions are referred and the basal dimension is about 5.0-mm diameter. In this analysis, Li and associates evaluated the larger end of the spectrum of choroidal nevi, those termed giant nevus, as their qualifying base was 10 mm or greater in diameter.

Many melanocytic tumors of 10 mm or greater are choroidal melanoma, not nevi. Melanoma tends to have thickness over 2 mm and shows related features of subretinal fluid, orange lipofuscin pigment, hemorrhage, and mushroom configuration. The thicker the melanoma, the more easily it is identified, but the worse the patient prognosis.[1] Nevi, on the other hand, tend to show little or absent subretinal fluid and rarely any of the other features.[2] Nevi more likely show retinal pigment epithelial alterations and drusen.

In this analysis, looking at "worst case scenario" large nevi, the authors found that growth into melanoma occurred in 18% by 10 years and into those that were more posterior in the eye and those with acoustic hollowness on B scan ultrasonography. These findings corroborate known risk factors for identification of small melanoma, as both features represent 2 of the 8 risk factors.[3] Any patient with a large or giant choroidal nevus should be examined by an ocular oncologist to determine if the mass indeed is a benign nevus, or if it could be a melanoma, particularly the ominous flat (diffuse) melanoma.[3]

C. L. Shields, MD

References

1. Shields CL, Furuta M, Thangappan A, et al. Metastasis of uveal melanoma millimeter-by-millimeter in 8033 consecutive eyes. *Arch Ophthalmol.* 2009;127: 989-998.
2. Shields CL, Furuta M, Berman EL, et al. Choroidal nevus transformation into melanoma: analysis of 2514 consecutive cases. *Arch Ophthalmol.* 2009;127: 981-987.
3. Shields CL, Shields JA, DePotter P, Cater J, Tardio D, Barrett J. Diffuse choroidal melanoma. Clinical features predictive of metastasis. *Arch Ophthalmol.* 1996;114: 956-963.

Intraocular Tumor-Associated Lymphangiogenesis: A Novel Prognostic Factor for Ciliary Body Melanomas with Extraocular Extension?

Heindl LM, Hofmann TN, Adler W, et al (Friedrich-Alexander Univ Erlangen-Nürnberg, Germany)
Ophthalmology 117:334-342, 2010

Purpose.—To evaluate whether intraocular tumor-associated lymphangiogenesis contributes to prognosis of ciliary body melanomas with extraocular extension and to study its association with other tumor characteristics.

Design.—Nonrandomized, retrospective case series.

Participants.—Twenty consecutive patients enucleated for a malignant melanoma of the ciliary body with extraocular extension.

Methods.—Lymphatic vessels were identified using lymphatic vascular endothelial-specific hyaluronic acid receptor-1 (LYVE-1) and podoplanin as specific immunohistochemical markers for lymphatic vascular endothelium. Baseline tumor characteristics included intra- and extraocular tumor size, 2009 tumor, node, metastasis (TNM) classification, route of extraocular spread, tumor cell type, mitotic rate, Ki-67 proliferation-index, microvascular patterns and density, tumor-infiltrating lymphocytes and macrophages, and expression of human leukocyte antigen (HLA) class I and insulin-like growth factor-1 receptor. Kaplan-Meier and Cox regression analyses of melanoma-specific survival were performed.

Main Outcome Measures.—Prevalence of intraocular LYVE-1⁺/podoplanin⁺ lymphatic vessels and association with intraocular tumor characteristics and metastasis-free survival.

Results.—Intraocular LYVE-1⁺ and podoplanin⁺ lymphatic vessels could be detected in 12 (60%) of 20 ciliary body melanomas with extraocular extension. Presence of intraocular LYVE-1⁺/podoplanin⁺ lymphatic vessels was significantly associated with larger intra- ($P = 0.002$) and extraocular tumor size ($P < 0.001$), higher TNM categories ($P = 0.004$), epithelioid cellularity ($P = 0.016$), higher mitotic rate ($P = 0.003$), higher Ki-67 proliferation-index ($P = 0.049$), microvascular networks ($P = 0.005$), higher microvascular density ($P = 0.003$), more tumor-infiltrating macrophages ($P = 0.002$), higher expression of HLA class I ($P = 0.046$), and insulin-like growth factor-1 receptor ($P = 0.033$), but not significantly with route of extraocular spread ($P = 0.803$), and tumorinfiltrating lymphocytes ($P = 0.069$). Melanoma-specific mortality rates increased significantly with the presence of intraocular LYVE-1$^+$/podoplanin$^+$ lymphatic vessels ($P = 0.008$). By multivariate Cox regression, tumor size (hazard ratio, 14.40; $P = 0.002$), and presence of intraocular lymphatic vessels (hazard ratio, 8.09; $P = 0.04$) were strong prognostic predictors of mortality.

Conclusions.—Intraocular peritumoral lymphangiogenesis seems to be associated with an increased mortality risk in patients with ciliary body melanomas and extraocular extension. This association may be primarily because of an association of intraocular lymphangiogenesis with greater tumor size and increased malignancy.

▶ Extrascleral extension of uveal melanoma occurs in approximately 8% of cases and is usually related to large tumor size and ciliary body location. The tumor gains access to the extrascleral space by egressing through a preformed emissary canal, not necessarily through gross invasion into the scleral fibers. In most cases, the extension appears as a circumscribed black or dark brown mass deep to Tenon fascia on the surface of the eye and with dilated episcleral vessels feeding into it. In rare instances, it can appear as a major ill-defined mass in the orbit, causing globe compression or even with black epiphora, termed melanodacryorrhea.[1]

The presence of extrascleral extension of uveal melanoma portends a poor life prognosis by direct and indirect findings. The tumor gains direct access to the orbital and conjunctival vascular tree with risk for hematogenous spread. Indirectly, this extension suggests a more aggressive larger malignancy with greater risk for metastatic disease. Rarely is it found that ocular melanoma metastasizes by lymphatic route. In this report, Heindl and associates studied 20 eyes with ciliary body melanoma and extrascleral extension to look for related lymphatic vessel development. Surprisingly, they found that 60% had related lymphatics, and this was associated with poor outcome factors like large tumor size, higher proliferation, and the presence of the lymphatics was a strong predictor of mortality. The authors speculate that antilymphangiogenic therapies such as bevacizumab could assist in reducing lymphatic development and protect the patient from metastasis in the long term.

C. L. Shields, MD

Reference

1. Ghassemi F, Shields CL, Palamar M, Eagle RC Jr, Shields JA. Black tears (melano-dacryorrhea) from uveal melanoma. *Arch Ophthalmol.* 2008;126:1166-1168.

Management of Acute Stevens-Johnson Syndrome and Toxic Epidermal Necrolysis Utilizing Amniotic Membrane and Topical Corticosteroids

Shammas MC, Lai EC, Sarkar JS, et al (New York—Presbyterian Hosp)
Am J Ophthalmol 149:203-213, 2010

Purpose.—To describe the results of a novel treatment approach to the acute ophthalmic management of Stevens-Johnson syndrome (SJS) and toxic epidermal necrolysis (TEN).

Design.—Retrospective interventional case series.

Methods.—Setting: Institutional.

Study Population: Sixteen eyes of 8 patients with acute, biopsy-proven SJS or TEN and significant ophthalmic involvement.

Interventional Procedure(s): Application of amniotic membrane to the ocular surface, either in the operating room or at the bedside, and short-term use of intensive topical corticosteroid medication.

Main Outcome Measures: Visual acuity, slit-lamp appearance of the ocular surface, and patients' subjective impression of ocular comfort.

Results.—Two patients expired during the hospitalization. Mean follow-up time for the surviving patients was 7.7 months. Four surviving patients in whom the entire ocular surface (ie, the cornea, bulbar and palpebral conjunctiva, and eyelid margins) was treated with amniotic membrane retained visual acuities of 20/40 or better and an intact ocular surface. In contrast, the initial 2 patients in the study who were treated with only a Prokera device or unsutured amniotic membrane sheets, leaving the palpebral conjunctiva and eyelid margins uncovered, developed more significant ocular surface abnormalities, and 1 developed a corneal perforation.

Conclusions.—Amniotic membrane coverage of the ocular surface in its entirety coupled with the use of intensive short-term topical corticosteroids during the acute phase of SJS and TEN is associated with the preservation of good visual acuity and an intact ocular surface. Partial amniotic membrane coverage of the ocular surface may not serve to minimize the cicatrizing ocular sequelae of SJS and TEN as effectively as complete coverage.

▶ Stevens Johnson syndrome (SJS) and toxic epidermal necrolysis (TEN) are a spectrum of rare, acute vesiculobullous disorders of skin and mucous membranes that result in sloughing and ultimate scarring. The exact pathogenesis is unclear, but it is believed that this results from exuberant immunologic response to some agent whether it be an antibiotic or infection. The conjunctiva and oropharynx are the most commonly affected mucosal surfaces, and they are reported to be involved in > 50% of patients with SJS and TEN.

Mucous membrane involvement starts as a conjunctivitis with membranes and later develops into sloughing. Chronically, cicatrization happens with formation of symblepharon, entropion, trichiasis, limbal stem cell deficiency, severe dry eye, and ultimately corneal ulcer with vision loss. In the past, this was treated with vigorous lubrication, topical antibiotics, as well as symblepharon lysis with long-term poor prognosis. More recently, the application of amniotic membrane has been more successful with improved outcomes. The addition of systemic pulsed corticosteroid application may be even more beneficial.

In this report, the authors explore the use of amniotic membrane (AM) coupled with intensive short-term topical corticosteroid medications in 8 patients with ophthalmic involvement in acute SJS or TEN. The AM was applied in the operating room to the lid margin, tarsal, bulbar, and corneal surface or at the bedside to the bulbar and corneal surface. The topical steroids were applied every 1 to 2 hours for 2 to 3 weeks until healing was underway. They found much improved outcomes with vision of 20/40 or better and intact surface in those who had extensive AM of the lid margin, tarsal, bulbar, and corneal surface. They concluded that partial coverage might not be sufficient. This is a tremendous improvement in outcome of this disease with a relatively simple approach.

C. L. Shields, MD

Rituximab Treatment of Patients with Severe, Corticosteroid-Resistant Thyroid-Associated Ophthalmopathy
Khanna D, Chong KKL, Afifiyan NF, et al (Univ of California at Los Angeles; Los Angeles Biomed Inst at Harbor-UCLA Med Ctr, Torrance)
Ophthalmology 117:133-139, 2010

Purpose.—To study the effectiveness of anti-CD20 (rituximab [RTX]; Rituxan; Genentech, Inc., South San Francisco, CA) therapy in patients with severe, corticosteroid (CS)-resistant thyroid-associated ophthalmopathy (TAO).

Design.—Retrospective, interventional case series.

Participants.—Six consecutive subjects with severe, progressive TAO unresponsive to CS.

Methods.—Electronic medical record review of consecutive patients receiving RTX during the previous 18 months. Responses to therapy were graded using standard clinical assessment and flow cytometric analysis of peripheral lymphocytes.

Main Outcome Measures.—Clinical activity score (CAS), proptosis, strabismus, treatment side effects, and quantification of regulatory T cells.

Results.—Six patients were studied. Systemic CS failed to alter clinical activity in all patients (mean CAS ± standard deviation, 5.3 ± 1.0 before vs. 5.5 ± 0.8 during therapy for 7.5 ± 6.4 months; $P = 1.0$). However, after RTX treatment, CAS improved from 5.5 ± 0.8 to 1.3 ± 0.5 at 2 months after treatment ($P<0.03$) and remained quiescent in all patients (CAS, 0.7 ± 0.8, $P<0.0001$) at a mean follow-up of 6.2 ± 4.5 months. Vision improved bilaterally in all 4 patients with dysthyroid optic neuropathy (DON). None of the 6 patients experienced disease relapse after RTX infusion, and proptosis remained stable (Hertel measurement, 24 ± 3.7 mm before therapy and 23.6 ± 3.7 mm after therapy; $P = 0.17$). The abundance of T regulatory cells, assessed in 1 patient, increased within 1 week of RTX and remained elevated at 18 months of follow-up.

Conclusions.—In progressive, CS-resistant TAO, rapid and sustained resolution of orbital inflammation and DON followed treatment with RTX.

▶ The standard treatment of the inflammatory portion of thyroid-associated ophthalmopathy involves systemic corticosteroids, external radiotherapy, or both. Neither approach is ideal. Evidence shows that both T cells and B cells are involved with thyroid-associated ophthalmopathy. B cells are found diffusely in this condition within the affected tissue and can produce local auto-antibodies as well as present antigens to T cells. There are new medications aimed to control B cells, and the most popular is rituximab. This monoclonal antibody targets CD20, a protein present on immature and mature B cells and not found on plasma cells. Rituximab is used to treat non-Hodgkin B cell lymphoma and even rheumatoid arthritis.

In this report, the authors found that rituximab was effective against the inflammatory component of thyroid-associated ophthalmopathy. In addition, this medication resolved dysthyroid optic neuropathy in 4 of 4 cases with notable vision improvement. Despite these good results, proptosis and lid retraction were not necessarily improved.

The authors suggest a prospective study to better evaluate the role of B cell depletion with rituximab for thyroid-associated ophthalmopathy. This report of 6 patients suggests that it may play an important role in inflammation control.

C. L. Shields, MD

Spectrum of CD30⁺ Lymphoid Proliferations in the Eyelid: Lymphomatoid Papulosis, Cutaneous Anaplastic Large Cell Lymphoma, and Anaplastic Large Cell Lymphoma
Sanka RK, Eagle RC Jr, Wojno TH, et al (Emory Univ School of Medicine, Atlanta, GA; Wills Eye Inst, Philadelphia, PA; et al)
Ophthalmology 117:343-351, 2010

Purpose.—To report the clinicopathologic features of 3 patients with CD30⁺ lymphoid proliferations of the eyelid.

Design.—Retrospective case series.

Participants.—Patients with cutaneous CD30⁺ lymphoproliferative lesions of the eyelid.

Methods.—Three patients with CD30⁺ non-mycosis fungoides T-cell lymphoid infiltrates of the eyelid were identified. The histories, clinical findings, pathologic features including immunohistochemical staining, treatments, and outcomes were reviewed and compared.

Main Outcome Measures.—Pathologic findings including immunohistochemical analysis.

Results.—The patients included an 81-year-old man, an 18-year-old man, and a 42-year-old woman with CD30⁺ lymphoid proliferations of the eyelid and adjacent soft tissue. The first patient had an isolated crateriform eyelid lesion that was classified as lymphomatoid papulosis (LyP). The second patient had an isolated multinodular lesion of the eyelid that was classified as cutaneous anaplastic large cell lymphoma (cALCL). The third patient presented with eyelid edema with an underlying mass and was found to have widely disseminated anaplastic large cell lymphoma (ALCL). Diagnoses were dependent on clinical findings.

Conclusions.—The CD30$^+$ lymphoid proliferations represent a spectrum of conditions ranging from indolent LyP, to moderately aggressive cALCL, to highly aggressive ALCL. Interpretation of the pathologic findings in CD30$^+$ lymphoid proliferations is based in part on clinical findings.

▶ Lymphoma represents among the most common malignancies of the conjunctiva and orbit. Most lymphomas in this region are B-cell lymphomas, notably mucosal-associated lymphoid tissue, and carry low-grade activity with relatively good long-term life prognosis. In the skin, lymphomas can be T cell and are represented by the well-known mycosis fungoides and the lesser known indolent lymphomatoid papulosis, primary cutaneous anaplastic large-cell lymphoma, and aggressive systemic anaplastic large-cell lymphoma, all of which are discussed in this report.

These lesser-known T-cell lymphomas all manifest CD30 surface marker and represent 30% of the skin lymphomas. In contrast, T-cell lymphomas are extremely rare in the ocular region, representing perhaps only 1% of lymphomas. In this report, the patients ranged in age from 18 to 81 years. The tumors were all deep to the surface of the eyelid and appeared a localized or diffuse nodule in all cases and with ulceration in 2 cases. One patient had diffuse markedly swollen upper and lower eyelids, suggestive of allergy or inflammation and not necessarily tumor.

The take-home point is that a patient with a deep nodule of the eyelid most likely harbors a chalazion or inflammation, but if it does not resolve, a biopsy to rule out underlying malignancy is critical.

C. L. Shields, MD

Topical Treatment for Capillary Hemangioma of the Eyelid Using β-Blocker Solution
Guo S, Ni N (Univ of Medicine and Dentistry of New Jersey—New Jersey Med School, Newark; Yale Univ School of Medicine, New Haven, CT)
Arch Ophthalmol 128:255-256, 2010

The prevalence of periorbital or eyelid hemangioma ranges from 1% to 3%. There are more than 1.5 million affected children in the United States. Amblyopia is the most common complication of capillary hemangioma of the eyelid in children, with an incidence of 60%. If it is not treated promptly, it may lead to irreversible blindness in young children. The treatment options include corticosteroids, interferon alfa-2a, laser therapy, embolization, immunomodulators, surgery, and systemic propranolol. All therapeutic options are associated with adverse effects, some of which are serious. The treatment of a large capillary hemangioma on a child's left upper eyelid using topical β-blocker solution is reported. The hemangioma significantly improved within a few weeks of the topical treatment.

▶ Cutaneous capillary hemangioma of infancy is found in 10% of infants. Children at risk for this tumor are premature babies and those of multiple births. In most instances, there is no need for treatment, as this tumor resolves slowly over 1 to 4 years, leaving thin skin and minimal cosmetic deformity. There are instances that require urgent treatment for this tumor, and this includes those babies with hemangioma in the nasopharynx, gastrointestinal tract, or the periocular region.

The treatment is most often corticosteroids, interferon, and more recently propranolol. All of these options carry risks. With propranolol, the child must be admitted for observation in the hospital while the drug is instituted to watch for side effects of bronchospasm, vasospasm, hypoglycemia, hypotension, bradycardia, congestive heart failure, and others. In this case, the 4-month-old baby was treated with topical application of β blocker eyedrop (timoptic 0.5%) that was dripped and rubbed into the hemangioma twice daily for 7 weeks. There was substantial reduction in tumor volume by age 5 months. This could be an exciting new option for treatment of hemangioma if it is superficially located.

C. L. Shields, MD

11 Pathology

Frequent Mutation of *BAP1* in Metastasizing Uveal Melanomas
Harbour JW, Onken MD, Roberson EDO, et al (Washington Univ School of Medicine, St Louis, MO)
Science 330:1410-1413, 2010

Metastasis is a defining feature of malignant tumors and is the most common cause of cancer-related death, yet the genetics of metastasis are poorly understood. We used exome capture coupled with massively parallel sequencing to search for metastasis-related mutations in highly metastatic uveal melanomas of the eye. Inactivating somatic mutations were identified in the gene encoding BRCA1- associated protein 1 (*BAP1*) on chromosome 3p21.1 in 26 of 31 (84%) metastasizing tumors, including 15 mutations causing premature protein termination and 5 affecting its ubiquitin carboxyl terminal hydrolase domain. One tumor harbored a frameshift mutation that was germline in origin, thus representing a susceptibility allele. These findings implicate loss of BAP1 in uveal melanoma metastasis and suggest that the BAP1 pathway may be a valuable therapeutic target (Figs 1 and 2).

▶ Improvements in survival of patients with uveal melanoma are unlikely to arise from new therapies for advanced metastatic disease but, rather, from adjuvant therapy before detection of metastatic disease or from therapies aimed at early detection and treatment of metastatic disease. Uveal melanomas are divided into class 1 (low metastatic risk) and class 2 (high metastatic risk) based on gene expression profile. However, the specific gene(s) involved in acquisition of metastatic potential by uveal melanoma have not been previously identified. The discovery of *BAP1* gene by Harbour et al. is, therefore, an exciting and promising development in uveal melanoma research.

BAP1 encodes a nuclear ubiquitin carboxy-terminal hydrolase (UCH), one of several classes of deubiquitinating enzymes. In addition to the UCH catalytic domain, *BAP1* contains a UCH37-like domain, binding domains for BRCA1 and BARD1, which form a tumor suppressor heterodimeric complex, and a binding domain for HCFC1, which interacts with histone-modifying complexes during cell division. *BAP1* also interacts with ASXL1 to form the Polycomb group repressive deubiquitinase complex, which is involved in stem cell pluripotency and other developmental processes. *BAP1* exhibits tumor suppressor activity in cancer cells, and *BAP1* mutations have been reported in a small number of breast and lung cancer samples.

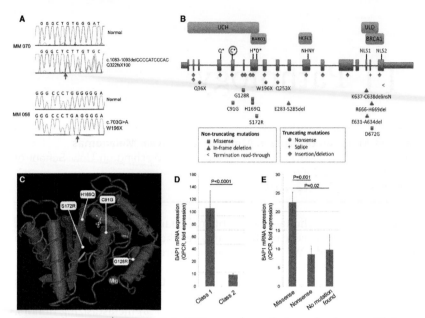

FIGURE 1.—Inactivating mutations in *BAP1* occur frequently in uveal melanomas. (A) Sanger sequence traces of MM 056 and MM 070 at the sites of the mutations. Location of mutated base in MM 056 and the start of the deletion of MM 070 are indicated (arrows). The noncoding *BAP1* strand is shown for MM 070. (B) Map of *BAP1* gene and location of *BAP1* mutations. *BAP1* contains 17 exons (shaded boxes) that encode a 728—amino acid protein. Introns are not to scale. Mutations are shown below the gene figure as indicated. The UCH domain [amino acids (aa) 1 to 188] and UCH37-like domain (ULD) (aa 635 to 693) are indicated (*12, 13*). The critical Q, C, H, and D residues of the active site (Gln[85], Cys[91], His[169], and Asp[184]) are indicated with asterisks. The catalytic cysteine is indicated with a circle. Also shown are the NHNY consensus sequence for interaction with HCFC1 (aa 363 to 365, exon 11), nuclear localization signals (NLS) at aa 656 to 661 (exon 15) and aa 717 to 722 (exon 17), the BARD1 binding domain within the region bounded by aa 182 to 240 (*13*), and the BRCA1 binding domain within aa 598 to 729 (*11*). (C) Location of *BAP1* missense mutations in the UCH domain aligned to the crystal structure of *UCH-L3* (*21*). Three-dimensional structure of *UCH-L3* was visualized with MMDB software (*22*). The small molecule near C91G, H169Q, and S172R represents a suicide inhibitor, illustrating the critical location of these mutations for catalytic activity. (D) *BAP1* mRNA levels measured by quantitative RT-PCR in 9 nonmetastasizing class 1 UMs and 28 metastasizing class 2 UMs. (E) Relationship between *BAP1* mRNA levels (measured by quantitative RT-PCR) and type of *BAP1* mutation in 9 UMs with nonsense and other truncating mutations, 10 UMs with missense mutations (together with small inframe deletions, splice acceptor, and stop codon read-through mutations), and 4 class 2 UMs in which no *BAP1* mutations were detected. Single-letter abbreviations for the amino acid residues are as follows: A, Ala; C, Cys; D, Asp; E, Glu; F, Phe; G, Gly; H, His; I, Ile; K, Lys; L, Leu; M, Met; N, Asn; P, Pro; Q, Gln; R, Arg; S, Ser; T, Thr; V, Val; W, Trp; and Y, Tyr. (From Harbour JW, Onken MD, Roberson ED, et al. Frequent mutation of *BAP1* in metastasizing uveal melanomas. *Science.* 2010;330:1410-1413. Reprinted with permission from AAAS.)

Harbour and colleagues identified *BAP1* mutations in 26 of 31 (84%) class 2 tumors, while only 1 of 26 class 1 tumors contained a *BAP1* mutation. This case may represent a transition state in which the tumor has sustained a *BAP1* mutation but has not yet converted to class 2, suggesting that *BAP1* mutations may precede the emergence of the class 2 signature and possibly explaining the infrequent development of metastatic disease in patients with class 1 tumors. One copy of chromosome 3 was missing in all 17 *BAP1*-mutant class 2 tumors

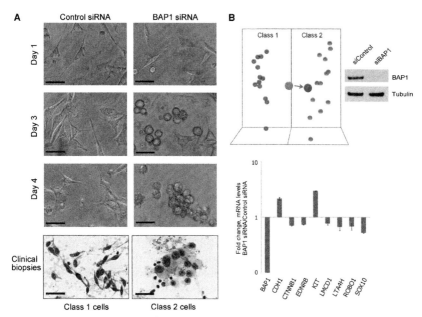

FIGURE 2.—UM cells depleted of BAP1 acquire properties that are typical of metastasizing class 2 tumor cells. (A) Phase-contrast photomicrographs of 92.1 uveal melanoma cells transfected with BAP1 or control siRNA at the indicated days. Bottom panels show representative examples of class 1 and class 2 uveal melanoma cells obtained from patient biopsy samples (Papanicolaou stain). Scale bars, 10 μm. (B) 92.1 cells transfected with BAP1 siRNA and evaluated after 5 days. BAP1 protein levels were efficiently depleted to less than 95% of control levels (see Western blot). Upper panel depicts principal component analysis to show the effect of BAP1 knockdown on gene expression signature. The small spheres represent the training set of known class 1 (blue) and class 2 (red) tumors. Large spheres represent the control-transfected (gray) and BAP1 siRNA−transfected (red) cells. The lower panel depicts mRNA levels measured by quantitative RT-PCR of a panel of melanocyte lineage genes, presented as relative change (fold change) in BAP1 siRNA/control siRNA−transfected cells. Results are representative of three independent experiments. For interpretation of the references to color in this figure legend, the reader is referred to web version of this article. (From Harbour JW, Onken MD, Roberson ED, et al. Frequent mutation of *BAP1* in metastasizing uveal melanomas. *Science*. 2010;330:1410-1413. Reprinted with permission from AAAS.)

for which cytogenetic data were available, consistent with chromosome 3 loss uncovering recessive *BAP1* mutations. There was no correlation between *GNAQ* (mutant gene identified in ∼50% of uveal melanomas in prior studies) and *BAP1* mutation status, confirming the existing evidence that *GNAQ* mutation is an early event in uveal melanoma development and is in itself not prognostically significant. The researchers have also investigated the effect of RNA interference−mediated knock down of *BAP1* in uveal melanoma cell line and found that *BAP1*-depleted cells developed epithelioid morphology, grew in discohesive fashion, and shifted gene expression profile into class 2 direction.

The discovery that mutational inactivation of *BAP1* could be the key event in the acquisition of metastatic competence in uveal melanoma may open the door to development of therapeutic modalities targeting *BAP1* and other deubiquitinating enzymes.

T. Milman, MD

MDM2 as a Modifier Gene in Retinoblastoma

Castéra L, Sabbagh A, Dehainault C, et al (Institut Curie, Paris, France; Université Paris Descartes, Paris, France)
J Natl Cancer Inst 102:1805-1808, 2010

Variability in the age of onset and number of tumors is occasionally described among retinoblastoma patients, and possible genetic modifiers might lie in the pRB or p53 pathways, both of which are involved in the development of retinoblastoma. MDM2, which increases p53 and pRB catabolism, is therefore a prominent candidate. The minor allele of *MDM2* that includes a 309T>G transversion (single-nucleotide polymorphism rs2279744) in the *MDM2* promoter is known to enhance MDM2 expression. Its genetic transmission was studied in 326 individuals including 212 *RB1* mutation carriers in 70 retinoblastoma families, and the marker genotype was tested for association with age at diagnosis and disease phenotype. In family-based association analyses, the *MDM2* 309G allele was found to be statistically significantly associated with incidence of bilateral or unilateral retinoblastoma among members of retinoblastoma families ($Z = 3.305$, two-sided exact $P = .001$) under a recessive model (ie, affected patients tend to be homozygous for the G allele); in transmission disequilibrium analyses using the recessive model, the association was also observed (estimated odds ratio $= 4.0$, 95% confidence interval $= 1.3$ to 12.0). The strong association of this genotype with retinoblastoma development designates *MDM2* as the first modifier gene to be identified among retinoblastoma patients and suggests that enhancement of pRB haploinsufficiency and/or resistance to p53-mediated apoptosis is critical to tumor formation.

▶ In accordance with Knudson's 2-hit hypothesis, most retinoblastoma families (carriers of germline *RB* gene mutation) demonstrate autosomal dominant inheritance with almost complete penetrance and high expressivity. However, in some families, a significant proportion of carriers remain unaffected (reduced penetrance), and many affected individuals have only unilateral retinoblastoma or benign retinocytomas (reduced expressivity). Various mechanisms for low-penetrance retinoblastoma have been proposed. A spectrum of qualitative or quantitative mutations in *RB1* gene may be implicated in pathogenesis of reduced penetrance retinoblastoma. Other proposed mechanisms include immunologic factors and infectious agents, DNA methylation, epigenetic mechanisms, delayed mutation, host resistance factors, a second retinoblastoma locus (such as *RB2*), and modulator genes. Castera et al further explored the potential role of modulator genes in pathogenesis of reduced penetrance retinoblastoma. The authors focused on the role of murine double minute (MDM) family proteins, such as MDM2 and MDM4, which are both expressed in retinoblastoma cells. MDM family proteins are key negative regulators of the p53 pathway: their amplification would be expected to inhibit p53-mediated transactivation activity targeting p53 for proteosomal degradation, thereby bypassing p53-mediated apoptosis and conferring a cell growth advantage when

RB1 expression has been lost. The authors found a strong association of MDM2 mutations and retinoblastoma, suggesting that enhancement of pRB haploinsufficiency and/or resistance to p53-mediated apoptosis is critical to tumor formation. These findings may have therapeutic implications since the inhibitors of MDM2 and MDM4 gene products, such as nutlin-3, have been identified. This article, along with the other recent studies, has shed the light on the complexity of genetics in retinoblastoma, which cannot be explained solely with the 2-hit hypothesis. For more information on this topic, please read the articles by Guo et al, Harbour et al, De Falco et al, and Hume et al.[1-4]

T. Milman, MD

References

1. Hume AJ, Kalejta RF. Regulation of the retinoblastoma proteins by the human herpesviruses. *Cell Div.* 2009;4:1.
2. De Falco G, Giordano A. pRb2/p130: a new candidate for retinoblastoma tumor formation. *Oncogene.* 2006;25:5333-5340.
3. Guo Y, Pajovic S, Gallie BL. Expression of p14ARF, MDM2 and MDM4 in human retinoblastoma. *Biochem Biophys Res Commun.* 2008;375:1-5.
4. Harbour JW. Molecular basis of low-penetrance retinoblastoma. *Arch Ophthalmol.* 2001;119:1699-1704.

Intraocular Lymphatics in Ciliary Body Melanomas With Extraocular Extension: Functional for Lymphatic Spread?
Heindl LM, Hofmann TN, Schrödl F, et al (Friedrich-Alexander Univ Erlangen-Nürnberg, Germany; Paracelsus Univ, Salzburg, Austria)
Arch Ophthalmol 128:1001-1008, 2010

Objective.—To assess the functional significance of intraocular tumor—associated lymphatic vessels in ciliary body melanomas with extraocular extension.

Methods.—Twelve consecutive patients enucleated for a malignant melanoma of the ciliary body with extraocular extension and immunohistochemical presence of intraocular LYVE-1—positive and podoplanin-positive lymphatic vessels were examined for proliferation status and tumor invasion into tumor-associated lymphatics. Proliferating lymphatic vessels were identified using LYVE-1 and podoplanin as specific lymphatic endothelial markers and Ki-67 as the proliferation marker. Tumor invasion into lymphatic vessels was assessed using Melan-A as the melanoma marker. Kaplan-Meier analyses of survival and metastasis were performed.

Results.—Intraocular proliferating lymphatic vessels were detected in all 12 ciliary body melanomas with extraocular extension. The ratio of proliferating lymphatics was significantly higher in the intraocular vs extraocular tumor compartment (*P* < .001). Extraocular lymphatic invasion by tumor cells was observed in 5 patients (42%), intraocular lymphatic invasion in 4 (33%), and synchronous intraocular and extraocular lymphatic invasion in 3 (25%). Detection of melanoma cells in intraocular and extraocular lymphatic vessels was significantly associated with higher risks of lymphatic spread ($P < .001$) and lower metastasis-free survival rates ($P = .03$).

Conclusions.—Intraocular tumor—associated lymphatic vessels contain proliferating endothelial cells and can be invaded by cancer cells in ciliary body melanomas with extraocular extension. Lymphatic invasion by tumor cells seems to be associated with an increased risk of lymphatic spread and mortality in these affected patients.

▶ The concept of recruitment of lymphatic channels by the tumors and intratumoral lymphatic channel proliferation is not new to general pathology, where associations between intratumoral lymphatic density and lymph node metastases were observed in cervical carcinoma. The recent studies by Heindl et al apply this knowledge to ophthalmic pathology and investigate the role of tumor-associated lymphangiogenesis in ocular malignancies, namely conjunctival squamous cell carcinoma and ciliary body melanoma. In these studies, the authors demonstrated the presence of proliferating lymphatic channels within the tumors and found that the presence and density of intratumoral lymphatics strongly correlate with previously reported prognostic factors, such as tumor size in conjunctival squamous cell carcinoma and tumor size and epithelioid cell type in ciliary body melanoma. In addition, intratumoral lymphatic density strongly correlated with the risk of local recurrence in conjunctival squamous cell carcinoma and with ciliary body melanoma specific mortality.

Additional prospective studies with larger sample size are needed to confirm the prognostic significance of intratumoral lymphangiogenesis in ocular malignancies. Furthermore, correlation of tumor-associated lymphangiogenesis and gene expression profiling in uveal melanoma may be of interest. Despite these limitations, the studies by Heindl and colleagues provide important information on biologic behavior of ocular malignancies and may suggest avenues for antiangiogenesis and antilymphangiogenesis therapies in management of these tumors.

T. Milman, MD

Intraocular Tumor-Associated Lymphangiogenesis: A Novel Prognostic Factor for Ciliary Body Melanomas with Extraocular Extension?

Heindl LM, Hofmann TN, Adler W, et al (Friedrich-Alexander Univ Erlangen-Nürnberg, Germany)

Ophthalmology 117:334-342, 2010

Purpose.—To evaluate whether intraocular tumor-associated lymphangiogenesis contributes to prognosis of ciliary body melanomas with extraocular extension and to study its association with other tumor characteristics.

Design.—Nonrandomized, retrospective case series.

Participants.—Twenty consecutive patients enucleated for a malignant melanoma of the ciliary body with extraocular extension.

Methods.—Lymphatic vessels were identified using lymphatic vascular endothelial-specific hyaluronic acid receptor-1 (LYVE-1) and podoplanin as specific immunohistochemical markers for lymphatic vascular endothelium. Baseline tumor characteristics included intra- and extraocular tumor size, 2009 tumor, node, metastasis (TNM) classification, route of extraocular spread, tumor cell type, mitotic rate, Ki-67 proliferation-index, microvascular patterns and density, tumor-infiltrating lymphocytes and macrophages, and expression of human leukocyte antigen (HLA) class I and insulin-like growth factor-1 receptor. Kaplan-Meier and Cox regression analyses of melanoma-specific survival were performed.

Main Outcome Measures.—Prevalence of intraocular LYVE-1⁺/podoplanin⁺ lymphatic vessels and association with intraocular tumor characteristics and metastasis-free survival.

Results.—Intraocular LYVE-1⁺ and podoplanin⁺ lymphatic vessels could be detected in 12 (60%) of 20 ciliary body melanomas with extraocular extension. Presence of intraocular LYVE-1⁺/podoplanin⁺ lymphatic vessels was significantly associated with larger intra- (P = 0.002) and extraocular tumor size (P<0.001), higher TNM categories (P = 0.004), epithelioid cellularity (P = 0.016), higher mitotic rate (P = 0.003), higher Ki-67 proliferation-index (P = 0.049), microvascular networks (P = 0.005), higher microvascular density (P = 0.003), more tumor-infiltrating macrophages (P = 0.002), higher expression of HLA class I (P = 0.046), and insulin-like growth factor-1 receptor (P = 0.033), but not significantly with route of extraocular spread (P = 0.803), and tumorinfiltrating lymphocytes (P = 0.069). Melanoma-specific mortality rates increased significantly with the presence of intraocular LYVE-1⁺/podoplanin⁺ lymphatic vessels (P = 0.008). By multivariate Cox regression, tumor size (hazard ratio, 14.40; P = 0.002), and presence of intraocular lymphatic vessels (hazard ratio, 8.09; P = 0.04) were strong prognostic predictors of mortality.

Conclusions.—Intraocular peritumoral lymphangiogenesis seems to be associated with an increased mortality risk in patients with ciliary body melanomas and extraocular extension. This association may be primarily because of an association of intraocular lymphangiogenesis with greater tumor size and increased malignancy.

▶ The concept of recruitment of lymphatic channels by the tumors and intratumoral lymphatic channel proliferation is not new to general pathology, where associations between intratumoral lymphatic density and lymph node metastases were observed in cervical carcinoma. The recent studies by Heindl et al apply this knowledge to ophthalmic pathology and investigate the role of tumor-associated lymphangiogenesis in ocular malignancies namely conjunctival squamous cell carcinoma and ciliary body melanoma. In these studies, the authors demonstrated the presence of proliferating lymphatic channels within the tumors and found that the presence and density of intratumoral lymphatics strongly correlate with previously reported prognostic factors, such as tumor size in conjunctival squamous cell carcinoma and tumor size and epithelioid cell type in ciliary body melanoma (Figs 1-5, squamous cell carcinoma article). In addition, intratumoral lymphatic density strongly correlated with the risk of local recurrence in conjunctival squamous cell carcinoma and with ciliary body melanoma—specific mortality.

Additional prospective studies with larger sample size are needed to confirm the prognostic significance of intratumoral lymphangiogenesis in ocular malignancies. Furthermore, correlation of tumor-associated lymphangiogenesis and gene expression profiling in uveal melanoma may be of interest. Despite these limitations, the studies by Heindl and colleagues provide important information on biological behavior of ocular malignancies and may suggest avenues for antiangiogenesis and antilymphangiogenesis therapies in management of these tumors.

T. Milman, MD

Tumor-Associated Lymphangiogenesis in the Development of Conjunctival Squamous Cell Carcinoma
Heindl LM, Hofmann-Rummelt C, Adler W, et al (Friedrich-Alexander Univ Erlangen-Nürnberg, Germany)
Ophthalmology 117:649-658, 2010

Purpose.—To analyze whether tumor-associated lymphangiogenesis accompanies the development from premalignant conjunctival intraepithelial neoplasia (CIN) into invasive squamous cell carcinoma (SCC) of the conjunctiva and to study its association with prognosis and other tumor characteristics.

Design.—Case-controlled, matched-pair cohort study.

Participants.—Twenty patients with invasive SCC were closely matched with 20 patients with high-grade CIN and 20 patients with low-grade CIN regarding tumor size, tumor location, tumor extension, and patients' age.

Methods.—Proliferating lymphatic vessels were identified using lymphatic vascular endothelial hyaluronan receptor-1 and podoplanin as specific lymphatic endothelial markers and Ki-67 as proliferation marker. Baseline tumor characteristics included tumor size, tumor-to-limbus distance, tumor-to-fornix distance, 2009 TNM classification, tumor cell type, mitotic rate, and Ki-67 proliferation index. Kaplan—Meier and Cox regression analyses of recurrence-free survival were performed.

Main Outcome Measures.—Lymphatic vascular density (LVD) and relative lymphatic vascular area (RLVA) of proliferating lymphatic vessels within the tumor mass (intratumoral) and within an area $\leq 500 \, \mu m$ from the tumor border (peritumoral), and its association with tumor characteristics and recurrence-free survival.

Results.—Intratumoral and peritumoral proliferating lymphatic vessels could be detected in all of the 60 conjunctival tumor samples. Invasive SCC revealed significantly higher values of intratumoral and peritumoral LVD and RLVA of proliferating lymphatics than high-grade or low-grade

CIN ($P \leq 0.001$). Higher intratumoral lymphatic densities were significantly associated with larger tumor size ($P=0.001$), lower tumor-to-limbus distance ($P=0.002$), lower tumor-to-fornix distance ($P=0.003$), and higher TNM categories ($P<0.001$). Recurrence-free survival rates decreased significantly with higher intratumoral lymphatic densities ($P<0.001$). By multivariate Cox regression, large tumor size (hazard ratio 1.68, $P=0.002$) and high intratumoral lymphatic density (hazard ratio 1.10, $P=0.046$) were significant prognostic predictors of local recurrence.

Conclusions.—Development of conjunctival SCC from premalignant lesions is accompanied by the outgrowth of new conjunctival lymphatic vessels. This active tumor-associated lymphangiogenesis seems to be associated with an increased risk of local recurrence in patients with CIN and conjunctival invasive SCC (Figs 1-5).

▶ The concept of recruitment of lymphatic channels by the tumors and intratumoral lymphatic channel proliferation is not new to general pathology, where associations between intratumoral lymphatic density and lymph node metastases were observed in cervical carcinoma. The recent studies by Heindl et al apply this knowledge to ophthalmic pathology and investigate the role of tumor-associated lymphangiogenesis in ocular malignancies, namely conjunctival squamous cell carcinoma and ciliary body melanoma. In these studies, the

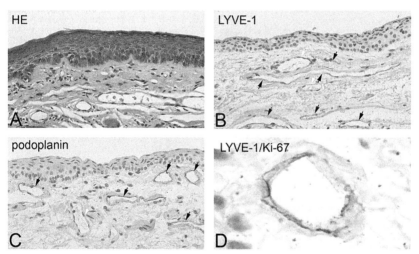

FIGURE 1.—Immunohistochemical identification of lymphatic vessels in normal conjunctiva: Underlying normal conjunctival epithelium (**A**, hematoxylineosin): large, irregularly shaped, thin-walled lymphatic vessels with an erythrocyte-free lumen (*black arrows*) were positively stained with LYVE-1 (**B**) and podoplanin (**C**). In contrast, erythrocyte-filled blood capillaries surrounded by smooth muscle (*white arrows*) did not react with the lymphatic endothelial-specific antibodies (**B, C**). By double staining for LYVE-1 (brown membrane staining) and the Ki-67 proliferation antigen (red nuclear staining), no newly dividing nuclei could be detected in the lymph vessel endothelia (**D**). (Magnification: A ×200, B ×200, C ×200, D ×800.) HE = hematoxylin-eosin. (Reprinted from Heindl LM, Hofmann-Rummelt C, Adler W, et al. Tumor-associated lymphangiogenesis in the development of conjunctival squamous cell carcinoma. *Ophthalmology.* 2010;117:649-658, copyright © 2010, with permission from the American Academy of Ophthalmology.)

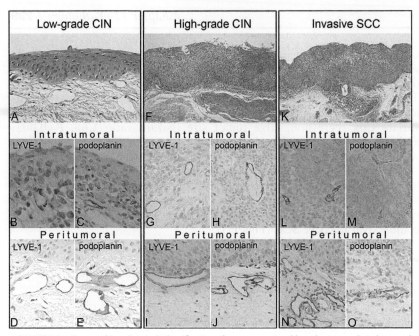

FIGURE 2.—Immunohistochemical identification of tumor-associated lymphatic vessels in low-grade CIN (A–E), high-grade CIN (F–J), and invasive SCC of the conjunctiva (K–O): Intratumoral LYVE-1+ (B, G, L) and podoplanin+ (C, H, M) lymphatic vessels increased in density from discrete hotspots concentrated within sheets of tumor cells in CIN (B, C, G, H) toward a branching network in invasive SCC (L, M). Peritumoral LYVE-1+ (D, I, N) and podoplanin+ (E, J, O) lymphatic vessels showed larger and more dilated lumina. (A, F, K, hematoxylin-eosin. Original magnification: A, D, E, F, K, L, M ×200; B, C, G, H, I, J, N, O ×400.) CIN = conjunctival intraepithelial neoplasia; SCC = squamous cell carcinoma. (Reprinted from Heindl LM, Hofmann-Rummelt C, Adler W, et al. Tumor-associated lymphangiogenesis in the development of conjunctival squamous cell carcinoma. *Ophthalmology.* 2010;117:649-658, copyright © 2010, with permission from the American Academy of Ophthalmology.)

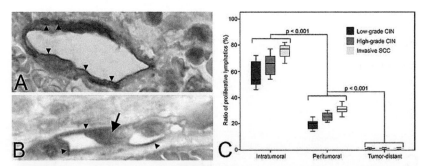

FIGURE 3.—Tumor-associated active lymphangiogenesis in low-grade CIN, high-grade CIN, and invasive SCC of the conjunctiva: A, By using LYVE-1/Ki-67 double staining (LYVE-1 brown, Ki-67 red), multiple lymphatic endothelial cells showing nuclear Ki-67 positivity (*arrowheads*) identified lymphatic vessels as active and proliferating. (Original magnification: ×800.) B, Note the tumor embolus (*arrow*) within this intratumoral proliferating lymphatic vessel showing Ki-67+ lymphatic endothelial cells (*arrowheads*). (LYVE-1/Ki-67; magnification: ×800.) C, Significantly more lymphatic vessels were found as proliferating (LYVE-1+/Ki-67+) within the tumor mass (intratumoral) compared with an area ≤ 500 μm from the tumor border (peritumoral) and a more distant area of conjunctiva (tumor-distant) (*P*<0.001 and *P*<0.001, Mann–Whitney *U* test). CIN = conjunctival intraepithelial neoplasia; SCC = squamous cell carcinoma. (Reprinted from Heindl LM, Hofmann-Rummelt C, Adler W, et al. Tumor-associated lymphangiogenesis in the development of conjunctival squamous cell carcinoma. *Ophthalmology.* 2010;117: 649-658, copyright © 2010, with permission from the American Academy of Ophthalmology.)

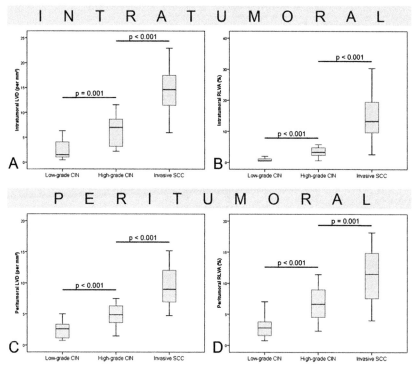

FIGURE 4.—Computer-assisted morphometric analysis of tumor-associated lymphangiogenesis in low-grade CIN, high-grade CIN, and invasive SCC of the conjunctiva: Invasive SCC demonstrated significantly higher intratumoral (A) and peritumoral (C) LVD, and significantly higher intratumoral (B) and peritumoral (D) RLVA of proliferating LYVE-1⁺/Ki-67⁺ lymphatic vessels compared with high-grade and low-grade CIN. CIN = conjunctival intraepithelial neoplasia; SCC = squamous cell carcinoma. (Reprinted from Heindl LM, Hofmann-Rummelt C, Adler W, et al. Tumor-associated lymphangiogenesis in the development of conjunctival squamous cell carcinoma. *Ophthalmology*. 2010;117:649-658, copyright © 2010, with permission from the American Academy of Ophthalmology.)

authors demonstrated the presence of proliferating lymphatic channels within the tumors and found that the presence and density of intratumoral lymphatics strongly correlate with previously reported prognostic factors, such as tumor size in conjunctival squamous cell carcinoma and tumor size in epithelioid cell type and ciliary body melanoma (Figs 1-5). In addition, intratumoral lymphatic density strongly correlated with the risk of local recurrence in conjunctival squamous cell carcinoma and with ciliary body melanoma—specific mortality.

Additional, prospective studies with larger sample size are needed to confirm the prognostic significance of intratumoral lymphangiogenesis in ocular malignancies. Furthermore, correlation of tumor-associated lymphangiogenesis and gene expression profiling in uveal melanoma may be of interest. Despite these limitations, the studies by Heindl and colleagues provide important information on biologic behavior of ocular malignancies and may suggest avenues

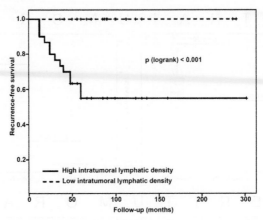

FIGURE 5.—Tumor-associated lymphangiogenesis and prognosis in ocular surface squamous neoplasia: There was a significantly lower recurrence-free survival rate in patients with tumors showing a high intratumoral lymphatic density (intratumoral LVD for proliferating LYVE-1+/Ki-67+ lymphatic vessels >7.9 per mm^2) than in those with a lower intratumoral lymphatic density ($P<0.001$, log-rank test). (Reprinted from Heindl LM, Hofmann-Rummelt C, Adler W, et al. Tumor-associated lymphangiogenesis in the development of conjunctival squamous cell carcinoma. *Ophthalmology.* 2010;117:649-658, copyright © 2010, with permission from the American Academy of Ophthalmology.)

for antiangiogenesis and antilymphangiogenesis therapies in management of these tumors.

T. Milman, MD

The molecular genetics underlying basal cell carcinoma pathogenesis and links to targeted therapeutics

Iwasaki JK, Srivastava D, Moy RL, et al (Dept of Dermatology of Henry Ford Health System, Detroit, MI; Univ of Texas Southwestern Med Ctr, Dallas; Univ of California at Los Angeles David Geffen School of Medicine, et al)
J Am Acad Dermatol 2010 [Epub ahead of print]

Mutations in the sonic hedgehog signaling pathway play a key role in the development of basal cell carcinomas. Specifically, mutations in the *PTCH1* (also known as *PTCH* or *PTC1*) and *SMO* genes cause tumor formation through constitutive activation of the pathway. Misregulation of the pathway has also been implicated in the nevoid basal cell carcinoma syndrome and other tumors. Understanding the function of the sonic hedgehog pathway has led to novel strategies for treatment. In this review we highlight the role of the pathway in the pathogenesis of basal cell carcinoma and review potential targeted therapies (Figs 1-4 and Table 1).

▶ In the recent years, the field of molecular genetics has been burgeoning with the articles on molecular mechanisms involved in pathogenesis of cutaneous malignancies. The article by Iwasaki and colleagues provides just a taste of

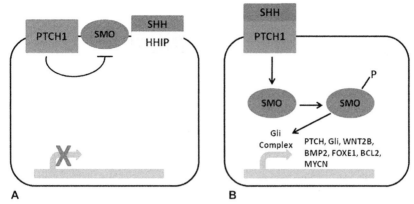

FIGURE 1.—Summary of the SHH signaling pathway. A, In the absence of SHH, PTCH1 constitutively represses SMO. B, Binding of SHH to PTCH1 releases inhibition of SMO, leading to transcriptional activation of GLI proteins and downstream target genes. (Reprinted from Iwasaki JK, Srivastava D, Moy RL, et al. The molecular genetics underlying basal cell carcinoma pathogenesis and links to targeted therapeutics. *J Am Acad Dermatol.* 2010;[Epub ahead of print], copyright 2010, with permission from the American Academy of Dermatology, Inc.)

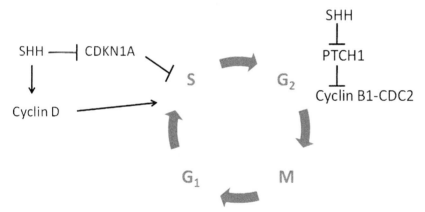

FIGURE 2.—Sonic hedgehog interactions with the cell cycle. PTCH1 inhibits cyclin B1 by preventing its translocation to the nucleus, thereby obstructing cell cycle progression at the G2/M checkpoint. SHH blocks CDKN1A (cyclin-dependent kinase inhibitor 1A, also known as p21)-induced growth arrest in keratinocytes and up-regulates cyclin D1 at the G1/S checkpoint, stimulating cell cycle progression. (Reprinted from Iwasaki JK, Srivastava D, Moy RL, et al. The molecular genetics underlying basal cell carcinoma pathogenesis and links to targeted therapeutics. *J Am Acad Dermatol.* 2010;[Epub ahead of print], copyright 2010, with permission from the American Academy of Dermatology, Inc.)

the complex molecular events involved in skin cancer development. In addition to elucidation of molecular pathways involved in pathogenesis of basal cell carcinoma (ie, sonic hedgehog signaling pathway and its target genes: platelet-derived growth factor receptor α, forkhead box proteins, β-catenin, *BCL-2* proto-oncogene, N-*myc* proto-oncogene, and *RUNX* gene family), advances have been made in genetics of other skin cancers. For example, it

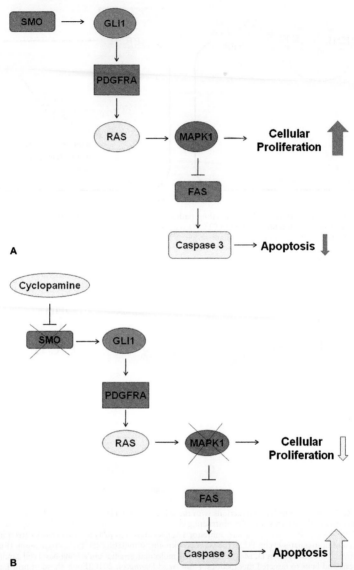

FIGURE 3.—A and B, Regulation of FAS expression by cyclopamine via the RAS-MAPK1 pathway (also known as the RAS-ERK pathway). Inhibition of SMO by cyclopamine leads to down-regulation of the RAS-MAPK1 pathway, activation of FAS, and ultimately apoptosis. (Reprinted from Iwasaki JK, Srivastava D, Moy RL, et al. The molecular genetics underlying basal cell carcinoma pathogenesis and links to targeted therapeutics. *J Am Acad Dermatol.* 2010;[Epub ahead of print], copyright 2010, with permission from the American Academy of Dermatology, Inc.)

has been recently discovered that in majority of cases, Merkel cell carcinoma development is preceded by the integration of genomic sequences of Merkel cell polyomavirus. High frequency of mutations in p53 gene has been recently

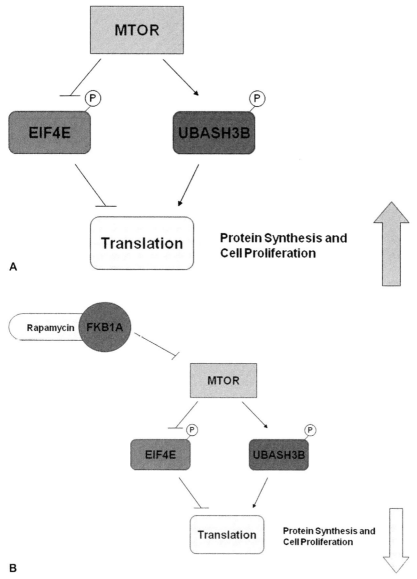

FIGURE 4.—A and B, The effect of rapamycin on MTOR, protein synthesis, and proliferation in GLI1-expressing cells. (Reprinted from Iwasaki JK, Srivastava D, Moy RL, et al. The molecular genetics underlying basal cell carcinoma pathogenesis and links to targeted therapeutics. *J Am Acad Dermatol.* 2010;[Epub ahead of print], copyright 2010, with permission from the American Academy of Dermatology, Inc.)

detected in sebaceous carcinoma of the eyelid. The variants within the key pigmentation gene, melanocortin receptor 1, have been linked with high-risk traits and both melanoma and nonmelanoma skin cancers. In search of potential

TABLE 1.—Novel Therapeutic Agents Target Specific Proteins in the SHH Pathway: Summary

Therapeutic Agent	SHH Pathway Target	Mechanism of Action	Current Uses
Cyclopamine	SMO	Binds and inactivates SMO by inducing a change in conformation Up-regulates FAS expression and apoptosis Down-regulates RAS-MAPK1 signaling	Phase 1 clinical by Genentech completed by using topical cyclopamine showed a reduction of advanced BCCs, Infinity to start Phase 1 testing of a semisynthetic cyclopamine analog
CUR61414	SMO	Synthetic aminoproline inhibitor of SMO Mechanism of action similar to that of cyclopamine	Topical CUR61414 eradicated BCCs in an ex vivo mouse model. However, the phase 1 clinical trial ended early because no clinical effect was seen.
GDC-0449	SMO	Small molecule inhibitor of SMO	Phase 1 clinical trial with oral GDC-0449 completed Phase 2 clinical trial began August 2009.
Statins	SMO	Binds SMO Effect uncertain; may regulate SMO localization to the cell membrane	No human studies yet
Vitamin D_3	SMO	Binds SMO and decreases GLI activity	No human studies yet
Recombinant HHIP	HHIP	HHIP fragments have been proposed as tumor-associated antigens that may be useful in a cancer vaccine.	No human studies yet
Rapamycin	Binds FKB1A, which inhibits proliferation of cells expressing GLI1 via MTOR	Inhibits MTOR in GLI1-transformed cells, leading to decreased cell protein synthesis and proliferation	No human studies yet
MYCN anti-sense oligonucleotides	MYCN	Anti-sense oligonucleotides inhibit MYCN expression.	No human studies yet

Please see Abbreviations Used box for expansion of abbreviations.

targeted therapeutics, recent studies have focused on various genes involved in an important cutaneous melanoma pathway, mitogen-activated protein kinase pathway. These new insights will potentially lead to development of molecular tests for both disease diagnosis and monitoring and to development of gene-specific targeted therapy. For more information on this topic, please refer to articles by Blokx et al,[1] Scherer and Kumar,[2] Houben et al,[3] and Kiyosaki et al.[4]

T. Milman, MD

References

1. Blokx WA, van Dijk MC, Ruiter DJ. Molecular cytogenetics of cutaneous melanocytic lesions - diagnostic, prognostic and therapeutic aspects. *Histopathology.* 2010;56:121-132.

2. Scherer D, Kumar R. Genetics of pigmentation in skin cancer—a review. *Mutat Res.* 2010;705:141-153.
3. Houben R, Schrama D, Becker JC. Molecular pathogenesis of Merkel cell carcinoma. *Exp Dermatol.* 2009;18:193-198.
4. Kiyosaki K, Nakada C, Hijiya N, et al. Analysis of p53 mutations and the expression of p53 and p21WAF1/CIP1 protein in 15 cases of sebaceous carcinoma of the eyelid. *Invest Ophthalmol Vis Sci.* 2010;51:7-11.

Adipophilin expression in sebaceous tumors and other cutaneous lesions with clear cell histology: an immunohistochemical study of 117 cases
Ostler DA, Prieto VG, Reed JA, et al (The Univ of Texas, Houston)
Mod Pathol 23:567-573, 2010

Adipophilin is a monoclonal antibody against a protein on the surface of intracellular lipid droplets, and it was recently shown to be expressed in sebocytes and sebaceous lesions. This study examines adipophilin expression in various sebaceous lesions and other cutaneous tumors with a clear cell histology that may mimic sebaceous differentiation. A total of 117 cutaneous clear cell lesions including 16 sebaceous adenomas, 25 sebaceous carcinomas, 8 basal cell carcinomas, 12 squamous cell carcinomas, 6 xanthomas, 10 xanthelasmas, 10 xanthogranulomas, 4 balloon cell nevi, 5 trichilemmomas, 8 clear cell hidradenomas, and 13 metastatic renal cell carcinomas were examined using immunohistochemistry for the expression of adipophilin. Of these 117 lesions, 42 (36%) were from the periocular region. Adipophilin was expressed in 16 of 16 (100%) sebaceous adenomas, 23 of 25 (92%) sebaceous carcinomas, 10 of 10 (100%) xanthelasmas, 9 of 10 (90%) xanthogranulomas, 6 of 6 (100%) xanthomas, and 9 of 13 (62.5%) metastatic renal cell carcinomas. The characteristic staining pattern differed between sebaceous and non-sebaceous tumors with the former showing a membranous vesicular pattern and the latter being more granular. Adipophilin expression was not seen in any of the other lesions with clear cell histology, basal cell carcinomas, or squamous cell carcinomas, including cases that had focal clear cell differentiation. Adipophilin can be valuable in an immunohistochemical panel when evaluating cutaneous lesions with clear cell histology as it identifies intracytoplasmic lipid vesicles in sebaceous and xanthomatous lesions. In periocular lesions, it is effective in helping to exclude basal cell carcinoma and squamous cell carcinoma when sebaceous carcinoma is under consideration. Adipophilin expression is not as useful for the differential diagnosis that includes metastatic renal cell carcinoma, a rare but important, diagnostic differential. The pattern of adipophilin reactivity is important to observe as membranous vesicular staining is suggestive of intracellular lipids whereas granular cytoplasmic reactivity is not (Figs 1-3, Tables 1-3).

▶ Histopathologic diagnosis of poorly differentiated sebaceous carcinoma can be diagnostically challenging. Traditionally, Oil Red O and Sudan Black IV special stains have been used to identify intracytoplasmic lipids in sebaceous

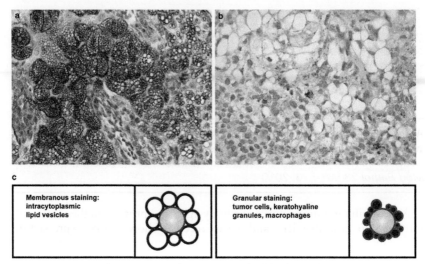

FIGURE 1.—(a) Membranous staining of intracytoplasmic lipid droplets in sebaceous adenoma (original magnification, 400×). (b) Nonspecific uptake of adipophilin by macrophages and rare tumor cells of a basal cell carcinoma with clear cell features (original magnification, 400×). This nonspecific uptake of antibody was also seen in association with keratohyalin bodies in squamous cells. (c) Depiction of positive vesicular staining pattern and nonspecific granular uptake of adipophilin antibody. (Reprinted from USCAP, Inc, from Ostler DA, Prieto VG, Reed JA, et al. Adipophilin expression in sebaceous tumors and other cutaneous lesions with clear cell histology: an immunohistochemical study of 117 cases. *Mod Pathol.* 2010;23:567-573, copyright 2010.)

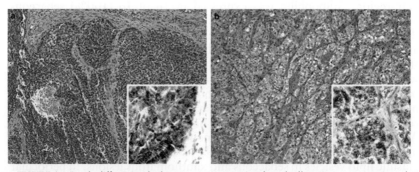

FIGURE 2.—Poorly differentiated sebaceous carcinoma (a) and renal cell carcinoma metastatic to the skin (b) with insets strong membranous staining of intracytoplasmic lipid vacuoles by adipophilin antibody. (Reprinted from USCAP, Inc, from Ostler DA, Prieto VG, Reed JA, et al. Adipophilin expression in sebaceous tumors and other cutaneous lesions with clear cell histology: an immunohistochemical study of 117 cases. *Mod Pathol.* 2010;23:567-573, copyright 2010.)

lesions in fresh frozen tissue. Standard permanent tissue processing extracts the intracellular lipids, rendering these approaches useless in formalin-fixed paraffin-embedded material. Thus, the search for immunohistochemical method(s) that will aid in the diagnosis of sebaceous carcinoma has been ongoing. Until recently, no sensitive or specific immunohistochemical markers for sebaceous carcinoma were available. Studies have shown that epithelial

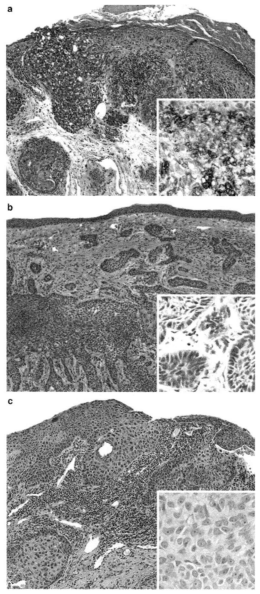

FIGURE 3.—Hematoxylin and eosin stains with insets showing adipophilin immunostains showing the strong membranous staining of intracytoplasmic lipid in sebaceous carcinoma (a) compared to basal cell carcinoma (b) and squamous cell carcinoma (c). (Reprinted with permission from USCAP, Inc, from Ostler DA, Prieto VG, Reed JA, et al. Adipophilin expression in sebaceous tumors and other cutaneous lesions with clear cell histology: an immunohistochemical study of 117 cases. *Mod Pathol*. 2010;23:567-573, copyright 2010.)

TABLE 1.—Clinical Data

Diagnostic Category (n)	Age (Range)	Sex (M:F)	Anatomic Sites
Sebaceous adenoma (16)	46—81 years	11:5	10 head, 1 neck, 3 upper extremity, 2 trunk
Sebaceous carcinoma (25)	36—93 years	3:2	21 periorbital region, 2 head, 1 upper extremity, 1 trunk
Basal cell carcinoma (8)	35—83 years	7:1	5 periorbital region
Squamous cell carcinoma (12)	62—88 years	5:1	5 periorbital region, 5 head, 1 neck, 1 lower extremity
Hidradenoma, clear cell (8)	31—81 years	1:1	4 head, 3 upper extremity, 1 trunk
Trichilemmoma (5)	52—74 years	4:1	5 head
Xanthelasma (10)	38—57 years	7:3	8 periorbital region, 1 nose, 1 upper extremity
Xanthogranuloma (10)	8 months—61 years	7:3	2 periorbital region, 5 head, 2 trunk, 1 lower extremity
Xanthoma (6)	9 months—67 years	1:1	2 head, 2 upper extremity, 2 trunk
Melanocytic nevus, balloon cell (4)	63—83 years	3:1	4 trunk
Renal cell carcinoma, metastatic (13)	41—79 years	9:4	6 head (3 scalp, 3 face), 1 neck, 3 upper extremity, 2 trunk, 1 lower extremity

TABLE 2.—Adipophilin Expression in Sebaceous Lesions and Other Cutaneous Lesions, Including Lesions with Clear Cell Histology

	Tumor Cells Staining (%)				Intensity of Staining			
	Negative (%)	1+ (%)	2+ (%)	3+ (%)	Negative (%)	1+ (%)	2+ (%)	3+ (%)
Sebaceous adenoma ($n = 16$)	0 (0)	0 (0)	0 (0)	16 (100)	0 (0)	0 (0)	0 (0)	16 (100)
Sebaceous carcinoma ($n = 25$)	2 (8)	0 (0)	11 (44)	12 (48)	2 (8)	1 (4)	6 (24)	17 (68)
Basal cell carcinoma ($n = 8$)	8 (100)	0 (0)	0 (0)	0 (0)	8 (100)	0 (0)	0 (0)	0 (0)
Basal cell carcinoma, clear cell type ($n = 3$)	3 (100)	0 (0)	0 (0)	0 (0)	3 (100)	0 (0)	0 (0)	0 (0)
Squamous cell carcinoma ($n = 12$)	12 (100)	0 (0)	0 (0)	0 (0)	12 (100)	0 (0)	0 (0)	0 (0)
Squamous cell carcinoma, clear cell type ($n = 5$)	3 (100)	0 (0)	0 (0)	0 (0)	3 (100)	0 (0)	0 (0)	0 (0)
Hidradenoma, clear cell ($n = 8$)	8 (100)	0 (0)	0 (0)	0 (0)	8 (100)	0 (0)	0 (0)	0 (0)
Trichilemmoma ($n = 5$)	5 (100)	0 (0)	0 (0)	0 (0)	5 (100)	0 (0)	0 (0)	0 (0)
Xanthelasma ($n = 10$)	0 (0)	0 (0)	0 (0)	10 (100)	0 (0)	0 (0)	0 (0)	10 (100)
Xanthogranuloma ($n = 10$)	1 (10)	0 (0)	5 (50)	4 (40)	0 (0)	1 (10)	1 (10)	8 (80)
Xanthoma ($n = 6$)	0 (0)	0 (0)	2 (33)	4 (66)	0 (0)	0 (0)	1 (17)	5 (83)
Melanocytic nevus, balloon cell ($n = 4$)	4 (100)	0 (0)	0 (0)	0 (0)	4 (100)	0 (0)	0 (0)	0 (0)
Renal cell carcinoma, metastatic ($n = 13$)	4 (31)	3 (23)	4 (31)	2 (15)	4 (31)	3 (23)	4 (30)	2 (15)

Percentage: 0, no labeling to 5%; 1+, labeling in 6—25% of cells; 2+, labeling in 26—75%; and 3+, labeling in more than 75% of clear cells in the lesion.

Intensity: 0, negative; 1+, weak; 2+, moderate; 3+, strong.

TABLE 3.—Eyelid Lesions: Grading of Adipophilin Staining Results

	Negative (%)	1+ (%)	2+ (%)	3+ (%)
Sebaceous carcinoma ($n = 21$)	2 (10)	0 (0)	9 (43)	10 (47)
Basal cell carcinoma ($n = 5$)	5 (100)	0 (0)	0 (0)	0 (0)
Squamous cell carcinoma ($n = 5$)	5 (100)	0 (0)	0 (0)	0 (0)
Xanthelasma ($n = 8$)	0 (0)	0 (0)	0 (0)	8 (100)
Xanthogranuloma ($n = 2$)	0 (0)	0 (0)	2 (100)	0 (0)

0, no labeling; 1+, labeling in 6–25% of cells; 2+, labeling in 26–75%; and 3+, labeling in more than 75% of clear cells in the lesion.

membrane antigen, cytokeratin 7, focally positive for low-molecular-weight cytokeratin, and androgen receptors can be used to suggest sebaceous differentiation with variable success. The discovery of adipophilin as a sensitive and specific marker of periocular sebaceous carcinoma is, therefore, an exciting development.

Adipophilin is an intracellular membrane protein involved in the packaging of intracytoplasmic lipids and not a specific marker of sebaceous or other type of differentiation. Mature sebaceous glands demonstrate a membranous vesicular staining for adipophilin, which can be used as an internal positive control in the biopsied tissue. Similar membranous staining pattern has been observed in sebaceous carcinomas and adenomas. In contrast, a nonspecific granular staining was noted in squamous and basal cell carcinomas containing keratohyalin granules, hidradenomas, trichilemmomas, and balloon cell nevi.

Vesicular immunostaining for adipophilin can also be observed in liposarcomas (but not in mature adipose tissue), renal cell carcinomas, and xanthomatous lesions, highlighting possible diagnostic pitfalls of relying purely on this immunostain. Nonetheless, the results of this and other recent studies will likely prompt a wider nonresearch use of adipophilin for diagnosis of sebaceous carcinoma in challenging cases.

T. Milman, MD

Ocular Adnexal IgG4-Related Lymphoplasmacytic Infiltrative Disorder
Kubota T, Moritani S, Katayama M, et al (Nagoya Med Ctr, Japan; et al)
Arch Ophthalmol 128:577-584, 2010

Objective.—To determine the clinicopathological characteristics of patients with infiltration of IgG4-positive plasma cells into the ocular adnexa.

Methods.—We designed a prospective study to evaluate 24 patients with ocular adnexal lymphoplasmacytic infiltrative lesions, including sclerosing inflammation and reactive lymphoid hyperplasia. We analyzed peripheral blood and biopsy specimens from all patients. The classification criteria for placement in the IgG4-related group included having both an elevated serum level of IgG4 of 135 mg/dL or greater and an IgG4:IgG ratio of infiltrating plasma cells of 30% or greater.

Results.—Ten patients met the classification criteria (IgG4-related group), 9 patients did not meet the criteria (IgG4-unrelated group), and 5 patients met 1 but not both criteria (indeterminate group). Patients in the IgG4-related group had significantly higher bilateral involvement ($P = .02$), a higher number of allergic diseases ($P = .01$), and elevated IgE serum levels ($P = .01$). Of the 10 patients in the IgG4-related group, 3 also had polyclonal hypergammaglobulinemia, 6 had systemic lymphadenopathy or salivary gland enlargement, and 1 developed autoimmune pancreatitis. Patients in the IgG4-unrelated group did not have these serum and/or systemic abnormalities.

Conclusion.—The IgG4-related and IgG4-unrelated groups have different patterns of tissue involvement and systemic disease associations and possibly different prognoses.

▶ Recent retrospective studies have focused on an association of ocular adnexal inflammatory lesions containing high numbers of IgG4-positive plasma cells with autoimmune disorders, such as autoimmune pancreatitis, sclerosing cholangitis, retroperitoneal fibrosis, and chronic sclerosing sialadenitis. The ocular adnexal IgG4-related disease predominantly involves the lacrimal gland and is typically bilateral. The histopathologic features are similar to those seen in other forms of IgG4-related diseases (lymphoplasmacytic lesions with lymphoid hyperplasia and fibrosis, although obliterative phlebitis is generally absent). Immunohistochemical stains for IgG4 reveal an elevated number of IgG4-positive plasma cells (greater than 10 per high-power field), with an elevated IgG4-to-IgG ratio (30%-50%). Serum IgG4 is typically elevated. Several studies have also demonstrated the presence of immunoglobulin heavy chain gene rearrangement in a background of IgG4-related chronic inflammation, and B-cell lymphomas arising from pre-existent IgG4-related sclerosing orbital inflammation.

The study by Kubota et al is a prospective study in which the authors attempt to further characterize and define the ocular adnexal IgG4-related lymphoplasmacytic infiltrative disorder. Similar to prior studies, the investigators noted a higher frequency of bilateral lacrimal gland involvement, an association with B-cell clonality, IgG4 serum abnormalities, and an association with autoimmune diseases in patients with IgG4-related orbital inflammatory disease. Although the results of the work by Kubota et al shed more light on this recently emerged subtype of orbital inflammatory disease, the study has several limitations. These include absence of refined criteria for diagnosis of IgG4-related orbital inflammatory disease. In addition, a larger number of patients and longer follow-up are needed to reach meaningful conclusions about the regional and systemic associations of IgG4-related orbital inflammatory disease.

For more information on this topic, please read the articles by Sato et al, Geyer et al, Cheuk et al, and Matsuo et al.[1-4]

T. Milman, MD

References

1. Matsuo T, Ichimura K, Sato Y, et al. Immunoglobulin G4 (IgG4)-positive or
-negative ocular adnexal benign lymphoid lesions in relation to systemic involvement. *J Clin Exp Hematop.* 2010;50:129-142.
2. Sato Y, Ohshima K, Ichimura K, et al. Ocular adnexal IgG4-related disease has
uniform clinicopathology. *Pathol Int.* 2008;58:465-470.
3. Cheuk W, Yuen HK, Chan AC, et al. Ocular adnexal lymphoma associated with
IgG4+ chronic sclerosing dacryoadenitis: a previously undescribed complication
of IgG4-related sclerosing disease. *Am J Surg Pathol.* 2008;32:1159-1167.
4. Geyer JT, Deshpande V. IgG4-associated sialadenitis. *Curr Opin Rheumatol.*
2011;23:95-101.

Retrocorneal Membranes: A Comparative Immunohistochemical Analysis of Keratocytic, Endothelial, and Epithelial Origins

Jakobiec FA, Bhat P (Massachusetts Eye and Ear Infirmary, Boston)
Am J Ophthalmol 150:230-242, 2010

Purpose.—To determine through the use of immunohistochemistry the
origins of retrocorneal cellular and fibrillar membranes.

Design.—Retrospective, clinicopathologic study using surgically removed
human corneal tissues.

Methods.—Clinical records of patients' ocular diseases and surgical
procedures were reviewed. Immunohistochemical staining was performed
on 5 enucleated control globes, 32 penetrating keratoplasty specimens, and
6 Descemet stripping endothelial keratoplasty specimens to analyze: (1) the
normal corneal epithelium, stroma, and endothelium; and (2) stromal
scars, endothelial abnormalities, and retrocorneal membranes. Paraffin
sections were stained with hematoxylin and eosin, periodic acid—Schiff,
and Masson trichrome methods, and immunohistochemical analyses
were performed with commonly available monoclonal and polyclonal antibodies for various cytokeratins (CKs), CD34, α-smooth muscle actin
(SMA), and vimentin.

Results.—Five subtypes among 28 retrocorneal membranes were characterized. Twelve fibrous (keratocytic) membranes of stromal origin had
coarse collagen and immunostained negatively for all CKs, but strongly
for vimentin and α-SMA, the last the only marker of diagnostic value.
Nine metaplastic endothelium-derived membranes produced delicate
collagenous matrices and immunoreacted with CK7, vimentin, and
α-SMA. Two epithelial multilaminar or monolaminar membranes reacted
with CK cocktail and wide-spectrum CK, mildly with CK7 (not observed
in orthotopic surface epithelium), and negatively for α-SMA and vimentin
The final 2 categories were indeterminate or nonimmunoreactive (3 specimens) and mixed (2 specimens).

Conclusions.—Immunohistochemistry can diagnose retrocorneal membranes of different provenances reliably in most cases. Clinical correlations
established that these membranes develop after serious inflammatory

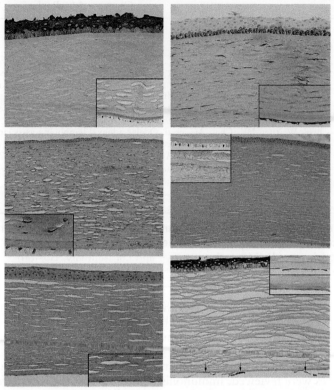

FIGURE 1.—Photomicrographs showing normal corneal layers and agonal endothelium. (Top left) Corneal specimen obtained from an enucleated eye of a 71-year-old woman with a posterior choroidal melanoma treated with proton beam radiation demonstrating heavy cytokeratin (CK) cocktail immunostaining of the suprabasilar epithelium situated on an intact Bowman membrane, whereas the stroma and diaphanous endothelium (inset) did not stain (immunoperoxidase method, diaminobenzidine chromogen, hematoxylin counterstain; ×200 magnification; inset, ×200 magnification). (Top right) The same corneal specimen immunoreacted with vimentin, which stains the basal epithelial cells, stromal keratocytes, and endothelial cells (inset; immunoperoxidase chromogen, diaminobenzidine chromogen, hematoxylin counterstain; ×200 magnification; inset, ×200 magnification). (Middle left) Corneal specimen obtained from an enucleated eye of a 56-year-old man with a blind eye resulting from multiple retinal detachments and subsequent surgeries discloses CD34 immunoreactivity of normal quiescent keratocytes but not of epithelial and endothelial cells (inset; immunoperoxidase method, diaminobenzidine chromogen, hematoxylin counterstain; ×100 magnification; inset, ×400 magnification). (Middle right) α-Smooth muscle actin (SMA) fails to decorate epithelium, keratocytes, and endothelium (also shown in top inset) of the same corneal specimen shown in Middle left. The bottom inset displays α-SMA immunoreactivity of keratocytes participating in a superficial stromal scar beneath the epithelium, seen in the corneal specimen of an 83-year-old woman with a history of Fuchs dystrophy, multiple penetrating keratoplasties, cataract surgery, and nonhealing persistent epithelial defects requiring a final penetrating keratoplasty (immunoperoxidase method, diaminobenzidine chromogen, hematoxylin counterstain; ×100 magnification; top inset, ×200 magnification; bottom inset, ×100 magnification). (Bottom left) Agonal (distressed) endothelial cells in a 68-year-old woman with Turner syndrome, cataract extraction, anterior chamber intraocular lens implantation, and pseudophakic endotheliopathy. The inset discloses widely separated nuclei with attenuated, faintly eosinophilic cytoplasm (hematoxylin and eosin; ×200 magnification; inset, ×400 magnification). (Bottom right) Agonal (injured) endothelial cells (arrows) from a corneal specimen of a 62-year-old woman with a history of trachoma, interstitial keratitis, scleritis, and uveitis stain positively with CK cocktail and CK 7 (top inset). The bottom inset reveals the absence of α-SMA within the endothelial cells of this specimen, whereas it was positive in other specimens with agonal cells. The suprabasilar corneal epithelium in the main panel immunoreacts with CK cocktail (immunoperoxidase reaction; ×200 magnification; top inset, ×200 magnification; bottom inset, ×200 magnification). (Reprinted from Jakobiec FA, Bhat P. Retrocorneal membranes: a comparative immunohistochemical analysis of keratocytic, endothelial, and epithelial origins. *Am J Ophthalmol.* 2010;150:230-242, with permission from Elsevier.)

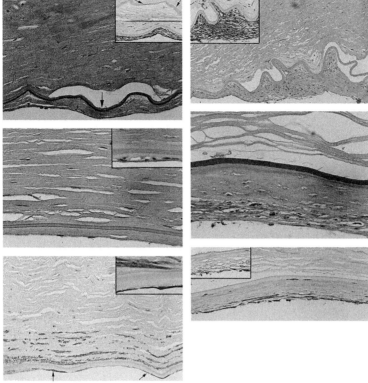

FIGURE 2.—Photomicrographs showing retrocorneal keratocytic and metaplastic endothelial membranes. (Top left) Corneal specimen from a 78-year-old male with multiple retinal detachment surgeries and eventual corneal opacification displays a moderately thick and mildly cellular membrane derived from stromal keratocytes on the back of a gently undulating Descemet membrane (arrow). The top inset shows cytokeratin (CK) 7 negativity of the multiple layers of cells adherent to the Descemet membrane (arrows). The bottom inset shows strong α-smooth muscle actin (SMA) positivity within the membrane (periodic acid−Schiff; ×200 magnification; top inset: immunoperoxidase reaction, diaminobenzidine chromogen, hematoxylin counterstain; ×100 magnification; bottom inset: ×100 magnification). (Top right) Hypercellular thick keratocytic retrocorneal membrane seen in the corneal specimen from a 68-year-old man with ocular trauma, limbus-to-limbus corneal laceration with repair, and later corneal opacification. The membrane has contracted to create striking folds in the Descemet membrane. The inset highlights strong α-SMA positivity of all the intramembranous cells. CK staining demonstrated negative results (not shown; hematoxylin and eosin; ×100 magnification; inset: immunoperoxidase reaction: ×100 magnification). (Middle left) A 50-year-old man had multiple retinal detachment surgeries, lensectomy, and silicone oil removal. There is a delicately fibrillar, thin, retro-Descemet membrane of endothelial metaplastic origin with a few surviving surface cells. The Descemet membrane is straight. The inset demonstrates focal mild eosinophilia of the cytoplasm of the covering cells (hematoxylin and eosin; ×200 magnification; inset: ×200 magnification). (Middle right) Corneal specimen from a 29-year-old woman with Peter anomaly, multiple penetrating keratoplasties, multiple retinal detachment, and filtration surgeries exhibiting a thick, multilaminar, endothelial metaplastic membrane containing cells at all levels. Note the presence of periodic acid−Schiff-positive strands in the matrix. The Descemet membrane is nonfolded (periodic acid−Schiff; ×400 magnification). (Bottom left) An 83-year-old woman had Fuchs dystrophy, multiple prior penetrating keratoplasties, and cataract surgery with an ensuing nonhealing epithelial defect requiring another corneal transplantation. Immunostaining disclosed α-SMA immunoreactivity focally present within the surviving endothelial cells (arrows) covering a thin retro-Descemet fibrillar membrane. Note the pre-Descemet deep stromal keratocytic α-SMA cytoplasmic positivity. The inset documents CK 7 positivity of the covering metaplastic endothelial cells (immunoperoxidase reaction; ×200 magnification; inset: ×200 magnification). (Bottom right) CK 7 vividly stains the multilaminar cells in the thick metaplastic membrane in the middle right panel. The surface cells are discontinuous, as also revealed in the inset with CK cocktail positive immunostaining (×200 magnification; inset: ×200 magnification). (Reprinted from Jakobiec FA, Bhat P. Retrocorneal membranes: a comparative immunohistochemical analysis of keratocytic, endothelial, and epithelial origins. *Am J Ophthalmol.* 2010;150:230-242, with permission from Elsevier.)

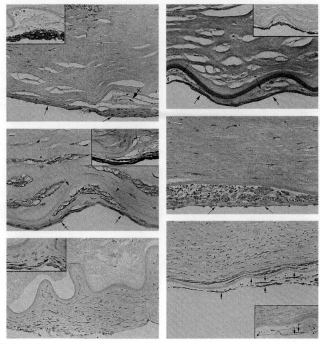

FIGURE 3.—Photomicrographs showing epithelial and mixed retrocorneal membranes. (Top left) A 47-year-old man with pseudophakic bullous keratopathy, multiple penetrating keratoplasties, corneal graft rejection, and epithelial downgrowth was treated with 5-flurouracil, pars plana vitrectomy, and cryotherapy. There is a multilaminar squamous epithelial retrocorneal membrane (arrows) with a subjacent focus of metaplastic endothelial cells producing a delicate matrix (crossed arrows). Mild stromal scarring and a small vessel are present at the top. The inset demonstrates cytokeratin (CK) cocktail immunostaining of the squamous cell membrane but not of the metaplastic endothelial cells interposed between it and the Descemet membrane (hematoxylin and eosin; ×200 magnification; inset: immunoperoxidase reaction, diaminobenzidine chromogen, hematoxylin counterstain; ×200 magnification). (Top right) Same specimen as in Top left. A stretched out monolayer or bilayer of squamous epithelium (arrows) covers a delicate matrix with strands of periodic acid–Schiff-positive material and scattered nuclei (crossed arrows) belonging to surviving metaplastic endothelial cells that were CK 7 and α-smooth muscle actin positive. The inset displays CK cocktail immunoreactivity of the attenuated layer of squamous epithelium (periodic acid–Schiff; ×400 magnification; inset: immunoperoxidase reaction; ×200 magnification). (Middle left) Same specimen as depicted in the Top right demonstrating α-SMA positive staining of the pre-Descemet deep stromal keratocytes and the metaplastic endothelial cells found on the other side of the Descemet membrane (arrows) beneath the membranous epithelial downgrowth membrane (crossed arrows). The endothelial cells were also CK 7 positive (not shown). The squamous epithelium (crossed arrows) is α-SMA negative and CK 7 positive (inset); the latter finding that is absent in nonmigrated surface epicorneal squamous epithelium (immunoperoxidase reaction; ×400 magnification; inset: ×200 magnification). (Middle right) A mixed vascular–keratocytic–endothelial membrane that is also inflamed developed in a 91-year-old woman with multiple retinal detachment surgeries and recurrent corneal perforations despite gluing. Note the continuous surface monolayer of endothelial cells (arrows), which was α-SMA and CK 7 positive. The subjacent spindle cells were α-SMA positive but CK 7 negative. The corneal stroma is lightly inflamed in this field (hematoxylin and eosin; ×200 magnification). (Bottom left) Same case as shown in the Middle right. A nonvascularized portion of the membrane demonstrates CK 7-positive metaplastic endothelial cells, also depicted in the inset. There are intermixed nonstaining keratocytes that instead manifest α-SMA positivity (immunoperoxidase reaction; ×200 magnification; inset: ×400 magnification). (Bottom right) A 61-year-old man had lattice corneal dystrophy, multiple penetrating keratoplasties, corneal graft rejection, and subsequent infectious corneal ulceration with group A streptococcus. Mixed membrane with prominent inflammatory component. α-SMA stains the keratocytic component (crossed arrows) of the mixed keratocytic–metaplastic–endothelial and loosely organized inflammatory membrane seen in the specimen. Note the pre-Descemet membrane (arrows) keratocytic actin-positivity and the stromal inflammation. The inset demonstrates surviving CK 7-positive endothelial cells (arrows) admixed with inflammatory cells (×200 magnification; inset: ×200 magnification). (Reprinted from Jakobiec FA, Bhat P. Retrocorneal membranes: a comparative immunohistochemical analysis of keratocytic, endothelial, and epithelial origins. *Am J Ophthalmol.* 2010;150:230-242, with permission from Elsevier.)

TABLE 1.—Immunohistochemical Probes and Their Targeted Ocular and Non-Ocular Tissues

Antibody	Common Nonocular and Ocular Specificities	Staining Pattern	Source	Dilution
CK,[a] CK 7[b]	Large number of simple glandular, lung, breast, complex, and transitional (urothelial) epithelia; mesothelia (but not normal corneal endothelium)	Cytoplasmic	Mouse monoclonal, IgG1/k[c]	Prediluted
CK 20[d]	Simple epithelia of intestines and stomach, Merkel cells	Cytoplasmic	Mouse monoclonal, IgG2a/k[c]	Prediluted
CK Cam5.2[e]	Basal cells of glandular epithelia, myoepithelia, and simple epithelia	Cytoplasmic	Mouse monoclonal, IgG2a[f]	1:80
CK Cocktail[g]	Basal cells of glandular epithelia, myoepithelia, simple and complex epithelia, and corneal epithelium	Cytoplasmic	Mouse monoclonal, IgG2a[f], and IgG1[h]	1:80; 1:160
CK wide spectrum[i]	Either suprabasal or all epidermal layers, all adnexal glandular cells	Cytoplasmic	Polyclonal rabbit[j]	1:900
CD[k] 34	Capillary endothelium, proliferating vessels, nonvascular spindle cell tumors, embryonic and a subpopulation of dermal fibroblasts, keratocytes	Membranous	Mouse monoclonal, IgG1[c]	Prediluted
Vimentin	Mesenchymal cells, anterior and posterior iridial pigmented epithelium, pigmented and nonpigmented ciliary epithelium, normal subcapsular lens, and cataractous epithelium (Wedl cells)	Cytoplasmic	Mouse monoclonal, IgG/k[c]	Prediluted
α-Smooth muscle actin	Smooth muscle cells of blood vessels, myofibroblasts, myoepithelial cells	Cytoplasmic	Mouse monoclonal, IgG[c]	Prediluted
EMA	Epithelial and mesothelial cells (indicative of epithelial differentiation as a supplement to cytokeratins)	Cytoplasmic + membranous	Mouse monoclonal, IgG2a/k[c]	Prediluted

CD = cluster of differentiation; CK = cytokeratin; EMA = epithelial membrane antigen; IgG = immunoglobulin G.
[a]Cytokeratins are a class of intermediate cytoplasmic filaments composed of heteropolymers with acidic and basic components encompassing over 25 subtypes, ranging from a low molecular weight of 40 kD to a high of 68 kD.
[b]CK 7, molecular weight of 54 kD.
[c]Ventana Medical Systems, Oro Valley, Arizona, USA.
[d]CK 20, molecular weight of 46 kD.
[e]CK Cam5.2 recognizes CK 8 (53 kD) and CK 18 (45 kD) exclusively.
[f]Becton Dickinson, San Jose, California, USA.
[g]CK cocktail recognizes both high and low molecular weight cytokeratins and is a combination of Cam5.2 and AE1/AE3 cytokeratins with 2 different classes of IgG and dilutions; AE1 recognizes type I acidic cytokeratins (CK 10, CK 13, CK 14, CK 15, CK 16, and CK 19, 56.5 to 40 kD), whereas AE3 recognizes type II basic cytokeratins (CK 1, CK 2, CK 3, CK 4, CK 5, CK 6, CK 7, and CK 8, 68 to 53 kD).
[h]Signet Laboratories, Dedham, Massachusetts, USA.
[i]Stains prominently cytokeratins with molecular weights 52, 56, and 58 kD, and less strongly stains cytokeratins with weights of 48, 51, and 60 kD.
[j]Dako Corporation, Carpinteria, California, USA.
[k]Class II.

disorders, prolonged wounding or ulcerations, and multiple surgeries (an average of 3.4 per patient) (Figs 1-3, Tables 1 and 2).

▶ Jakobiec and Bhat performed a systematic analysis of immunohistochemical phenotypes of retrocorneal membranes. As the authors indicate, this is not the

TABLE 2.—Immunohistochemical Characterization of Controls, Normal Regions of Cellular Corneal Layers, Scarred Stromas, Agonal (Damaged) Endothelium, and 28 Retrocorneal Membranes

Tissue	No. of Specimens	CK 7	CK 20	CK Cam5.2	CK Cocktail	CK Wide Spectrum	EMA	CD34	α-SMA	Vimentin
Normal components of corneal layers										
Epithelium	27[a]	–	–	–	+++	+++	–	–	–	+[b]
Stromal keratocytes	32[c]	–	–	–	–	–	–	+++	–	+++
Endothelium	5[d]	–	–	–	–	–	–	–	–	+++
Pathologic alterations in corneal layers										
Keratocytes in or near stromal scar	19[e]	–	–	–	+/++	+	–	–	+++	+++
Agonal (damaged) endothelium	10[f]	+++	–	++	+/++	+	–	–	+/–[g]	++
Retrocorneal membrane origins										
Fibrous (keratocytic)	12[h]	–	–	–	–	–	–	–	+++	++
Metaplastic (endothelial)	9[i]	+++	–	–/+	+/++	+/++	–	–	++	++
Epithelial	2	+	–	–	+++	++	–	–	–	–
Indeterminate	3[j]	–	–	–	–	–	–	–	–	–
Mixed	2[k]	see Results for immunostaining								

– = nonstaining; + = mild staining; ++ = moderate staining; +++ = strong staining; α-SMA = α-smooth muscle actin; CD = cluster of differentiation, class II; CK = cytokeratin; DSEK = Descemet stripping endothelial keratoplasty; EMA = epithelial membrane antigen; PK = penetrating keratoplasty.

[a]Normal corneal epithelium of 5 enucleated eyeballs and regions with unaffected epithelium and intact Bowman membrane in 22 of 32 pathologic PK procedures.

[b]Focal staining of the basal epithelial layer in half of the specimens.

[c]Normal corneas of 5 enucleated eyes and nondiseased stromal regions of 27 PK procedures that were immunoreactive.

[d]Normal endothelium of 5 enucleated eyeballs.

[e]PK specimens with focal scars and wounds in which keratocytes manifested strong cytoplasmic α-SMA and vimentin positivity.

[f]Five PK procedures and 5 DSEK procedures with distressed endothelium but without a membrane.

[g]Agonal (damaged or marginally viable) endothelium without a membrane may or may not stain for α-SMA (seen in half the specimens).

[h]Ten purely fibrous and 2 predominantly fibrous membranes covered focally by metaplastic endothelium with appropriate staining characteristics.

[i]Eight PK procedures and 1 DSEK, the latter obtained from 1 case of toxic anterior segment syndrome.

[j]Totally nonstaining: probably 2 fibrous and 1 metaplastic, based on trichrome staining characteristics of matrix and Descemet ruptures in the former.

[k]One vascularized and 1 inflammatory keratocytic–metaplastic–endothelial composite membrane, each example exhibiting 3 cellular elements.

first study on this topic. Other studies have provided us with similar information regarding the histological, immunohistochemical, and ultrastructural characteristics of retrocorneal membranes. This study, however, puts it all together, giving the reader clear-cut guidelines for retrocorneal membrane immunophenotyping. The authors also confirm previous observations that corneal endothelium can undergo epithelial metaplasia in a variety of degenerative conditions, in addition to well-characterized iridocorneal endothelial syndrome and posterior polymorphous dystrophy. Thus, the distinction between these entities cannot rely solely on immunohistochemical features. Conversely, immunophenotyping can help distinguish epithelial downgrowth from metaplastic endothelium in cases when histology is inconclusive.

T. Milman, MD

Clinicopathologic Review of Enucleated Eyes After Intra-arterial Chemotherapy With Melphalan for Advanced Retinoblastoma

Vajzovic LM, Murray TG, Aziz-Sultan MA, et al (Bascom Palmer Eye Inst, Miami, FL; Univ of Miami/Jackson Memorial Hosp, FL; et al)
Arch Ophthalmol 128:1619-1623, 2010

Retinoblastoma is a rare disease with only 250 to 300 cases diagnosed per year in the United States. Over the last 15 to 20 years, the long-term survival rates have been up to 99% in the developed world with aggressive treatment including systemic chemotherapy combined with focal laser therapy. Newer treatment techniques are focused on globe conservation while minimizing toxic systemic adverse effects such as myelosuppression, need for blood transfusions, infections, and increased incidence of secondary tumors.[1] One of these newer treatment techniques includes intra-arterial chemotherapy infusion of melphalan. This supraselective intra-ophthalmic artery chemotherapeutic drug delivery has been shown to be successful by Yamane et al[2] and Abramson et al[3] in advanced intraocular retinoblastoma (Reese-Ellsworth group V) cases. Herein, we report the clinicopathologic finding of 3 eyes of 3 patients diagnosed with advanced retinoblastoma, Reese-Ellsworth group Vb, or International Classification of Retinoblastoma group D, treated with supraselective intra-ophthalmic artery infusion of melphalan at our institution by a technique previously described by Abramson et al.[3] The patients underwent enucleation for evidence of tumor progression.

▶ In an attempt to avoid enucleation, the oncologists tried to manage Reese-Ellsworth group V eyes with either primary external beam irradiation or systemic multiagent chemotherapy followed by focal treatments and/or external beam irradiation. These treatment modalities have significant side effects, including increased risk of second cancers in the field of external beam irradiation and hematopoietic toxicity from systemic chemotherapy. Not surprisingly, the search for alternative treatment modalities focused on globe conservation while minimizing the risk of second malignancies and toxic systemic effects has been ongoing.

In a recent article by Abramson et al, the authors reported their successful treatment of 23 patients (28 eyes) with intra-arterial chemotherapy infusions, with only 1 eye developing progressive disease, leading to enucleation. The results of pathologic evaluation of the enucleated eye are not stated.[1] A prior smaller pilot study by Abramson et al showed that the 2 eyes enucleated after intra-arterial chemotherapy had no viable tumor.[2]

The article by Vajzovic and colleagues provides additional insight into the pathology of enucleated eyes previously treated with superselective intra-arterial chemotherapy. They documented viable tumor in all 3 enucleated eyes, with progressive disease after superselective intra-arterial melphalan infusion. Moreover, 2 of 3 cases had a viable tumor with high-risk characteristics for the development of metastatic disease on histopathologic evaluation, thus suggesting the potential benefit of systemic chemotherapy in these patients. Other, as yet unpublished, data from other ophthalmic pathology groups demonstrate that intra-arterial chemotherapy can be associated with other pathologically identifiable complications, such as foreign body emboli in the branches of ophthalmic artery and choroidal infarcts. These findings suggest the need for more evidence-based data before embracing intra-arterial chemotherapy as a miracle cure for retinoblastoma.

T. Milman, MD

References

1. Abramson DH, Dunkel IJ, Brodie SE, Marr B, Gobin YP. Superselective ophthalmic artery chemotherapy as primary treatment for retinoblastoma (chemosurgery). *Ophthalmology*. 2010;117:1623-1629.
2. Abramson DH, Dunkel IJ, Brodie SE, Kim JW, Gobin YP. A phase I/II study of direct intraarterial (ophthalmic artery) chemotherapy with melphalan for intraocular retinoblastoma initial results. *Ophthalmology*. 2008;115:1398-1404.

Evisceration in Unsuspected Intraocular Tumors
Rath S, Honavar SG, Naik MN, et al (LV Prasad Eye Inst, Bhubaneswar, India; LV Prasad Eye Inst, Hyderabad, India; et al)
Arch Ophthalmol 128:372-379, 2010

Background.—Disfigured or painful blind eyes can be either enucleated or eviscerated. Although these two approaches produce functionally and esthetically similar outcomes, evisceration is preferred by most clinicians because of ease of surgery, better implant and prosthesis motility, preserved orbital anatomy (fewer complications), and the scleral barrier that avoids implant migration and extrusion. However, when an intraocular malignancy is suspected, enucleation is required. Sometimes pathologists find clinically unsuspected intraocular tumors during histopathologic assessment of eviscerated eyes. The most common lesions are uveal melanoma, although other malignancies are also reported. Six cases in which unsuspected intraocular tumors were found after evisceration were reported, noting lessons that can be learned from these cases.

Methods.—The case series included six patients ranging in age from 8 to 70 years (median age 18 years). Medical records were reviewed for symptoms, initial clinical findings, initial clinical diagnosis, imaging, previous treatment, indication for evisceration, intraoperative findings, histopathology, postevisceration management, and final outcome with respect to tumor recurrence and metastasis. Guidelines for treatment were developed based on the outcomes of these cases.

Results.—Three patients had preoperative ultrasound B-scan that showed no obvious evidence of an intraocular mass. One patient had a preoperative computed tomographic (CT) scan that was also unrevealing. Four patients had painful blind eye, one had a cosmetic concern, and one had a perforated hypotonus eye with uveal prolapse. On histopathologic evaluation, retinoblastoma was identified in two patients, uveal melanoma in one, adenocarcinoma of the ciliary body in one, choroidal ganglioneuroma in one, and conjunctival squamous cell carcinoma with intraocular invasion in one. The patients with retinoblastoma required high-dose chemotherapy, orbital exenteration, and external beam radiotherapy; the one with uveal melanoma had orbital exenteration and external beam radiotherapy; the one with adenocarcinoma of the ciliary body required enucleation and external beam radiotherapy; the patient with benign choroidal ganglioneuroma was observed; and the patient with intraocular invasion of conjunctival squamous cell carcinoma had orbital exenteration. None had developed local recurrence or systemic metastasis up to 28 months later.

Conclusions.—Six steps were suggested to prevent surprises with evisceration and its consequences. A thorough clinical history and diligent examination are essential. Appropriate imaging and adequate analysis and interpretation of results contribute significantly. Enucleation should be chosen rather than evisceration when reasonable clinical measures cannot rule out the presence of an intraocular tumor. Unusual appearing or feeling intraocular contents should be carefully assessed intraoperatively, with surgery modified as necessary. All eviscerated tissues should undergo histopathologic evaluation. Should a malignant intraocular tumor be found, appropriate treatment should be undertaken to avoid local recurrence or systemic metastases.

▶ The authors add another 6 cases of eviscerated blind eyes with unsuspected intraocular tumors to the recently described series of 7 similar cases by Eagle et al.[1] These data provide additional evidence about the necessity of meticulous preoperative, intraoperative, and pathologic evaluation of the eviscerated eyes. It is heartening to know that with an appropriate postoperative management, none of the patients in this case series, including the child with retinoblastoma, developed local recurrence or metastasis. For additional information on this topic, please read the article by Eagle et al.[1]

T. Milman, MD

Reference

1. Eagle RC Jr, Grossniklaus HE, Syed N, Hogan RN, Lloyd WC 3rd, Folberg R. Inadvertent evisceration of eyes containing uveal melanoma. *Arch Ophthalmol.* 2009;127:141-145.

Direct Scanning of Pathology Specimens Using Spectral Domain Optical Coherence Tomography: A Pilot Study

Fine JL, Kagemann L, Wollstein G, et al (Univ of Pittsburgh School of Medicine, PA)
Ophthalmic Surg Lasers Imaging 41:S58-S64, 2010

Background and Objective.—Digital pathology has thus far focused on producing digital images of glass microscope slides. Spectral domain optical coherence tomography (SD-OCT) can be used to directly scan tissue blocks to produce three-dimensional histology images, potentially bypassing glass slide workflow.

Materials and Methods.—Formalin-fixed paraffin-embedded tissue blocks were scanned using SD-OCT and resulting images were compared with corresponding areas on microscope slides.

Results.—Low-magnification features were recognizable, including tissue outlines, fat, vessels, and outlines of colonic mucosal crypts. Subtle textures that were suggestive of benign breast lobules and ovarian tumor features were also visible. Initial SD-OCT images lacked resolution and contrast relative to traditional microscopy, but the image content suggests that additional features of interest are present and may be revealed with improved SD-OCT resolution and more post-processing experience. Elucidation of three-dimensional histology and pathology are also future tasks.

Conclusion.—Eventual availability of diagnostic-quality three-dimensional histology would have a profound impact on anatomic pathology.

▶ In this article, Fine et al further expand the frontiers of digital pathology by exploring the potential applications of spectral domain optical coherence tomography (SD-OCT) to directly scan tissue blocks to produce 3-dimensional histology images. The investigators have used SD-OCT to scan the paraffin-embedded tissue and image-processing software to create a 3-dimensional histology image. Although the images obtained in this study lack the resolution of routine histopathologic sections prepared on glass slide, the technique can potentially be refined to produce a higher quality image rapidly and relatively inexpensively. Despite these promising results, at the present time routine histology methods are still superior, so don't throw away your microtome and hematoxylin-eosin stainer just yet!

T. Milman, MD

12 Socio-Economics

Morphine Use after Combat Injury in Iraq and Post-Traumatic Stress Disorder

Holbrook TL, Galarneau MR, Dye JL, et al (Naval Health Res Ctr, San Diego, CA)

N Engl J Med 362:110-117, 2010

Background.—Post-traumatic stress disorder (PTSD) is a common adverse mental health outcome among seriously injured civilians and military personnel who are survivors of trauma. Pharmacotherapy in the aftermath of serious physical injury or exposure to traumatic events may be effective for the secondary prevention of PTSD.

Methods.—We identified 696 injured U.S. military personnel without serious traumatic brain injury from the Navy—Marine Corps Combat Trauma Registry Expeditionary Medical Encounter Database. Complete data on medications administered were available for all personnel selected. The diagnosis of PTSD was obtained from the Career History Archival Medical and Personnel System and verified in a review of medical records.

Results.—Among the 696 patients studied, 243 received a diagnosis of PTSD and 453 did not. The use of morphine during early resuscitation and trauma care was significantly associated with a lower risk of PTSD after injury. Among the patients in whom PTSD developed, 61% received morphine; among those in whom PTSD did not develop, 76% received morphine (odds ratio, 0.47; P<0.001). This association remained significant after adjustment for injury severity, age, mechanism of injury, status with respect to amputation, and selected injury-related clinical factors.

Conclusions.—Our findings suggest that the use of morphine during trauma care may reduce the risk of subsequent development of PTSD after serious injury.

▶ This article shows that immediate morphine for pain control after war injuries in Iraq significantly reduced posttraumatic stress disorder, even after controlling other factors relating to the nature and severity of the injury. Similar results have been found in patients with burns. Morphine provides not only pain relief but also suppresses adronorgic activity. Trauma without pain may benefit from anti-adrenergic treatment with propanolol or clonidine with regard to the development of posttraumatic stress. These seem like relatively easy interventions to prevent long-term sequelae of trauma, well worth investigating.

E. J. Cohen, MD

Preventing Surgical-Site Infections in Nasal Carriers of *Staphylococcus aureus*

Bode LGM, Kluytmans JAJW, Wertheim HFL, et al (Erasmus Univ Med Ctr, Rotterdam, the Netherlands; Amphia Hosp, Breda, the Netherlands; et al)
N Engl J Med 362:9-17, 2010

Background.—Nasal carriers of *Staphylococcus aureus* are at increased risk for health care–associated infections with this organism. Decolonization of nasal and extranasal sites on hospital admission may reduce this risk.

Methods.—In a randomized, double-blind, placebo-controlled, multicenter trial, we assessed whether rapid identification of *S. aureus* nasal carriers by means of a real-time polymerase-chain-reaction (PCR) assay, followed by treatment with mupirocin nasal ointment and chlorhexidine soap, reduces the risk of hospital-associated *S. aureus* infection.

Results.—From October 2005 through June 2007, a total of 6771 patients were screened on admission. A total of 1270 nasal swabs from 1251 patients were positive for *S. aureus*. We enrolled 917 of these patients in the intention-to-treat analysis, of whom 808 (88.1%) underwent a surgical procedure. All the *S. aureus* strains identified on PCR assay were susceptible to methicillin and mupirocin. The rate of *S. aureus* infection was 3.4% (17 of 504 patients) in the mupirocin–chlorhexidine group, as compared with 7.7% (32 of 413 patients) in the placebo group (relative risk of infection, 0.42; 95% confidence interval [CI], 0.23 to 0.75). The effect of mupirocin–chlorhexidine treatment was most pronounced for deep surgical-site infections (relative risk, 0.21; 95% CI, 0.07 to 0.62).

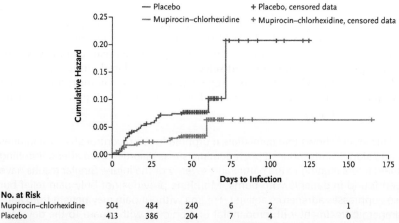

No. at Risk

Mupirocin–chlorhexidine	504	484	240	6	2	1
Placebo	413	386	204	7	4	0

FIGURE 3.—Kaplan–Meier Curves Showing Cumulative Hazard of Hospital-Acquired *Staphylococcus Aureus* Infection in the Study Groups. Data were censored at the end of the follow-up period or at the time of death. (Reprinted from Bode LGM, Kluytmans JAJW, Wertheim HFL, et al. Preventing surgical-site infections in nasal carriers of *Staphylococcus aureus*. N Engl J Med. 2010;362:9-17, copyright © 2010 Massachusetts Medical Society. All rights reserved.)

TABLE 2.—Relative Risk of Hospital-Acquired *Staphylococcus aureus* Infection and
Characteristics of Infections (Intention-to-Treat Analysis)

Variable	Mupirocin—Chlorhexidine (N = 504) *no. (%)*	Placebo (N = 413)	Relative Risk (95% CI)*
S. aureus infection	17 (3.4)	32 (7.7)	0.42 (0.23—0.75)
Source of infection[†]			
Endogenous	12 (2.4)	25 (6.1)	0.39 (0.20—0.77)
Exogenous	4 (0.8)	6 (1.5)	0.55 (0.16—1.92)
Unknown	1 (0.2)	1 (0.2)	
Localization of infection			
Deep surgical site[‡]	4 (0.9)	16 (4.4)	0.21 (0.07—0.62)
Superficial surgical site[‡]	7 (1.6)	13 (3.5)	0.45 (0.18—1.11)
Lower respiratory tract	2 (0.4)	2 (0.5)	0.82 (0.12—5.78)
Urinary tract	1 (0.2)	0	
Bacteremia	1 (0.2)	1 (0.2)	
Soft tissue	2 (0.4)	0	

*Relative risks are for *S. aureus* infection in the mupirocin—chlorhexidine group.
[†]The source of the *S. aureus* infections was determined by comparing nasal strains with strains isolated from the infection site by pulsed-field gel electrophoresis.
[‡]Data are for surgical patients only: 441 in the mupirocin—chlorhexidine group and 367 in the placebo group.

There was no significant difference in all-cause in-hospital mortality between the two groups. The time to the onset of nosocomial infection was shorter in the placebo group than in the mupirocin—chlorhexidine group (P = 0.005).

Conclusions.—The number of surgical-site *S. aureus* infections acquired in the hospital can be reduced by rapid screening and decolonizing of nasal carriers of *S. aureus* on admission. (Current Controlled Trials number, ISRCTN56186788.) (Fig 3, Table 2).

▶ This article reports a significant reduction in postoperative infections caused by *Staphylococcus aureus* following detection of nasal carriers by polymerase chain reaction (PCR) and treatment with nasal mupirocin twice daily for 5 days and use of chlorhexidine soap for bathing. This may be of interest in the prevention of postoperative eye infections, which are known to be often caused by endogenous flora, especially coagulase-negative *Staphylococcus*. The accompanying editorial describes studies showing greater efficacy of chlorhexidine scrubs compared with povidone-iodine. In ophthalmology, this can be considered for the skin, but povidone-iodine is necessary for the ocular surface because of the toxicity of chlorhexidine. Topical povidone-iodine has been shown to decrease postoperative endophthalmitis and is more effective than topical antibiotics for prophylaxis.

E. J. Cohen, MD

Article Index

Chapter 1: Cataract Surgery

Chapter 2: Refractive Surgery

Chapter 3: Glaucoma

Chapter 4: Cornea

Chapter 5: Retina

Chapter 6: Oculoplastic Surgery

Chapter 7: Pediatric Ophthalmology

Chapter 8: Neuro-ophthalmology

Chapter 9: Imaging

Chapter 10: Ocular Oncology

Chapter 11: Pathology

Chapter 12: Socio-Economics

Author Index

Printed and bound by CPI Group (UK) Ltd, Croydon, CR0 4YY

08/05/2025

01864677-0005